2012
YEAR BOOK OF
PSYCHIATRY AND
APPLIED MENTAL HEALTH®

The 2012 Year Book Series

Year Book of Anesthesiology and Pain Management™: Drs Chestnut, Abram, Black, Gravlee, Lien, Mathru, and Roizen

Year Book of Cardiology®: Drs Gersh, Cheitlin, Elliott, Gold, Graham, and Thourani

Year Book of Critical Care Medicine®: Drs Dellinger, Parrillo, Balk, Dorman, Dries, and Zanotti-Cavazzoni

Year Book of Dermatology and Dermatologic Surgery™: Dr Del Rosso

Year Book of Diagnostic Radiology®: Drs Elster, Abbara, Oestreich, Offiah, Rosado de Christenson, Stephens, and Strickland

Year Book of Emergency Medicine®: Drs Hamilton, Bruno, Handly, Minczak, Mullin, Quintana, and Ramoska

Year Book of Endocrinology®: Drs Schott, Apovian, Clarke, Eugster, Ludlam, Meikle, Oetjen, Schteingart, and Toth

Year Book of Gastroenterology™: Drs Talley, DeVault, Harnois, Murray, Pearson, Philcox, Picco, and Smith

Year Book of Hand and Upper Limb Surgery®: Drs Yao and Steinmann

Year Book of Medicine®: Drs Barker, Garrick, Gersh, Khardori, LeRoith, Panush, Talley, and Thigpen

Year Book of Neonatal and Perinatal Medicine®: Drs Fanaroff, Benitz, Donn, Neu, Papile, Polin, and Van Marter

Year Book of Neurology and Neurosurgery®: Drs Klimo, Minagar, Breningstall, Gandhi, House, Kevill, Liu, Mazia, Panagariya, Ragel, Riesenburger, Shafazand, Uhm, and Yang

Year Book of Obstetrics, Gynecology, and Women's Health®: Drs Dungan and Shulman

Year Book of Oncology®: Drs Arceci, Bauer, Chiorean, Gordon, Lawton, Murphy, Thigpen, and Tsao

Year Book of Ophthalmology®: Drs Rapuano, Cohen, Flanders, Hammersmith, Milman, Myers, Nagra, Nelson, Penne, Pyfer, Sergott, Shields, Talekar, and Vander

Year Book of Orthopedics®: Drs Morrey, Huddleston, Swiontkowski, and Trigg

Year Book of Otolaryngology-Head and Neck Surgery®: Drs Sindwani, Balough, Franco, Gapany, and Mitchell

Year Book of Pathology and Laboratory Medicine®: Drs Raab, Parwani, Bejarano, and Bissell

Year Book of Pediatrics®: Dr Stockman

Year Book of Plastic and Aesthetic Surgery™: Drs Miller, Gosman, Gurtner, Gutowski, Ruberg, Salisbury, and Smith

Year Book of Psychiatry and Applied Mental Health®: Drs Talbott, Ballenger, Buckley, Frances, Krupnick, and Mack

Year Book of Pulmonary Disease®: Drs Barker, Jones, Maurer, Spradley, Tanoue, and Willsie

Year Book of Sports Medicine®: Drs Shephard, Cantu, Feldman, Galea, Jankowski, Janssen, Lebrun, and Nieman

Year Book of Surgery®: Drs Copeland, Behrns, Daly, Eberlein, Fahey, Huber, Klodell, Mozingo, and Pruett

Year Book of Urology®: Drs Andriole and Coplen

Year Book of Vascular Surgery®: Drs Moneta, Gillespie, Starnes, and Watkins

2012

The Year Book of PSYCHIATRY AND APPLIED MENTAL HEALTH®

Editor in Chief
John A. Talbott, MD
Professor, Department of Psychiatry, University of Maryland School of Medicine, Baltimore, Maryland

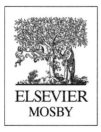

ELSEVIER
MOSBY

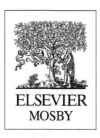

ELSEVIER
MOSBY

Vice President, Continuity: Kimberly Murphy
Developmental Editor: Sarah Barth
Production Supervisor, Electronic Year Books: Donna M. Skelton
Electronic Article Manager: Emily Ogle
Illustrations and Permissions Coordinator: Dawn Vohsen

2012 EDITION

Printed and bound by CPI Group (UK) Ltd, Croydon, CR0 4YY

Transferred to Digital Print 2011

Editorial Office:
Elsevier
Suite 1800
1600 John F. Kennedy Blvd.
Philadelphia, PA 19103-2899

International Standard Serial Number: 0084-3970
International Standard Book Number: 978-0-323-08892-3

Editors

James C. Ballenger, MD
Retired Professor and Chairman, Department of Psychiatry and Behavioral Sciences; Director, Institute of Psychiatry, Medical University of South Carolina; Private Practice, Charleston, South Carolina

Peter F. Buckley, MD
Dean, Medical College of Georgia, Georgia Health Sciences University, Augusta, Georgia

Richard J. Frances, MD
Clinical Professor of Psychiatry, New York University Medical School, New York, New York; Director of Professional and Public Education, Silver Hill Hospital, New Canaan, Connecticut

Janice L. Krupnick, PhD
Professor of Psychiatry and Director of the Trauma and Loss Program, Department of Psychiatry, Georgetown University, Washington, District of Columbia; Private Practice, Chevy Chase, Maryland

Avram H. Mack, MD
Associate Professor of Psychiatry and Director of Medical Student Education, Department of Psychiatry, Georgetown University, Washington, District of Columbia

Table of Contents

Journals Represented

Journals represented in this YEAR BOOK are listed below.

Acta Paediatrica
Acta Psychiatrica Scandinavica
American Journal on Addictions
American Journal of Epidemiology
American Journal of Human Genetics
American Journal of Medicine
American Journal of Obstetrics and Gynecology
American Journal of Preventive Medicine
American Journal of Psychiatry
American Journal of Psychotherapy
American Journal of Public Health
Archives of General Psychiatry
Archives of Pediatrics & Adolescent Medicine
Biological Psychiatry
British Journal of Psychiatry
British Medical Journal
Canadian Journal of Psychiatry
Clinical Pediatrics
Clinical Pharmacology & Therapeutics
Diabetes Care
Drugs
Endocrinology
Epilepsia
European Heart Journal
European Journal of Obstetrics & Gynecology and Reproductive Biology
European Journal of Paediatric Neurology
Genome Medicine
Headache
Hypertension
Journal of Adolescent Health
Journal of Affective Disorders
Journal of Child Psychology and Psychiatry
Journal of Clinical Psychiatry
Journal of Consulting and Clinical Psychology
Journal of Pain and Symptom Management
Journal of the American Academy of Child & Adolescent Psychiatry
Journal of the American Academy of Psychiatry and the Law
Journal of the American Geriatrics Society
Journal of the American Medical Association
Journal of the Canadian Academy of Child and Adolescent Psychiatry
Journal of Clinical Psychiatry
Journal of Clinical Psychopharmacology
Journal of Consulting and Clinical Psychology
Journal of Emergency Medicine
Journal of Nervous and Mental Disease
Journal of Neurosurgery
Journal of Nuclear Medicine

Journal of Pain
Journal of Pain and Symptom Management
Journal of Pediatric Gastroenterology and Nutrition
Journal of Plastic, Reconstructive & Aesthetic Surgery
Journal of Trauma
Medical Care
Medicine and Science in Sports and Exercise
Metabolism Clinical and Experimental
Morbidity and Mortality Weekly Report Surveillance Summaries
Neurology
Neuropsychopharmacology
New England Journal of Medicine
Pain
Pediatric Neurology
Pediatrics
Psychiatric Services
Psychologie Medicale
Schizophrenia Bulletin
Schizophrenia Research
Seizures

STANDARD ABBREVIATIONS

The following terms are abbreviated in this edition: acquired immunodeficiency syndrome (AIDS), cardiopulmonary resuscitation (CPR), central nervous system (CNS), cerebrospinal fluid (CSF), computed tomography (CT), deoxyribonucleic acid (DNA), electrocardiography (ECG), health maintenance organization (HMO), human immunodeficiency virus (HIV), intensive care unit (ICU), intramuscular (IM), intravenous (IV), magnetic resonance (MR) imaging (MRI), ribonucleic acid (RNA).

NOTE

The YEAR BOOK OF PSYCHIATRY AND APPLIED MENTAL HEALTH® is a literature survey service providing abstracts of articles published in the professional literature. Every effort is made to assure the accuracy of the information presented in these pages. Neither the editors nor the publisher of the YEAR BOOK OF PSYCHIATRY AND APPLIED MENTAL HEALTH® can be responsible for errors in the original materials. The editors' comments are their own opinions. Mention of specific products within this publication does not constitute endorsement.

To facilitate the use of the YEAR BOOK OF PSYCHIATRY AND APPLIED MENTAL HEALTH® as a reference tool, all illustrations and tables included in this publication are now identified as they appear in the original article. This change is meant to help the reader recognize that any illustration or table appearing in the YEAR BOOK OF PSYCHIATRY AND APPLIED MENTAL HEALTH® may be only one of many in the original article. For this reason, figure and table numbers will often appear to be out of sequence within the YEAR BOOK OF PSYCHIATRY AND APPLIED MENTAL HEALTH®.

1 Child and Adolescent Psychiatry

Introduction

As a field, child and adolescent psychiatry has marked various milestones in the past year, including the 50th anniversary of the main journal of the field, *Journal of the American Academy of Child & Adolescent Psychology*. But it reminds us that the field will need to continue to advance. Yet it must be done at its own pace and with attention to specific areas that differ from other segments of psychiatry. This year included few publications that represented major advances in child psychopharmacology this year. On the other hand, there were many, many important publications on substance use, gene x environment interactions, and brain imaging. Evidence continues to solidify the need to separate bipolar disorder from other mood dysregulation; there may be a PANDAS (pediatric autoimmune neuropsychiatric disorders associated with streptococcal infections), but under a different mechanism than had been asserted; children of parents serving in the military experience additional degrees of individual and family psychopathology. These are disparate findings, but they all are important to our practice and our research.

Avram H. Mack, MD

Risk and Etiologic Factors

A Systematic Review of Secretin for Children With Autism Spectrum Disorders

Krishnaswami S, McPheeters ML, Veenstra-VanderWeele J (Vanderbilt Univ, Nashville, TN)
Pediatrics 127:e1322-e1325, 2011

Context.—As many as 1 in every 110 children in the United States has an autism spectrum disorder (ASD). Secretin is 1 of many medical treatments studied for treating the symptoms of ASDs, but there is currently no consensus regarding which interventions are most effective.

Objective.—To systematically review evidence regarding the use of secretin in children with ASDs who are aged 12 years and younger.

1

Methods.—We searched the Medline, PsycINFO, and ERIC (Education Resources Information Center) databases from 2000 to May 2010 and reference lists of included articles. Two reviewers independently assessed each study against predetermined inclusion/exclusion criteria. Two reviewers independently extracted data regarding participant and intervention characteristics, assessment techniques, and outcomes and assigned overall quality and strength-of-evidence ratings on the basis of predetermined criteria.

Results.—Evidence from 7 randomized controlled trials supports a lack of effectiveness of secretin for the treatment of ASD symptoms including language and communication impairment, symptom severity, and cognitive and social skill deficits. No studies have resulted in significantly greater improvements in measures of language, cognition, or autistic symptoms when compared with placebo; study authors who reported improvement over time did so equally for both the intervention and placebo groups.

Conclusions.—Secretin has been studied extensively in multiple randomized controlled trials, and there is clear evidence that it lacks benefit. The studies of secretin included in this review uniformly point to a lack of significant impact of secretin in the treatment of ASD symptoms. Given the high strength of evidence for a lack of effectiveness, secretin as a treatment approach for ASDs warrants no further study.

▶ This article and its 2 companion articles[1,2] provide us with perhaps the most extensive review of treatments for autism this year (as well as in several past years). We are interested, of course, not only in what does work, but also in what does not work and what might be more dangerous than potentially helpful—secretin is one such substance. This systematic review found no evidence that it is helpful. Information at that level must be reviewed by anyone whose practice has anything to do with children with pervasive developmental disorders. After all, even if the physician is not the prescriber of the medication, dangerous conditions have resulted when patients and their parents seek specific medications that are said to be of potential benefit but in fact are dangerous. We should all be aware of these findings.

A. H. Mack, MD

References

1. Warren Z, McPheeters ML, Sathe N, Foss-Feig JH, Glasser A, Veenstra-Vanderweele J. A systematic review of early intensive intervention for autism spectrum disorders. *Pediatrics.* 2011;127:e1303-e1311.
2. McPheeters ML, Warren Z, Sathe N, et al. A systematic review of medical treatments for children with autism spectrum disorders. *Pediatrics.* 2011;127:e1312-e1321.

Aberrant Brain Activation During a Response Inhibition Task in Adolescent Eating Disorder Subtypes
Lock J, Garrett A, Beenhakker J, et al (Stanford Univ School of Medicine, CA)
Am J Psychiatry 168:55-64, 2011

Objective.—Behavioral and personality characteristics associated with excessive inhibition and disinhibition are observed in patients with eating disorders, but neural correlates of inhibitory control have not been examined in adolescents with these disorders.

Method.—Thirteen female adolescents with binge eating and purging behaviors (i.e., bulimia nervosa or anorexia nervosa, binge eating/purging type);14 with anorexia nervosa, restricting type; and 13 healthy comparison subjects performed a rapid, jittered event-related go/no-go task. Functional magnetic resonance images were collected using a 3 Tesla GE scanner and a spiral pulse sequence. A whole-brain three-group analysis of variance in SPM5 was used to identify significant activation associated with the main effect of group for the comparison of correct no-go versus go trials. The mean activation in these clusters was extracted for further comparisons in SPSS.

Results.—The binge eating/purging group showed significantly greater activation than the healthy comparison group in the bilateral precentral gyri, anterior cingulate cortex, and middle and superior temporal gyri as well as greater activation relative to both comparison and restricting type anorexia subjects in the hypothalamus and right dorsolateral prefrontal cortex. Within-group analysis found that only the restricting type anorexia group showed a positive correlation between the percent correct on no-go trials and activation in posterior visual and inferior parietal cortex regions.

Conclusions.—The present study provides preliminary evidence that during adolescence, eating disorder subtypes may be distinguishable in terms of neural correlates of inhibitory control. This distinction is consistent with differences in behavioral impulsivity in these patient groups.

▶ This study was performed to examine the neurobiological components of adolescents with anorexia nervosa (AN) and bulimia nervosa (BN), particularly in terms of the impulsive or disinhibited personality characteristics that occur in these patients. This is a small study of female patients with an eating disorder, and it poses questions about the pathology that is AN and BN. After all, aren't there impulse control aspects inherent in bulimia—is it neurochemical? There are findings that bulimic patients have poor executive function findings on go/no-go tasks, and perhaps the opposite has been elicited among those with AN. Here they grouped together the AN binging type and the BN group and compared them with those who were normal. Some studies suggest these neural/neuropsychological findings persist after the disease has been treated. Here the use of imaging should be considered with care, given that these are later adolescents. Those in the binge-purge group showed increased activation in the right dorso-lateral prefrontal cortex as well as increased hypothalamic function. So perhaps cognitive behavioral therapy is the answer here?

A. H. Mack, MD

Addiction as a Systems Failure: Focus on Adolescence and Smoking
Baler RD, Volkow ND (Natl Insts of Health, Bethesda, MD)
J Am Acad Child Adolesc Psychiatry 50:329-339, 2011

Objective.—Scientific advances in the field of addiction have forever debunked the notion that addiction reflects a character flaw under voluntary control, demonstrating instead that it is a bona fide disease of the brain. The aim of this review is to go beyond this consensus understanding and explore the most current evidence regarding the vast number of genetic, developmental, and environmental factors whose complex interactions modulate addiction risk and trajectory.

Method.—Focusing on childhood and adolescent smoking as a paradigm, we review the important risk factors for the development of addictions, starting at the level of genetics and closing with a focus on sociocultural and policy factors.

Results.—A critical review of the pertinent literature provides a detailed view of the cumulative power of risk and protection factors across different phenomenological levels to modulate the risk of undesirable outcomes, particularly for young people. The result represents a compelling argument for the need to engage in comprehensive, multilevel approaches to promoting health.

Conclusions.—Today, the field of medicine understands more about disease than about health; however it need not be that way. The view of drug addiction as a systems failure should help refocus our general approach to developing dynamic models and early comprehensive interventions that optimize the ways in which we prevent and treat a complex, developmental disorder such as drug addiction.

▶ This article is a blueprint for the public-level approach to adolescent addiction written by the leadership of the National Institute on Drug Abuse. It brings together a plethora of knowledge about the development of addiction or substance use, framing it in terms of "systems" or conceptual portions of the individual's life: from genetic factors through several layers of one's ecology—social relationships, living conditions, neighborhoods, institutions, and policies. The report highlights the perspective on epigenetics, which is a pragmatic approach to the idea of gene x environment interaction: environment effects changes in gene expression at distal time points. The authors are careful to make distinctions between substance use and a substance use disorder. A telling example is the relating of the findings that adolescents who exercise regularly have significantly lower rates of drug use. Parents of adolescent substance users frequently tell me that their concerns about substance use are heightened when their teen is not engaged in physical activity. I used to think they were focusing on this to excess; maybe they were right on target—or at least right that this is among the many systems and layers in the adolescent's life. It is not simply genetics—it is many systems altogether.

A. H. Mack, MD

Cannabis Use and Earlier Onset of Psychosis: A Systematic Meta-analysis
Large M, Sharma S, Compton MT, et al (Prince of Wales Hosp, Sydney, Australia; Emory Univ School of Medicine, Atlanta, GA; et al)
Arch Gen Psychiatry 68:555-561, 2011

Context.—A number of studies have found that the use of cannabis and other psychoactive substances is associated with an earlier onset of psychotic illness.

Objective.—To establish the extent to which use of cannabis, alcohol, and other psychoactive substances affects the age at onset of psychosis by meta-analysis.

Data Sources.—Peer-reviewed publications in English reporting age at onset of psychotic illness in substance-using and non–substance-using groups were located using searches of CINAHL, EMBASE, MEDLINE, PsycINFO, and ISI Web of Science.

Study Selection.—Studies in English comparing the age at onset of psychosis in cohorts of patients who use substances with age at onset of psychosis in non–substance-using patients. The searches yielded 443 articles, from which 83 studies met the inclusion criteria.

Data Extraction.—Information on study design, study population, and effect size were extracted independently by 2 of us.

Data Synthesis.—Meta-analysis found that the age at onset of psychosis for cannabis users was 2.70 years younger (standardized mean difference = −0.414) than for nonusers; for those with broadly defined substance use, the age at onset of psychosis was 2.00 years younger (standardized mean difference = −0.315) than for nonusers. Alcohol use was not associated with a significantly earlier age at onset of psychosis. Differences in the proportion of cannabis users in the substance-using group made a significant contribution to the heterogeneity in the effect sizes between studies, confirming an association between cannabis use and earlier mean age at onset of psychotic illness.

Conclusions.—The results of meta-analysis provide evidence for a relationship between cannabis use and earlier onset of psychotic illness, and they support the hypothesis that cannabis use plays a causal role in the development of psychosis in some patients. The results suggest the need for renewed warnings about the potentially harmful effects of cannabis.

▶ It is hoped that we all can agree adolescent cannabis exposure is dangerous and a signal of several potential problems for the regular adolescent user. There is also an ongoing set of data that describe use to be associated with the development of psychosis. For several years, there has been conflict over whether this is an association solely or whether the intoxication experience is causative of psychosis. To answer this question, the authors compared adolescents exposed to cannabis with those exposed to alcohol. Their sources of data were articles (see figure in the original article) that used a variety of methods. It is difficult to resolve the debate over whether, in predisposed adolescents and young adults, cannabis allows for psychosis to "bloom" or whether the experience of use with whichever peer group allows the adolescent to use with peer pressure. It is likewise challenging to tease out the question, and the current answers include the illegality of those substances and the real potential that it is hard to protect against publication bias in this sense.

A. H. Mack, MD

Child μ-Opioid Receptor Gene Variant Influences Parent–Child Relations

Copeland WE, Sun H, Costello EJ, et al (Duke Univ Med Ctr, Durham, NC; NIH/NIAAA/LNG, Bethesda, MD)
Neuropsychopharmacology 36:1165-1170, 2011

Variation in the μ-opioid receptor gene has been associated with early social behavior in mice and rhesus macaques. The current study tested whether the functional *OPRM1* A118G predicted various indices of social relations in children. The sample included 226 subjects of self-reported European ancestry (44% female; mean age 13.6, SD = 2.2) who were part of a larger representative study of children aged 9–17 years in rural North Carolina. Multiple aspects of recent (past 3 months) parent–child relationship were assessed using the Child and Adolescent Psychiatric Assessment. Parent problems were coded based upon a lifetime history of mental health problems, substance abuse, or criminality. Child genotype interacted with parent behavior such that there were no genotype

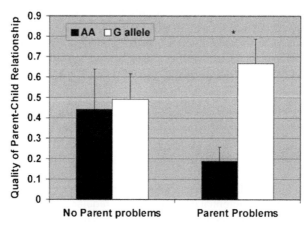

FIGURE 1.—Results of the Poisson multiple regression analyses estimating the association between parent problems and enjoyment of parent–child interactions as a function of the *OPRM1* A118G genotype. The overall main effect for genotype was significant ($\chi^2(1) = 4.3$, $p = 0.04$, MR = 2.0, 95% CI = 1.0, 3.8), but not for parent problems ($\chi^2(1) = 0.7$, $p = 0.40$, MR = 1.31, 95% CI = 0.7, 2.5). The interaction term (genotype by parent problems) interaction term was also significant ($\chi^2(1) = 6.6$, $p = 0.01$). For those with no parent problems, genotype status is not significant ($\chi^2(1) = 0.04$, $p = 0.84$, MR = 1.1, 95% CI = 0.4, 3.1), whereas for those with parent problems, genotype predicts enjoyment of parent–child interactions ($\chi^2(1) = 9.5, p = 0.002$, MR = 3.5, 95% CI = 1.6, 8.0). (Reprinted by permission from Macmillan Publishers Ltd: Neuropsychopharmacology. Copeland WE, Sun H, Costello EJ, et al. Child μ-opioid receptor gene variant influences parent-child relations. *Neuropsychopharmacology.* 2011;36:1165-1170, copyright 2011.)

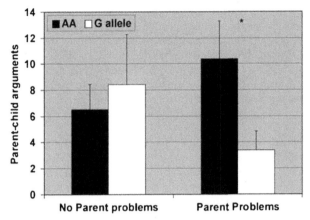

FIGURE 2.—Results of the Poisson multiple regression analyses estimating the association between parent problems and parent–child arguments as a function of the *OPRM1* A118G genotype. Neither of the main effects were significant (genotype: $\chi^2(1) = 1.1$, $p = 0.30$, MR $= 1.5$, 95% CI $= 0.7$, 3.5; parent problems: $\chi^2(1) = 0.4$, $p = 0.54$, MR $= 1.2$, 95% CI $= 0.6$, 2.5). The interaction term (genotype by parent problems) interaction term was also significant ($\chi^2(1) = 4.7$, $p = 0.03$). For those with no parent problems, genotype status is not significant ($\chi^2(1) = 0.21$, $p = 0.65$, MR $= 0.8$, 95% CI $= 0.2$, 2.4), whereas for those with parent problems, genotype predicts enjoyment of parent–child interactions ($\chi^2(1) = 4.5$, $p = 0.03$, MR $= 3.1$, 95% CI $= 1.1$, 8.9). (Reprinted by permission from Macmillan Publishers Ltd: Neuropsychopharmacology. Copeland WE, Sun H, Costello EJ, et al. Child μ-opioid receptor gene variant influences parent-child relations. *Neuropsychopharmacology.* 2011;36:1165-1170, copyright 2011.)

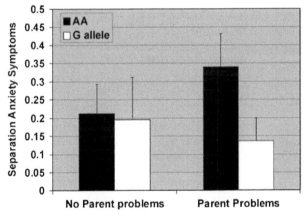

FIGURE 3.—Results of the Poisson multiple regression analyses estimating the association between parent problems and separation anxiety symptoms as a function of the *OPRM1* A118G genotype. Neither of the main effects were significant (genotype: $\chi^2(1) = 1.3$, $p = 0.25$, MR $= 1.6$, 95% CI $= 0.7$, 4.0; parent problems: $\chi^2(1) = 0.0$, $p = 0.90$, MR $= 0.9$, 95% CI $= 0.4$, 2.3). The interaction term (genotype by parent problems) interaction term was not statistically significant ($\chi^2(1) = 2.0$, $p = 0.16$). For those with no parent problems, genotype status is not significant ($\chi^2(1) = 0.0$, $p = 0.91$, MR $= 1.1$, 95% CI $= 0.3$, 4.3), and for those with parent problems, genotype showed a trend toward predicting enjoyment of parent–child interactions ($\chi^2(1) = 2.9$, $p = 0.09$, MR $= 2.5$, 95% CI $= 0.9$, 7.4). (Reprinted by permission from Macmillan Publishers Ltd: Neuropsychopharmacology. Copeland WE, Sun H, Costello EJ, et al. Child μ-opioid receptor gene variant influences parent-child relations. *Neuropsychopharmacology.* 2011;36:1165-1170, copyright 2011.)

differences for those with low levels of parent problems; however, when a history of parent problems was reported, the G allele carriers had more enjoyment of parent–child interactions (mean ratio (MR) = 3.5, 95% CI = 1.6, 8.0) and fewer arguments (MR = 3.1, 95% CI = 1.1, 8.9). These findings suggest a role for the *OPRM1* gene in the genetic architecture of social relations in humans. In summary, a variant in the μ-opioid receptor gene (118G) was associated with improved parent–child relations, but only in the context of a significant disruption in parental functioning (Figs 1-3).

▶ This article was selected not only because it covers the important area of gene-environment interaction but also because it was produced by a group that continues to create high-quality work. They have evaluated for the significance of a specific gene in the μ-opioid receptor and have demonstrated differences in their relations with their mother based much on gene. With Figs 1-3 as a basis, one can see that in certain areas of problem interaction there is a relationship to the normal or the abnormal gene one figures for each problem. The study's biggest drawback is its small size, but further study is needed because of the serious potential applications of this information. Countless children who simply do or do not get along with parents may benefit from more intensive assessment. This is one of several articles this year that combine psychiatry and human genome. Ideally, there will be further ease in doing such a study.

A. H. Mack, MD

Childhood CBCL bipolar profile and adolescent/young adult personality disorders: A 9-year follow-up

Halperin JM, Rucklidge JJ, Powers RL, et al (Queens College of the City Univ of New York; Univ of Canterbury, Christchurch, New Zealand; The Graduate Ctr of the City Univ of New York; et al)
J Affect Disord 130:155-161, 2011

Background.—To assess the late adolescent psychiatric outcomes associated with a positive Child Behavior Checklist-Juvenile Bipolar Disorder Phenotype (CBCL-JBD) in children diagnosed with ADHD and followed over a 9-year period.

Methods.—Parents of 152 children diagnosed as ADHD (ages 7–11 years) completed the CBCL. Ninety of these parents completed it again 9 years later as part of a comprehensive evaluation of Axis I and II diagnoses as assessed using semi-structured interviews. As previously proposed, the CBCL-JBD phenotype was defined as T-scores of 70 or greater on the Attention Problems, Aggression, and Anxiety/Depression subscales.

Results.—The CBCL-JBD phenotype was found in 31% of those followed but only 4.9% of the sample continued to meet the phenotype criteria at follow-up. Only two of the sample developed Bipolar Disorder by late adolescence and only one of those had the CBCL-JBD profile in childhood. The proxy did not predict any Axis I disorders. However, the CBCL-JBD proxy was highly predictive of later personality disorders.

Limitations.—Only a subgroup of the original childhood sample was followed. Given this sample was confined to children with ADHD, it is not known whether the prediction of personality disorders from CBCL scores would generalize to a wider community or clinical population.

Conclusions.—A positive CBCL-JBD phenotype profile in childhood does not predict Axis I Disorders in late adolescence; however, it may be prognostic of the emergence of personality disorders.

▶ This report was intended to add further data to the efforts to establish that nature and definition of bipolar disorder in children and adolescents. Rather than attempt to reanalyze the current diagnosis, this study provides longitudinal follow-up with diagnostic outcomes. The sample happens to be a group of adults who had attention-deficit/hyperactivity disorder and for whom Child Behavior Checklist (CBCL) data were available. The authors applied the definition of the CBCL juvenile bipolar disorder phenotype (a T score of greater than 70 on the attention problems, aggression, and anxiety/depression scales) to find cases and followed up with them 9 years later, finding more personality disorder diagnoses than bipolar disorder. Therefore, this calls into question the value of the CBCL bipolar phenotype. These data are not devoid of clinical value—the high rate of ultimate personality disorder diagnosis is encapsulated by the closing words of the report, "the CBCL-JBD phenotype may be a useful prognostic indicator that is merely in need of a name change."

A. H. Mack, MD

Childhood history of behavioral inhibition and comorbidity status in 256 adults with social phobia
Rotge J-Y, Grabot D, Aouizerate B, et al (Charles Perrens Hosp, Bordeaux, France; et al)
J Affect Disord 129:338-341, 2011

Background.—Behavioral inhibition (BI), a heritable temperament, predisposes one to an increased risk of social phobia. Recent investigations have reported that BI may also be a precursor to anxiety as well as depressive and alcohol-related disorders, which are frequently comorbid with social phobia. In the present study, we explored the relationship between BI and psychiatric disorders in 256 adults with a primary diagnosis of social phobia.

Methods.—BI severity was retrospectively assessed with the Retrospective Self-Report of Inhibition (RSRI). The severity of social phobia and the presence of comorbid diagnoses were evaluated with the Liebowitz Social Anxiety Scale (LSAS) and the Mini-International Neuropsychiatric Interview, respectively.

Results.—The RSRI score was significantly and positively correlated with both the LSAS score and the occurrence of a major depressive

TABLE 1.—Correlations Between the RSRI Global Score and Lifetime Comorbidities in Social Phobia (n = 256)

Lifetime Comorbidity	ORs[a]	IC 95%	Wald's Chi-Square Test χ^2	df	p
Major Depressive Disorder[b] (n = 196)	1.88	1.08–3.29	4.95	4	<0.05
Panic Disorder (n = 86)	1.34	0.85–2.12	1.56	4	0.21
Agoraphobia (n = 81)	1.51	0.94–2.41	2.93	4	0.09
Generalized Anxiety Disorder (n = 78)	1.47	0.91–2.37	2.47	4	0.12
Obsessive–Compulsive Disorder (n = 32)	1.01	0.99–1.01	0.87	4	0.35
Alcohol abuse (n = 30)	1.39	0.70–2.77	0.89	4	0.35
Alcohol dependence (n = 44)	1.69	0.94–3.05	3.10	4	0.08
Substance abuse (n = 14)	0.46	0.01–73.29	0.09	4	0.77
Substance dependence (n = 24)	0.79	0.37–1.69	0.35	4	0.55
Avoidant Personality Disorder[b] (n = 183)	1.99	1.12–3.54	5.54	4	<0.05

OR: Odds Ratio, IC 95%: 95% confidence interval, df: degrees of freedom.
[a]Adjustments were made for age, sex and LSAS score.
[b]IC 95% excluded 1.

disorder. No significant association was found with other anxiety and substance-related disorders.

Limitation.—The assessment of BI was retrospective and self-reported.

Conclusion.—A childhood history of BI was associated with an increased risk of depressive comorbidity in social phobia.

▶ This is an additional study on the relationship between childhood status and adult outcomes. It is of interest that it reports on adult depressive and anxiety conditions (see Table 1 for odds ratios of the various adult disorders). It is also valuable that the authors have used standardized instruments in making the current diagnoses. It is questionable how they were able to attempt to recreate or relate the reality of their childhoods; the Retrospective Self-Report of Inhibition is a tool that is not in mainstream use, and its reliance on self-report is a problem. One may also wonder why the Munich scale was used, except to help with language barriers. Nonetheless, continued attention to the relationship between childhood conditions and adult outcomes is of great interest, and this study assists in that plan. The findings shown in Table 1 suggest that many adult conditions may follow this state and a more streamlined process would be to their benefit.

A. H. Mack, MD

Childhood Trauma and Children's Emerging Psychotic Symptoms: A Genetically Sensitive Longitudinal Cohort Study
Arseneault L, Cannon M, Fisher HL, et al (King's College London, UK; the Inst of Psychiatry, London, UK; Beaumont Hosp, Dublin; Ireland; et al)
Am J Psychiatry 168:65-72, 2011

Objective.—Using longitudinal and prospective measures of trauma during childhood, the authors assessed the risk of developing psychotic symptoms associated with maltreatment, bullying, and accidents in a nationally representative U.K. cohort of young twins.

Method.—Data were from the Environmental Risk Longitudinal Twin Study, which follows 2,232 twin children and their families. Mothers were interviewed during home visits when children were ages 5, 7, 10, and 12 on whether the children had experienced maltreatment by an adult, bullying by peers, or involvement in an accident. At age 12, children were asked about bullying experiences and psychotic symptoms. Children's reports of psychotic symptoms were verified by clinicians.

Results.—Children who experienced maltreatment by an adult (relative risk=3.16, 95% CI=1.92—5.19) or bullying by peers (relative risk=2.47, 95% CI=1.74—3.52) were more likely to report psychotic symptoms at age 12 than were children who did not experience such traumatic events. The higher risk for psychotic symptoms was observed whether these events occurred early in life or later in childhood. The risk associated with childhood trauma remained significant in analyses controlling for children's gender, socioeconomic deprivation, and IQ; for children's early symptoms of internalizing or externalizing problems; and for children's genetic liability to developing psychosis. In contrast, the risk associated with accidents was small (relative risk=1.47, 95% CI=1.02—2.13) and inconsistent across ages.

Conclusions.—Trauma characterized by intention to harm is associated with children's reports of psychotic symptoms. Clinicians working with children who report early symptoms of psychosis should inquire about traumatic events such as maltreatment and bullying.

▶ This is a rich study that provides the literature with contributions on many different levels. It uses a large twin study, and at the age-12 assessment, almost all eligible subjects presented themselves for assessment. The central finding is that of excessive psychotic symptoms being related to harm, which is a basic finding seen in Fig 1 in the original article. The assumption was that each type of childhood exposure was more or less associated with an intention to harm. By that logic, it is helpful that the authors included information on those who had been in severe accidents, given the assumption that those were least intended to harm the child. One other important feature of the study was the use of prospective assessments of the effects of trauma. The comparison of the mothers' and victims' view of the significance of the trauma is an important finding that supports the concept that parent reports differ from child reports, especially during adolescence.

A. H. Mack, MD

Children's Problems Predict Adults' *DSM-IV* Disorders Across 24 Years

Reef J, van Meurs I, Verhulst FC, et al (Erasmus Med Ctr—Sophia Children's Hosp, Rotterdam, the Netherlands)
J Am Acad Child Adolesc Psychiatry 49:1117-1124, 2010

Objective.—The goal of this study was to determine continuities of a broad range of psychopathology from childhood into middle adulthood in a general population sample across a 24-year follow-up.

Method.—In 1983, parent ratings of children's problems were collected with the Child Behavior Checklist (CBCL) in a general population sample of 2,076 children and young adolescents aged 4 to 16 years. In 2007, 24 years later, 1,339 of these individuals were reassessed with the CIDI, a standardized *DSM-IV* interview. We used univariate logistic regression analyses to determine the associations between children's problems and adults' psychiatric disorders.

Results.—Parent reported total problems scores in the deviant range (>85th percentile) predicted disruptive disorders in adulthood (odds ratio [OR] = 1.7, 95% confidence interval [95% CI] = 1.1−2.8). Adjusted for sex, age, and socioeconomic status in all analyses, deviant levels of parent-reported childhood anxiety predicted anxiety disorders in middle adulthood (OR = 1.6, 95% CI = 1.0−2.5). Conduct problems (i.e., cruelty to animals, lies) predicted both mood disorders (OR = 2.3, 95% CI = 1.1−4.8) and disruptive disorders (OR 2.1, 95% CI = 1.3−3.4), whereas oppositional defiant problems predicted only mood disorders (OR = 2.3, 95% CI = 1.0−5.2). Attention-deficit/hyperactivity problems did not predict any of the *DSM-IV* disorders in adulthood (OR = 0.8, 95% CI = 0.5−1.2).

Conclusions.—Children with psychopathology are at greater risk for meeting criteria for *DSM-IV* diagnoses in adulthood than children without psychopathology, even after 24 years. Moreover, different types of continuities of children's psychopathology exist across the lifespan. We found that anxious children, oppositional defiant children, and children with conduct problems are at greater risk for adult psychopathology. Effective identification and treatment of children with these problems may reduce long-term continuity of psychopathology (Fig 2).

▶ There were many reports in the past year about the long-term outcomes of those with psychiatric disorders during childhood, including others cited in this article, on cases of abuse, neglect, or bullying. But this report (along with its companion piece[1]) use findings and data for a clinical population—at least one that was originally a clinical population. This report by Reef used Child Behavior Checklist (CBCL) information on individuals ranging from 4 to 16 years of age and now followed up with them after 24 years. This is a remarkable achievement in itself. Predictive significance of conduct, oppositional, and anxiety conditions were high, as well as the fact that adult mood disorders were predicted by childhood anxiety or oppositional conditions. The outcomes of conduct disordered behavior included a variety of adult conditions, however. This actually is an important consideration about the validity of conduct disorder

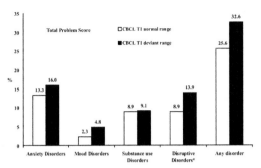

FIGURE 2.—*DSM-IV* disorders in adulthood for participants with scores in normal range or in deviant range on the Child Behavior Checklist Total Problem Scale. *Note:* *Significant ($p < .05$) difference in prevalence rates for childhood scores in normal range and in deviant range derived from univariate logistic regression analysis. (Reprinted from Journal of the American Academy of Child and Adolescent Psychiatry, Reef J, van Meurs I, Verhulst FC, et al. Children's problems predict adults' *DSM-IV* disorders across 24 years. *J Am Acad Child Adolesc Psychiatry*. 2010;49:1117-1124. Copyright 2010 with permission from Elsevier.)

and whether we ought to continue to view it with skepticism as a final common pathway disorder. Nevertheless, as seen in Fig 2, the relationships between adult disorders and abnormal CBCL findings during childhood were significant and deserve attention, and parents (and the children) should be given assessments of their prognosis when possible.

A. H. Mack, MD

Reference

1. Althoff RR, Verhulst FC, Rettew DC, Hudziak JJ, van der Ende J. Adult outcomes of childhood dysregulation: a 14-year Follow-up study. *J Am Acad Child Adolesc Psychiatry*. 2010;49:1105-1116.

Clinical and Psychosocial Predictors of Suicide Attempts and Nonsuicidal Self-Injury in the Adolescent Depression Antidepressants and Psychotherapy Trial (ADAPT)

Wilkinson P, Kelvin R, Roberts C, et al (Cambridge Univ, England; Manchester Univ, England; Royal Manchester Children's Hosp, Pendlebury, UK)
Am J Psychiatry 168:495-501, 2011

Objective.—The authors assessed whether clinical and psychosocial factors in depressed adolescents at baseline predict suicide attempts and nonsuicidal self-injury over 28 weeks of follow-up.

Method.—Participants were 164 adolescents with major depressive disorder taking part in the Adolescent Depression Antidepressants and Psychotherapy Trial (ADAPT). Clinical symptoms, family function, quality of current personal friendships, and suicidal and nonsuicidal self-harm were assessed at baseline. Suicidal and nonsuicidal self-harm thoughts and behaviors were assessed during 28 weeks of follow-up.

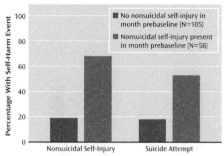

FIGURE 1.—Effects of Baseline Nonsuicidal Self-Injury on Risk of Harm Events in Adolescents with Major Depression Over 28 Weeks of Follow-Up. For nonsuicidal self-injury, $\chi^2=39$, df=1, p<0.0005; for suicide attempt, $\chi^2=22$, df=1, p<0.0005. (Reprinted with permission from the American Journal of Psychiatry, Wilkinson P, Kelvin R, Roberts C, et al. Clinical and psychosocial predictors of suicide attempts and nonsuicidal self-injury in the Adolescent Depression Antidepressants and Psychotherapy Trial (ADAPT). *Am J Psychiatry.* 2011;168:495-501. © 2011. American Psychiatric Association.)

Results.—High suicidality, nonsuicidal self-injury, and poor family function at entry were significant independent predictors of suicide attempts over the 28 weeks of follow-up. Nonsuicidal self-injury over the follow-up period was independently predicted by nonsuicidal self-injury, hopelessness, anxiety disorder, and being younger and female at entry.

Conclusions.—Both suicidal and nonsuicidal self-harm persisted in depressed adolescents receiving treatment in the ADAPT study. A history of nonsuicidal self-injury prior to treatment is a clinical marker for subsequent suicide attempts and should be as carefully assessed in depressed youths as current suicidal intent and behavior (Fig 1).

▶ This report provides valuable information as well as guidance regarding the treatment of adolescents who have had prior suicide attempts. It also provides reliable information on those adolescents who have a history of nonsuicidal self-injury, and it concludes that adolescents with a history of nonsuicidal self-injury are as much at risk of a suicide attempt in the future as are those with a prior suicide attempt. It also finds that family dysfunction is an important risk factor as well. The source of these data is the Adolescent Depression Antidepressants and Psychotherapy Trial, which is a British large-N study on treatment effectiveness of medications with and without cognitive behavioral therapy intervention. The results are consistent with those determined in other large studies of adolescent depression, such as the TORDIA study. One important point is that the population studied here included those with major depressive disorder only, rather than a not-otherwise-specified diagnosis or another mood disorder. Clinicians and investigators will take keen notice of these data to emphasize areas of clinical history taking or assessment sometimes not fully addressed and also to continue to determine the basis for these findings. The study created a composite score of family functioning, and one may wonder if other scoring systems would replicate their findings of dysfunction at the family level being associated with suicide. Nevertheless, the journal chose this article as one to provide clinical guidance, and one will learn a great deal from reviewing these data and the background behind them. Fig 1 displays the findings that nonsuicidal self-harm in the month before baseline was associated with a greater risk of suicidal behavior than a history of a suicide attempt in the prior month. The report does provide support for a reduced risk of nonsuicidal self-injury associated with depression treatment overall, however, which is an important vantage point.

A. H. Mack, MD

Correlates of At-Risk/Problem Internet Gambling in Adolescents

Potenza MN, Wareham JD, Steinberg MA, et al (Yale School of Medicine, New Haven, CT; Connecticut Council on Problem Gambling, Clinton; et al)
J Am Acad Child Adolesc Psychiatry 50:150-159, 2011

Objective.—The Internet represents a new and widely available forum for gambling. However, relatively few studies have examined Internet gambling in adolescents. This study sought to investigate the correlates of at-risk or problem gambling in adolescents acknowledging or denying gambling on the Internet.

Method.—Survey data from 2,006 Connecticut high school student gamblers were analyzed using χ^2 and logistic regression analyses.

Results.—At-risk/problem gambling was found more frequently in adolescent Internet gamblers than in non-Internet gamblers. Compared with at-risk/problem gambling in the non-Internet gambling group, at-risk/problem gambling in the Internet gambling group was more strongly associated with poor academic performance and substance use (particularly current heavy alcohol use; odds ratio 2.99; $p = .03$) and less strongly associated with gambling with friends (odds ratio 0.32; $p = .0003$). At-risk/problem gambling in the Internet and non-Internet gambling groups, respectively, was associated at $p < .05$, each with multiple adverse measurements including dysphoria/depression (odds ratios 1.76 and 1.96), getting into serious fights (odds ratios 2.50 and 1.93), carrying weapons (odds ratios 2.11 and 1.90), and use of tobacco (odds ratios 2.05 and 1.88 for regular use), marijuana (odds ratios 2.02 and 1.39), and other drugs (odds ratios 3.24 and 1.67).

Conclusions.—Clinically, it is important to assess for teenagers' involvement in Internet gambling, particularly because adolescent at-risk/problem Internet gambling appears specifically associated with nonpeer involvement, heavy alcohol use, and poor academic functioning.

▶ Gambling as a psychiatric disorder, that is, pathological gambling (PG), remains new and unfamiliar to many in the field. It is specifically placed in the disorders of impulse control, rather than in the substance use disorders section. Whatever the long-term outcome of gambling as an individual disorder, it has opened a new and fruitful avenue for understanding behavior and the associated problems with PG. This study is not intended to be the final word on the etiology of PG or whether it should be considered a disorder, but a discussion of what the features are of those youth who have problems. Independent substance use disorders are frequent among those with PG; is it the same for nondiagnostic gambling? This statewide review is helpful, although it is self-report only. More health problems were found in the at-risk group that used the Internet for gambling. This relationship was not replicated for dysphoria or depression. As a result, in a nondiagnostic group, at-risk gambling was a critical component. Hopefully we can also address family concerns about Internet use.

A. H. Mack, MD

Cortical Development in Typically Developing Children With Symptoms of Hyperactivity and Impulsivity: Support for a Dimensional View of Attention Deficit Hyperactivity Disorder

Shaw P, Gilliam M, Liverpool M, et al (Natl Inst of Mental Health, Bethesda, MD; McGill Univ, Montreal, Quebec, Canada)
Am J Psychiatry 168:143-151, 2011

Objective.—There is considerable epidemiological and neuropsychological evidence that attention deficit hyperactivity disorder (ADHD) is best considered dimensionally, lying at the extreme end of a continuous distribution of symptoms and underlying cognitive impairments. The authors investigated whether cortical brain development in typically developing children with symptoms of hyperactivity and impulsivity resembles that found in the syndrome of ADHD. Specifically, they examined whether a slower rate of cortical thinning during late childhood and adolescence, which they previously found in ADHD, is also linked to the severity of symptoms of hyperactivity and impulsivity in typically developing children.

Method.—In a longitudinal analysis, a total of 193 typically developing children with 389 neuroanatomic magnetic resonance images and varying levels of symptoms of hyperactivity and impulsivity (measured with the Conners' Parent Rating Scale) were contrasted with 197 children with ADHD with 337 imaging scans. The relationship between the rates of regional cortical thinning and severity of symptoms of hyperactivity/impulsivity was determined.

Results.—Youth with higher levels of hyperactivity/impulsivity had a slower rate of cortical thinning, predominantly in prefrontal cortical regions, bilaterally in the middle frontal/premotor gyri, extending down the medial prefrontal wall to the anterior cingulate; the orbitofrontal cortex; and the right inferior frontal gyrus. For each increase of one point in the hyperactivity/impulsivity score, there was a decrease in the rate of regional cortical thinning of 0.0054 mm/year (SE=0.0019 mm/year). Children with ADHD had the slowest rate of cortical thinning.

Conclusions.—Slower cortical thinning during adolescence characterizes the presence of both the symptoms and syndrome of ADHD, providing neurobiological evidence for dimensionality of the disorder.

▶ The study by Shaw et al is a milestone in the understanding of attention-deficit/ hyperactivity disorder (ADHD). It is an important finding about the developmental biology of the condition: that the rate of cortical thinning is slower in youth with ADHD-like signs who are not diagnosed with ADHD than in those with no ADHD signs or symptoms. And, more impressively, they demonstrate the distinction between those with no ADHD symptoms or signs and those who meet full diagnostic criteria, which strengthens the basis for a neurobiological basis of the diagnosis, but more importantly, which shows a continuum of neurobiological findings (Fig 3 in the original article). This had been shown many years ago, but only in ADHD-diagnosed groups. Now we're seeing a narrower perspective by focusing on hyperactivity and impulsivity. One should wonder why or how these children are not diagnosed with ADHD in an era when it is of such low threshold. Here they are using neuroimaging to gather data and showed (Fig 3 in the original article) a continuum of inverse rate of thinning related to ADHD symptoms, especially in prefrontal cortical regions. Regardless of its place in the diagnosis of ADHD, this is an important step toward understanding it.

A. H. Mack, MD

Distinguishing Between Major Depressive Disorder and Obsessive-Compulsive Disorder in Children by Measuring Regional Cortical Thickness

Fallucca E, MacMaster FP, Haddad J, et al (Wayne State Univ, Detroit, MI)
Arch Gen Psychiatry 68:527-533, 2011

Context.—Cortical abnormalities have been noted in previous studies of major depressive disorder (MDD).

Objective.—To hypothesize differences in regional cortical thickness among children with MDD, children with obsessive-compulsive disorder (OCD), and healthy controls.

Design.—Cross-sectional study of groups.

Setting.—Children's Hospital of Michigan in Detroit.

Participants.—A total of 24 psychotropic drug—naive pediatric patients with MDD (9 boys and 15 girls), 24 psychotropic drug—naive pediatric outpatients with OCD (8 boys and 16 girls), and 30 healthy controls (10 boys and 20 girls).

Intervention.—Magnetic resonance imaging.

Main Outcome Measure.—Cortical thickness.

Results.—In the right hemisphere of the brain, the pericalcarine gyrus was thinner in patients with MDD than in outpatients with OCD ($P = .002$) or healthy controls ($P = .04$), the postcentral gyrus was thinner in patients with MDD than in outpatients with OCD ($P = .002$) or healthy controls ($P = .02$), and the superior parietal gyrus was thinner in patients with MDD than in outpatients with OCD ($P = .008$) or healthy controls ($P = .03$). The outpatients with OCD and the healthy controls did not differ in these regions of the brain. The temporal pole was thicker in patients with MDD than in outpatients with OCD ($P < .001$) or healthy controls ($P = .01$), both of which groups did not differ in temporal pole thickness. The cuneus was thinner in patients with MDD than in outpatients with OCD ($P = .008$), but it did not differ from that in healthy controls. In the left hemisphere, the supramarginal gyrus was thinner in both patients with MDD ($P = .04$) and outpatients with OCD ($P = .01$) than in healthy controls, and the temporal pole was thicker in patients withMDDthan in both healthy controls and outpatients with OCD ($P < .001$).

Conclusions.—To our knowledge, this is the first study to explore cortical thickness in pediatric patients with MDD. Although differences in some regions of the brain would be expected given neurobiological models of MDD, our study highlights some unexpected regions (ie, supramarginal and superior parietal gyri) that merit further investigation. These results underscore the need to expand exploration beyond the frontal-limbic circuit.

▶ Here is another study that demonstrates tangible findings of neuroanatomy using magnetic resonance imaging. The research team not only used morphometry but specific software that assists in optimizing the calculation of cortical thickness. The study's findings need replication, but they should be stated now. They determined some distinctions in cortical thickness in some specific sites between medication-naive pediatric patients with major depressive disorder, obsessive-compulsive disorder (OCD), and healthy controls. One can see from the figure in the original article that the differences are discernible between all 3 groups. The left supramarginal gyrus marks an area of distinction between patients with OCD and controls. The authors hypothesized that differences would be found in the anterior cingulate lobe, the orbitofrontal area, and the dorsal prefrontal lobe; these were not detected in this study, which was a surprise. It is unknown if this is because of the age of these subjects or if there is a pathophysiology that is universal to these disorders. However, this study not only deserves replication but may be the starting point for considering new approaches to the neuroanatomy of these disorders.

A. H. Mack, MD

Early Brain Overgrowth in Autism Associated With an Increase in Cortical Surface Area Before Age 2 Years
Hazlett HC, Poe MD, Gerig G, et al (Univ of North Carolina, Chapel Hill; Univ of Utah, Salt Lake City)
Arch Gen Psychiatry 68:467-476, 2011

Context.—Brain enlargement has been observed in 2-year-old children with autism, but the underlying mechanisms are unknown.

Objective.—To investigate early growth trajectories in brain volume and cortical thickness.

Design.—Longitudinal magnetic resonance imaging study.

Setting.—Academic medical centers.

Participants.—Fifty-nine children with autism spectrum disorder (ASD) and 38 control children.

Intervention.—Children were examined at approximately 2 years of age. Magnetic resonance imaging was repeated approximately 24 months later (when aged 4-5 years; 38 children with ASD; 21 controls).

Main Outcome Measures.—Cerebral gray and white matter volumes and cortical thickness.

Results.—We observed generalized cerebral cortical enlargement in individuals with ASD at both 2 and 4 to 5 years of age. Rate of cerebral cortical growth across multiple brain regions and tissue compartments in children with ASD was parallel to that seen in the controls, indicating that there was no increase in rate of cerebral cortical growth during this interval. No cerebellar differences were observed in children with ASD. After controlling for total brain volume, a disproportionate enlargement in temporal lobe white matter was observed in the ASD group. We found no significant differences in cortical thickness but observed an increase in an estimate of surface area in the ASD group compared with controls for all cortical regions measured (temporal, frontal, and parieto-occipital lobes).

Conclusions.—Our longitudinal magnetic resonance imaging study found generalized cerebral cortical enlargement in children with ASD, with a disproportionate enlargement in temporal lobe white matter. There was no significant difference from controls in the rate of brain growth for this age interval, indicating that brain enlargement in ASD results from an increased rate of brain growth before age 2 years. The presence of increased cortical volume, but not cortical thickness, suggests that early brain enlargement may be associated with increased cortical surface area. Cortical surface area overgrowth in ASD may underlie brain enlargement and implicates a distinct set of pathogenic mechanisms.

▶ There are many different lines of investigation regarding the pathophysiology of autism, ranging from genetics to neural connections in the brain. Here is an approach that combines the use of our most advanced technical tools (volumetric analysis of the brain) with basic questions about the size of the brain. One should note the high threshold for diagnosis and entry into this study, particularly the reliance on the Autism Diagnostic Observation Schedule scale. There has been painstaking research to demonstrate abnormality in brain weight and head circumference. This study takes it a step further in finding which areas of the brain have this abnormal growth. The findings of specific difference in the temporal lobes are helpful (Fig 2 in the original article). However, overall, the findings that demonstrate the distinction between excess cortical thickness versus increased cortical surface area are both fascinating and important as a determination of a new area for neuroanatomical study of autism and, with its relationship to the timing of autism and its localization, perhaps a direction for the study of autism as a whole.

A. H. Mack, MD

Genetically Informative Research on Adolescent Substance Use: Methods, Findings, and Challenges
Lynskey MT, Agrawal A, Heath AC (Washington Univ School of Medicine, St Louis, MO)
J Am Acad Child Adolesc Psychiatry 49:1202-1214, 2010

Objective.—To provide an overview of the genetic epidemiology of substance use and misuse in adolescents.

Method.—A selective review of genetically informative research strategies, their limitations, and key findings examining issues related to the heritability of substance use and substance use disorders in children and adolescents is presented.

Results.—Adoption, twin, and extended-family designs have established there is a strong heritable component to liability to nicotine, alcohol, and illicit drug dependence in adults. However, shared environmental influences are relatively stronger in youth samples and at earlier stages of substance involvement (e.g., use). There is considerable overlap in the genetic influences associated with the abuse/dependence across drug classes, and shared genetic influences contribute to the commonly observed associations between substance-use disorders and externalizing and, to a lesser extent, internalizing psychopathology. Rapid technologic advances have made the identification of specific gene variants that influence risks for substance-use disorders feasible, and linkage and association (including genomewide association studies) have identified promising candidate genes implicated in the development of substance-use disorders.

Conclusions.—Studies using genetically informative research designs, including those that examine aggregate genetic factors and those examining specific gene variants, individually and in interaction with environmental influences, offer promising avenues not only for delineating genetic effects on substance-use disorders but also for understanding the unfolding of risk across development and the interaction between environmental and genetic factors in the etiology of these disorders.

▶ When we consider the import of genetics on all of psychiatry, or all of medicine for that matter, we should be able to grasp the wide application that this modality has. It presents many opportunities. This report is a compilation of what is known about substance use and genetics among youth. Of course, the main point is that there are shared, or heritable, risks that arise in some very basic aspects of mental state and vulnerability for misuse. Furthermore, although there may be wide support for genetic risks among adults, for some time, the best indicator for adolescent use has been peer group and its pressures. So genetic transmission may be a quite real phenomenon, but it does not and cannot determine all aspects of human behavior; we have to continue to seek manners in which this vulnerability does not become real use.

A. H. Mack, MD

Hurtful Words: Association of Exposure to Peer Verbal Abuse With Elevated Psychiatric Symptom Scores and Corpus Callosum Abnormalities
Teicher MH, Samson JA, Sheu Y-S, et al (McLean Hosp, Boston, MA; Harvard Med School, Boston, MA)
Am J Psychiatry 167:1464-1471, 2010

Objective.—Previous studies have shown that exposure to parental verbal abuse in childhood is associated with higher rates of adult psychopathology and alterations in brain structure. In this study the authors sought to examine the symptomatic and neuroanatomic effects, in young adulthood, of exposure to peer verbal abuse during childhood.

Method.—A total of 848 young adults (ages 18—25 years) with no history of exposure to domestic violence, sexual abuse, or parental physical abuse rated their childhood exposure to parental and peer verbal abuse and completed a self-report packet that included the Kellner Symptom Questionnaire, the Limbic Symptom Checklist—33, and the Dissociative Experiences Scale. Diffusion tensor images were collected for a subset of 63 young adults with no history of abuse or exposure to parental verbal abuse selected for varying degrees of exposure to peer verbal abuse. Images were analyzed using tract-based spatial statistics.

Results.—Analysis of covariance revealed dose-dependent effects of peer verbal abuse on anxiety, depression, anger-hostility, dissociation, "limbic irritability," and drug use. Peer and parental verbal abuse were essentially equivalent in effect size on these ratings. Path analysis indicated that peer verbal abuse during the middle school years had the most significant effect on symptom scores. Degree of exposure to peer verbal abuse correlated with increased mean and radial diffusivity and decreased fractional anisotropy in the corpus callosum and the corona radiata.

Conclusions.—These findings parallel results of previous reports of psychopathology associated with childhood exposure to parental verbal abuse and support the hypothesis that exposure to peer verbal abuse is an aversive stimulus associated with greater symptom ratings and meaningful alterations in brain structure.

▶ The past several years have included a literature replete with findings about bullying that coalesced with discoveries on the dose-dependent poor outcomes of childhood maltreatment generally. However, what is the overall mechanism or are there specific mechanisms that affect these outcomes one by one? There have been findings that there are neurobiological effects of adverse experiences, but here is an advance whereby neurobiological abnormal findings specifically in cases of a history of peer verbal abuse are documented. The significant findings of dose-dependent increases in drug use, dissociation, and limbic symptoms were seen, mainly in equal degrees of both sexes. The neurobiological findings included increased diffusivity of the splenium of the corpus callosum.

The importance of these findings is matched by the methodological strengths of the study. Some findings regarding symptoms were made using the data from a large community sample of young adults. Of the group selected for neuroimaging, there were more than 60 participants who underwent MRI scanning; and their exposure to past peer verbal abuse was measured using an instrument that had been shown to have reliability. In addition, they used standard scales for dissociation and limbic symptoms (Fig 1 in the original article). The exclusion of those who had experienced physical bullying or other forms of maltreatment is of further value, as is the exclusion of those with other psychiatric disorders.

These findings are interesting but also of great potential use in advancing our understanding of the psychopathology of those who have suffered from adverse experiences, ideally leading to hope in improved secondary prevention or treatment. The main concerns are, as identified by the authors, the possibilities of bias in these self-reports. In addition, there are the risks that these participants had inherent psychological qualities that have shaped all of their experiences and perspectives.

A. H. Mack, MD

Infant Media Exposure and Toddler Development
Tomopoulos S, Dreyer BP, Berkule S, et al (New York Univ School of Medicine—Bellevue Hosp Ctr)
Arch Pediatr Adolesc Med 164:1105-1111, 2010

Objective.—To determine whether duration and content of media exposure in 6-month-old infants are associated with development at age 14 months.

Design.—Longitudinal analysis of 259 mother-infant dyads participating in a long-term study related to early child development, from November 23, 2005, through January 14, 2008.

Setting.—An urban public hospital.

Participants.—Mothers with low socioeconomic status and their infants.

Main Exposure.—Duration and content of media exposure at age 6 months.

Main Outcome Measures.—Cognitive and language development at age 14 months.

Results.—Of 259 infants, 249 (96.1%) were exposed to media at age 6 months, with mean (SD) total exposure of 152.7 (124.5) min/d. In unadjusted and adjusted analyses, duration of media exposure at age 6 months was associated with lower cognitive development at age 14 months (unadjusted: $r=-0.17$, $P<.01$; adjusted: $\beta=-0.15$, $P=.02$) and lower language development ($r=-0.16$, $P<.01$; $\beta=-0.16$, $P<.01$). Of 3 types of content assessed, only 1 (older child/adult—oriented) was associated with lower cognitive and language development at age 14 months. No significant associations were seen with exposure to young child—oriented educational or noneducational content.

Conclusions.—This study is the first, to our knowledge, to have longitudinally assessed associations between media exposure in infancy and subsequent developmental outcomes in children from families with low socioeconomic status in the United States. Findings provide strong evidence in support of the American Academy of Pediatrics recommendations of no media exposure prior to age 2 years, although further research is needed.

▶ This study reviewed infant exposure to television and documented statistically significant declines in IQ as measure on the Bayley III Scales of Development and also the Preschool Language Scale in a form directly related to amount of TV. The conclusion emphasizes the American Academy of Pediatrics recommendation against any media exposure before age 2. Although this may well be a worthwhile conclusion and practice, readers will miss much in this article if not attentive to detail. First, it is a longitudinal study of mother-child dyads, so there is no control. Second is the baseline status of the mothers: the sample group was collected at a large urban public hospital with mothers who on average had not graduated from high school. The measurement was on TV exposure at age 6 months. To have a child "watching" television at 6 months suggests many negative assumptions about the mother, and one could easily make assumptions about the overall ecology in which the 6 month old lives or shall live. The study's attempt to stratify risk of developmental delay by the content of the program was not able to show differences among 2 of the 3 groups. In all, this is an important finding to add to the extant literature on the subject.

A. H. Mack, MD

Neuroanatomical Abnormalities That Predate the Onset of Psychosis: A Multicenter Study
Mechelli A, Riecher-Rössler A, Meisenzahl EM, et al (King's College London, UK; Univ Hosp Basel, Switzerland; Ludwig-Maximilians-Univ, Munich, Germany; et al)
Arch Gen Psychiatry 68:489-495, 2011

Context.—People experiencing possible prodromal symptoms of psychosis have a very high risk of developing the disorder, but it is not possible to predict, on the basis of their presenting clinical features, which individuals will subsequently become psychotic. Recent neuroimaging studies suggest that there are volumetric differences between individuals at ultra-high risk (UHR) for psychosis who later develop psychotic disorder and those who do not. However, the samples examined to date have been small, and the findings have been inconsistent.

Objective.—To assess brain structure in individuals at UHR for psychosis in a larger and more representative sample than in previous studies by combining magnetic resonance imaging data from 5 different scanning sites.

Design.—Case-control study.

Setting.—Multisite.

Participants.—A total of 182 individuals at UHR and 167 healthy controls. Participants were observed clinically for a mean of 2 years. Forty-eight individuals (26.4%) in the UHR group developed psychosis and 134 did not.

Main Outcome Measures.—Magnetic resonance images were acquired from each participant. Group differences in gray matter volume were examined using optimized voxel-based morphometry.

Results.—The UHR group as a whole had less gray matter volume than did controls in the frontal regions bilaterally. The UHR subgroup who later developed psychosis had less gray matter volume in the left parahippocampal cortex than did the UHR subgroup who did not.

Conclusions.—Individuals at high risk for psychosis show alterations in regional gray matter volume regardless of whether they subsequently develop the disorder. In the UHR population, reduced left parahippocampal volume was specifically associated with the later onset of psychosis. Alterations in this region may, thus, be crucial to the expression of illness. Identifying abnormalities that specifically predate the onset of psychosis informs the development of clinical investigations designed to predict which individuals at high risk will subsequently develop the disorder.

▶ Our interest in finding probable cases of schizophrenia continues unabated, and this study provides further data around the issues of neurological abnormalities that predate the diagnosis of schizophrenia. This is akin to, but not the same as, the neurological "soft signs" that have tantalized the biologists in us but have failed to provide help to the clinicians in us.

This is not to say that study of any prodromal group is easy; here the population of study are those at "ultra high risk," which used a polythetic criteria set. The authors assessed volumetric differences between ultra-high-risk subjects and made comparisons among those who would later develop schizophrenia and those who do not by combining magnetic resonance imaging data. Although there were some other differences noted, the central results indicated that reduced left parahippocampal volume is specifically associated with the later onset of psychosis. This is a regional variation that must be analyzed further. In addition, all of the ultra-high-risk patients displayed some alterations in regional gray matter, which was an important finding as well.

A. H. Mack, MD

Posttraumatic Stress Without Trauma in Children
Copeland WE, Keeler G, Angold A, et al (Duke Univ Med Ctr, Durham, NC)
Am J Psychiatry 167:1059-1065, 2010

Objective.—It remains unclear to what degree children show signs of posttraumatic stress disorder (PTSD) after experiencing low-magnitude stressors, or stressors milder than those required for the DSM-IV extreme stressor criterion.

Method.—A representative community sample of 1,420 children, ages 9, 11, and 13 at intake, was followed annually through age 16. Low-magnitude and extreme stressors as well as subsequent posttraumatic stress symptoms were assessed with the Child and Adolescent Psychiatric

Assessment. Two measures of posttraumatic stress symptoms were used: having painful recall, hyperarousal, and avoidance symptoms (subclinical PTSD) and having painful recall only.

Results.—During any 3-month period, low-magnitude stressors occurred four times as often as extreme stressors (24.0% compared with 5.9%). Extreme stressors elicited painful recall in 8.7% of participants and subclinical PTSD in 3.1%, compared with 4.2% and 0.7%, respectively, for low-magnitude stressors. Because of their higher prevalence, however, low-magnitude stressors accounted for two-thirds of cases of painful recall and half of cases of subclinical PTSD. Moreover, exposure to low-magnitude stressors predicted symptoms even among youths with no prior lifetime exposure to an extreme stressor.

Conclusions.—Relative to low-magnitude stressors, extreme stressors place children at greater risk for posttraumatic stress symptoms. Nevertheless, a sizable proportion of children manifesting posttraumatic stress symptoms experienced only a low-magnitude stressor.

▶ The Great Smoky Mountains Study is the basis for further excellent epidemiologically based assessments. In this instance, the study reviews the prevalence of posttraumatic stress disorder (PTSD) in children and especially the traumas associated with the disorder. The authors begin by citing a recent meta-analysis that suggests PTSD is as rare as 0.6% of all children; they use this as the basis for asking whether or not the current Diagnostic and Statistical Manual of Mental Disorders, Fourth Edition, criteria for PTSD are valid in children. This report comes as our classification is being revised, and of course there are some who argue that the current criteria for PTSD are insufficiently attuned to children. The study did not assess for a relationship with PTSD itself but rather PTSD symptoms. The authors defined subthreshold PTSD as the simple presence of painful recall, hyperarousal, and avoidance and linked low-magnitude events (which did not meet the threshold for criterion A of the PTSD definition) with this definition. However, the content of these components of the syndrome, as defined, are unclear and may well represent typical or expected responses to adverse events, rather than a syndrome of PTSD as we expect to occur in adults. The question is should the DSM have a specific PTSD definition for kids and why?

A. H. Mack, MD

Psychiatric Symptoms in Bereaved Versus Nonbereaved Youth and Young Adults: A Longitudinal Epidemiological Study
Kaplow JB, Saunders J, Angold A, et al (Univ of Michigan Med School, Ann Arbor; RAND Corporation, Ann Arbor, MI; Duke Univ, Durham NC)
J Am Acad Child Adolesc Psychiatry 49:1145-1154, 2010

Objective.—To examine potential differences in psychiatric symptoms between parentbereaved youth (N = 172), youth who experienced the death of another relative (N = 815), and nonbereaved youth (N = 235), aged 11 to 21 years, above and beyond antecedent environmental and individual risk factors.

Method.—Sociodemographics, family composition, and family functioning were assessed one interview wave before the death. Child psychiatric symptoms were assessed during the wave in which the death was reported and one wave before and after the death. A year was selected randomly for the nonbereaved group.

Results.—The early loss of a parent was associated with poverty, previous substance abuse problems, and greater functional impairment before the loss. Both bereaved groups of children were more likely than nonbereaved children to show symptoms of separation anxiety and depression during the wave of the death, controlling for sociodemographic factors and prior psychiatric symptoms. One wave following the loss, bereaved children were more likely than nonbereaved children to exhibit symptoms of conduct disorder and substance abuse and to show greater functional impairment.

Conclusions.—The impact of parental death on children must be considered in the context of pre-existing risk factors. Even after controlling for antecedent risk factors, both parent-bereaved children as well as those who lost other relatives were at increased risk for psychological and behavioral health problems.

▶ An estimated 4% of children in Western nations experience the loss of a parent—and there is the loss of friends and nonparent family. So bereavement is not novel. There is an inconsistency in terms of the number of symptoms or disorders after loss. Consider the long termination up to the death whether by illness or poverty. Many studies have retrieval bias. Here is the largest epidemiological sample: the Great Smoky Mountain Study has 1420 participants, and 172 had lost a parent or parental figure; 815 lost a nonparent figure during the study. Their interest was in comparing those 2 groups with those who were not bereaved. Both bereaved groups were more likely to demonstrate separation anxiety; there were no differences in posttraumatic stress disorder symptoms (albeit not eliciting the disorder itself). A prior study had focused on those whose parents died from sudden deaths.[1] In terms of depression, there was no likelihood that the parent-bereaved or nonbereaved group had more symptomatology, but there was an excess among the other-bereaved, for various possible reasons, such as lesser degrees of support or the experience of the parent as bereaving. Conduct disorder symptoms were also present in the bereaved group, and the same occurred for substance abuse. Finally, in terms of global functioning, both groups experienced a decrease.

A. H. Mack, MD

Reference

1. Melhem NM, Walker M, Moritz G, Brent DA. Antecedents and sequelae of sudden parental death in offspring and surviving caregivers. *Arch Pediatr Adolesc Med.* 2008;162:403-410.

Secondhand Smoke Exposure and Mental Health Among Children and Adolescents

Bandiera FC, Richardson AK, Lee DJ, et al (Univ of Miami, FL; Legacy, Washington, DC; et al)
Arch Pediatr Adolesc Med 165:332-338, 2011

Objective.—To examine a potential association between biologically confirmed secondhand smoke exposure and symptoms of *Diagnostic and Statistical Manual of Mental Disorders* (Fourth Edition) (*DSM-IV*) major depressive disorder, generalized anxiety disorder, panic disorder, attention-deficit/hyperactivity disorder, and conduct disorder using a nationally representative sample of US children and adolescents.

Design.—Nationally representative cross-sectional survey of the United States.

Setting.—Continental United States.

Participants.—Children and adolescents aged 8 to 15 years who participated in the National Health and Nutrition Examination Survey from 2001 to 2004.

Intervention.—Measurement of serum cotinine level to assess secondhand smoke exposure among nonsmokers.

Main Outcome Measures.—The *DSM-IV* symptoms were derived from selected modules of the National Institute of Mental Health's Diagnostic Interview Schedule for Children Version IV, a structured diagnostic interview administered by trained lay interviewers.

Results.—Among nonsmokers, serum cotinine level was positively associated with symptoms of *DSM-IV* major depressive disorder, generalized anxiety disorder, attention-deficit/hyperactivity disorder, and conduct disorder after adjusting for survey design, age, sex, race/ethnicity, poverty, migraine, asthma, hay fever, maternal smoking during pregnancy, and allostatic load. Associations with serum cotinine level were more apparent for boys and for participants of non-Hispanic white race/ethnicity.

Conclusions.—Our results are consistent with a growing body of research documenting an association between secondhand smoke exposure and mental health outcomes. Future research is warranted to establish the biological or psychological mechanisms of association.

▶ There have been many uses of the data from the National Health and Nutrition Examination Survey, which assessed more than 2900 youths aged 8 to 15, including a Diagnostic Interview Schedule for Children and serum cotinine levels. This study pursued the association between secondhand smoke and specific psychiatric symptoms of syndromes. One may notice that an association between serum cotinine was associated with syndromes, such as those of depression or anxiety. It is important to emphasize, however, that these were not findings on actual psychiatric diagnoses. In fact, this study reviewed cotinine for disorders, but even with attention-deficit/hyperactivity disorder, the authors were unable to find a significant association. Nonetheless, this is an important area of research and should be pursued. We will need to tease apart whether there are direct physiologic efforts regardless whether or not the psychology of the smoking parent is found to be reasonable. These questions will be pondered sooner or later (hopefully sooner).

A. H. Mack, MD

Streptococcal Upper Respiratory Tract Infections and Exacerbations of Tic and Obsessive-Compulsive Symptoms: A Prospective Longitudinal Study
Leckman JF, King RA, Gilbert DL, et al (Yale Univ School of Medicine, New Haven, CT; Univ of Cincinnati, OH; et al)
J Am Acad Child Adolesc Psychiatry 50:108-118, 2011

Objective.—The objective of this blinded, prospective, longitudinal study was to determine whether new group A β hemolytic streptococcal (GABHS) infections are temporally associated with exacerbations of tic or obsessive-compulsive (OC) symptoms in children who met published criteria for pediatric autoimmune neuropsychiatric disorders associated with streptococcal infections (PANDAS). A group of children with Tourette syndrome and/or OC disorder without a PANDAS history served as the comparison (non-PANDAS) group.

Method.—Consecutive clinical ratings of tic and OC symptom severity were obtained for 31 PANDAS subjects and 53 non-PANDAS subjects. Clinical symptoms and laboratory values (throat cultures and streptococcal antibody titers) were evaluated at regular intervals during a 25-month period. Additional testing occurred at the time of any tic or OC symptom exacerbation. New GABHS infections were established by throat swab cultures and/or recent significant rise in streptococcal antibodies. Laboratory personnel were blinded to case or control status, clinical (exacerbation or not) condition, and clinical evaluators were blinded to the laboratory results.

Results.—No group differences were observed in the number of clinical exacerbations or the number of newly diagnosed GABHS infections. On only six occasions of a total of 51 (12%), a newly diagnosed GABHS infection was followed, within 2 months, by an exacerbation of tic and/ or OC symptoms. In every instance, this association occurred in the non-PANDAS group.

Conclusions.—This study provides no evidence for a temporal association between GABHS infections and tic/OC symptom exacerbations in children who meet the published PANDAS diagnostic criteria.

▶ This is a study of children who met the criteria for pediatric autoimmune neuropsychiatric disorders associated with streptococcal infections (PANDAS), but does it study PANDAS as it has been conceptualized? It would be so interesting and heuristic to determine that some auto-antibody actually directly causes certain specific neuropsychiatric signs or symptoms. However, over more than a decade, the realization of that mechanism in certain cases of obsessive-compulsive disorder (OCD), Tourette syndrome, or other neuropsychiatric syndromes has been elusive, and many children may have been needlessly exposed to immunosuppressive therapies or antibiotics, putting them and the public health at risk.

So Leckman et al provide a basic evaluation: to assess prospectively for neuropsychiatric signs and symptoms in a blinded manner with a substantial regimen of prospective serum evaluations. Subjects included those with these neuropsychiatric signs whether they were assumed to be PANDAS or not. Of the groups, serum evaluations addressed whether there were alterations in ASO or other autoantibodies during periods of clinical exacerbation. The answer was no, there was not. It was important that all analyses were referred to the same laboratory.

So could it be other agents rather than those from strep? Could it be a systemic reaction to strep? Other infectious agents have been known to cause neuropsychiatric findings—why have they been excluded?[1] Ultimately, the lack of association between group A β hemolytic streptococcal and tic or OCD exacerbations should be encouragement for clinicians to reduce unnecessary tests and treatments and to focus on these conditions in their usual conceptualization.

A. H. Mack, MD

Reference

1. Cardoso F. Infectious and Transmissible Movement Disorders. In: Jakovic J, Tolosa E, eds. *Parkinson's Disease and Movement Disorders.* 4th ed. Baltimore, MD: Williams and WIlkins; 2002:930-940.

Trends in the Use of Standardized Tools for Developmental Screening in Early Childhood: 2002–2009

Radecki L, Sand-Loud N, O'Connor KG, et al (American Academy of Pediatrics, IL; Dartmouth Med School and Dartmouth Hitchcock Med Ctr, Lebanon, NH)
Pediatrics 128:14-19, 2011

Background.—Early identification of developmental delays is essential for optimal early intervention. An American Academy of Pediatrics (AAP) 2002 Periodic Survey of Fellows found <25% of respondents consistently used appropriate screening tools. Over the past 5 years, new research and education programs promoted screening implementation. In 2006, the AAP issued a revised policy statement with a detailed algorithm. Since the 2002 Periodic Survey, no national surveys have examined the effectiveness of policy, programmatic, and educational enhancements.

Objective.—The goal of this study was to compare pediatricians' use of standardized screening tools from 2002 to 2009.

Methods.—A national, random sample of nonretired US AAP members were mailed Periodic Surveys (2002: $N = 1617$, response rate: 55%; 2009: $N = 1620$, response rate: 57%). χ^2 analyses were used to examine responses across survey years; a multivariate logistic regression model was developed to compare differences in using ≥ 1 formal screening tools across survey years while controlling for various individual and practice characteristics.

Results.—Pediatricians' use of standardized screening tools increased significantly between 2002 and 2009. The percentage of those who self-reported always/almost always using ≥1 screening tools increased over time (23.0%–47.7%), as did use of specific instruments (eg, Ages & Stages Questionnaire, Parents' Evaluation of Developmental Status). No differences were noted on the basis of physician or practice characteristics.

Conclusions.—The percentage of pediatricians who reported using ≥1 formal screening tools more than doubled between 2002 and 2009. Despite greater attention to consistent use of appropriate tools, the percentage remains less than half of respondents providing care to patients younger than 36 months. Given the critical importance of developmental screening in early identification, evaluation, and intervention, additional research is needed to identify barriers to greater use of standardized tools in practice.

▶ There are 2 issues that arise in reading this study; the first is concern that perhaps developmental screening, when it is performed, is not using standardized instruments. The second is the rate of screening: although it can be assumed that most pediatricians made use of a developmental study, few actually used these scales. As a result, it is of higher import that child mental health specialists are trained in and use available screens. There is no harm in redundancy. At the same time, one simply needs to be concerned not with eliciting developmental delays or concerns but on a degree of added vigilance. Likely these physicians do perform screens, but not in a standardized manner. If they did the outcomes and data would be stronger.

A. H. Mack, MD

Validity of Evidence-Derived Criteria for Reactive Attachment Disorder: Indiscriminately Social/Disinhibited and Emotionally Withdrawn/Inhibited Types
Gleason MM, Fox NA, Drury S, et al (Tulane Univ School of Medicine, New Orleans, LA; Univ of Maryland; et al)
J Am Acad Child Adolesc Psychiatry 50:216-231, 2011

Objective.—This study examined the validity of criteria for indiscriminately social/disinhibited and emotionally withdrawn/inhibited reactive attachment disorder (RAD).

Method.—As part of a longitudinal intervention trial of previously institutionalized children, caregiver interviews and direct observational measurements provided continuous and categorical data used to examine the internal consistency, criterion validity, construct validity, convergent and discriminant validity, association with functional impairment, and stability of these disorders over time.

Results.—As in other studies, the findings showed distinctions between the two types of RAD. Evidence-derived criteria for both types of RAD showed acceptable internal consistency and criterion validity. In this study, rates of indiscriminately social/disinhibited RAD at baseline and at 30, 42, and 54 months were 41/129 (31.8%), 22/122 (17.9%), 22/122 (18.0%), and 22/125 (17.6%), respectively. Signs of indiscriminately social/disinhibited RAD showed little association with caregiving quality. Nearly half of children with indiscriminately social/disinhibited RAD had organized attachment classifications. Signs of indiscriminately social/disinhibited RAD were associated with signs of activity/impulsivity and of attention-deficit/hyperactivity disorder and modestly with inhibitory control but were distinct from the diagnosis of attention-deficit/hyperactivity disorder. At baseline, 30, 42, and 54 months, 6/130 (4.6%), 4/123 (3.3%), 2/125 (1.6%), and 5/122 (4.1%) of children met criteria for emotionally withdrawn/inhibited RAD. Emotionally withdrawn/inhibited RAD was moderately associated with caregiving at the first three time points and strongly associated with attachment security. Signs of this type of RAD were associated with depressive symptoms, although two of the five children with this type of RAD at 54 months did not meet criteria for major depressive disorder. Signs of both types of RAD contributed independently to functional impairment and were stable over time.

Conclusions.—Evidence-derived criteria for indiscriminately social/disinhibited and emotionally withdrawn/inhibited RAD define two statistically and clinically cohesive syndromes that are distinct from each other, shows stability over 2 years, have predictable associations with risk factors and attachment, can be distinguished from other psychiatric disorders, and cause functional impairment.

▶ Reactive attachment disorder (RAD) is a condition that has seemed so obviously a part of the psychiatric classification, yet there has been a dearth of good research on it, particularly in establishing its validity. This report presents data from the Bucharest Early Intervention Project in which ongoing attention is being focused on toddlers previously reared in institutions in Romania. The authors, highly regarded researchers in infant and toddler psychiatry, were interested in demonstrating validity by several measures, hewing to the concepts of Robins and Guze. The study was also concerned with the distinction between the 2 putative subtypes of RAD: (1) indiscriminately social/disinhibited RAD and (2) emotionally withdrawn/inhibited RAD. Several measures were made and they were able to control for various conditions. The data were presented to demonstrate a number of findings that showed significant associations between the diagnosis and findings on objective measures. These included assessments of attachment such as the "stranger at the door" test, a modified strange situation, as well as the Disturbances of Attachment Interview, Preschool Age Psychiatric Assessment, the Observational Record of the Caregiving Environment, the Wechsler Preschool and Primary Scale of Intelligence, the Infant Toddler Social Emotional Assessment, and the Bear-Dragon test (which is of inhibitory control and has been shown to have high interrater reliability and consistency with other tests of inhibition.[1] Table 6 shows infant measures of depression as a sign of validity using the Infant-Toddler Social Emotional Assessment and Preschool Age Psychiatric Assessment depression scales. One problem

TABLE 6.—Convergent Validity: Correlation between Emotionally Withdrawn/Inhibited
Reactive Attachment Disorder and Depressive Signs

	ITSEA Depression	PAPA Depression
Baseline (n = 121)	0.44***	
30 mo (n = 123)	0.35***	
42 mo (n = 126)	0.72***	
54 mo		0.62*

Note: ITSEA = Infant Toddler Social Emotional Assessment; PAPA = Preschool Age Psychiatric Assessment.
*p ≤ 05.
***p ≤ .001.

is that there were few exclusion criteria other than "genetic syndromes," "dysmorphic features of fetal alcohol syndrome," or "microcephaly." This is important
given the authors' ideas that there may be syndromal overlap between Williams
syndrome (based on chromosome 7) and RAD. Overall, this is a tremendous
advance in the understanding of RAD, and further studies are needed.

A. H. Mack, MD

Reference

1. Carlson SM, Moses LJ. Individual differences in inhibitory control and children's
theory of mind. *Child Dev.* 2001;72:1032-1053.

Assessment and Diagnosis

Cumulative Prevalence of Psychiatric Disorders by Young Adulthood: A Prospective Cohort Analysis From the Great Smoky Mountains Study

Copeland W, Shanahan L, Costello EJ, et al (Duke Univ Med Ctr, Durham NC; Univ of North Carolina at Greensbor)
J Am Acad Child Adolesc Psychiatry 50:252-261, 2011

Objective.—No longitudinal studies beginning in childhood have estimated the cumulative prevalence of psychiatric illness from childhood
into young adulthood. The objective of this study was to estimate the
cumulative prevalence of psychiatric disorders by young adulthood and
to assess how inclusion of not otherwise specified diagnoses affects cumulative prevalence estimates.

Method.—The prospective, population-based Great Smoky Mountains
Study assessed 1,420 participants up to nine times from 9 through 21 years
of age from 11 counties in the southeastern United States. Common psychiatric disorders were assessed in childhood and adolescence (ages 9 to
16 years) with the Child and Adolescent Psychiatric Assessment and in
young adulthood (ages 19 and 21 years) with the Young Adult Psychiatric
Assessment. Cumulative prevalence estimates were derived from multiple
imputed datasets.

Results.—By 21 years of age, 61.1% of participants had met criteria for
a well-specified psychiatric disorder. An additional 21.4% had met criteria

for a not otherwise specified disorder only, increasing the total cumulative prevalence for any disorder to 82.5%. Male subjects had higher rates of substance and disruptive behavior disorders compared with female subjects; therefore, they were more likely to meet criteria for a well-specified disorder (67.8% vs 56.7%) or any disorder (89.1% vs 77.8%). Children with a not otherwise specified disorder only were at increased risk for a well-specified young adult disorder compared with children with no disorder in childhood.

Conclusions.—Only a small percentage of young people meet criteria for a *DSM* disorder at any given time, but most do by young adulthood. As with other medical illness, psychiatric illness is a nearly universal experience.

▶ It is vital for practicing clinicians to understand the fundamentals of diagnosis, and there is no better place to start than in appreciation of the utility of our diagnostic system in terms of epidemiologic studies. The findings by this study demand understanding of psychiatric nosology. In this review of Great Smoky Mountain Study (GSMS) data, the authors have compiled diagnoses to prepare a figure of cumulative prevalence up to age 21, and they found rates of diagnosis far in excess of other retrospective and cross-sectional duties. Their use of cumulative prevalence is important, and when they move from specific disorders to not otherwise specified (NOS) categories, the rate goes from 61.1% to 82.5%. These are high rates indeed. What can be said about the addition of the NOS groups? Since the GSMS uses a standardized instrument, the NOS diagnoses did not represent inadequate effort or skill in diagnosis. One difference may be that this study used prospective diagnosis rather than retrospective diagnosis. Additionally, it is a study of a specific group. Cross-sectional studies that have lower prevalence rates of disorders may be less powerful than prospective studies (such as this one) given recall bias. Then again, retrospective analysis is how psychiatrists work. Perhaps Copeland et al are correct in their findings based on DSM-IV diagnosis. These findings are important for kids because, as the authors point out, two thirds of all cases have onset by age 14 and three quarters by age 24. And while use of NOS is sufficient, what would be the effect of removing NOS from the DSM altogether? The authors do acknowledge that the population in the GSMS is not fully representative of the United States today, but it is hard to consider how a population that is more diverse could be greatly different.

A. H. Mack, MD

Prevalence of bipolar disorder in children and adolescents with attention-deficit hyperactivity disorder
Hassan A, Agha SS, Langley K, et al (Cardiff Univ, UK)
Br J Psychiatry 198:195-198, 2011

Background.—Some research suggests that children with attention-deficit hyperactivity disorder (ADHD) have a higher than expected risk of bipolar affective disorder. No study has examined the prevalence of bipolar disorder in a UK sample of children with ADHD.

Aims.—To examine the prevalence of bipolar disorder in children diagnosed with ADHD or hyperkinetic disorder.

Method.—Psychopathology symptoms and diagnoses of bipolar disorder were assessed in 200 young people with ADHD (170 male, 30 female; age 6–18 years, mean 11.15, s.d. = 2.95). Rates of current bipolar disorder symptoms and diagnoses are reported. A family history of bipolar disorder in parents and siblings was also recorded.

Results.—Only one child, a 9-year-old boy, met diagnostic criteria for both ICD–10 hypomania and DSM-IV bipolar disorder not otherwise specified.

Conclusions.—In a UK sample of children with ADHD a current diagnosis of bipolar disorder was uncommon.

▶ This is a relatively small, yet important, report. It is drawn from the findings of another study on attention-deficit/hyperactivity disorder (ADHD), and the findings are that bipolar disorder is rarely seen in children with ADHD, despite claims to the contrary by several in the field. That participants were those accepted into a study on ADHD is important as well. Indeed, there have always been good ways to differentiate ADHD from bipolar disorder, but this study (and others before it) provide clear indications that there is not necessarily a symptomatic or syndromic overlap, which has implications for understanding ADHD to be a separate neurodevelopmental disorder and the need for specific treatments. After all, treatments for these 2 conditions now differ in terms of efficacy, but too many clinicians (of all professions) seem to be confused about which is which. This study will help because it covers the specific criteria for mania and other mood conditions.

A. H. Mack, MD

Self-, parent-, and teacher-reported behavioral symptoms in youngsters with Tourette syndrome: A case-control study

Termine C, Selvini C, Balottin U, et al (Univ of Insubria, Varese, Italy; Univ of Pavia, Italy; et al)

Eur J Paediatr Neurol 15:95-100, 2011

Aims.—Tourette syndrome (TS) is a neurodevelopmental disorder characterized by multiple tics and associated with co-morbid behavioral problems (TS-plus). We investigated the usefulness of self-report *versus* parent- and teacher-report instruments in assisting the specialist assessment of TS-plus in a child/adolescent population.

Methods.—Twenty-three patients diagnosed with TS (19 males; age 13.9 ± 3.7 years) and 69 matched healthy controls participated in this study. All recruited participants completed a standardized psychometric battery, including the Children's Depression Inventory (CDI), the Self Administrated Psychiatric Scales for Children and Adolescents (SAFA) and the State-Trait Anger Expression Inventory (STAXI). Parents completed the Child Behavior Checklist (CBCL) and Conners' Parent Rating Scales-Revised (CPRS-R). Participants' teachers completed the Conners' Teacher Rating Scales-Revised (CTRS-R). Results were compared with similar data obtained from controls.

Results.—Nineteen patients (82.6%) fulfilled DSM-IV-TR criteria for at least one co-morbid condition: obsessive-compulsive disorder (OCD, $n = 8$; 34.8%); attention deficit-hyperactivity disorder (ADHD, $n = 6$; 26.1%); OCD + ADHD ($n = 5$; 21.7%). Scores on self-report instruments failed to show any significant differences between TS and controls. Most subscores of the CPRS-R, CTRS-R, and CBCL were significantly higher for the TS group than controls. The TS + OCD subgroup scored significantly higher than the TS-OCD subgroup on the CBCL-Externalizing, Anxious/Depressed and Obsessive-Compulsive subscales.

Conclusions.—Self-report instruments appear to have limited usefulness in assisting the assessment of the behavioral spectrum of young patients with TS. However, proxy-rated instruments differentiate TS populations from healthy subjects, and the CBCL can add relevant information to the clinical diagnosis of co-morbid OCD.

▶ This report from clinics in Italy provides evidence that will be helpful in assessing and diagnosing tics and Tourette syndrome. The conclusions that there are differences between parent report and self-report are not necessarily novel, but here too are reports from teachers, all of which show that the affected individual teenagers have less insight and concern, at least using these measures, than do parents. This is an interesting finding, and it is akin to trends that occur among children and adolescents who have externalizing disorders, such as conduct disorder, oppositional defiant disorder, or attention deficit hyperactivity disorder. Is there some way in which the tics disorders may one day be seen as externalizing disorders? Do they affect parents more than the affected individuals? That study remains to be seen, but this study demonstrates that the symptoms at least are differentially noticed by these reporters. Unfortunately, this is a small study and its findings cannot, thus, be seen as robust, but further investigation seems warranted. Their use of standardized instruments is welcome.

A. H. Mack, MD

Severe Mood Dysregulation, Irritability, and the Diagnostic Boundaries of Bipolar Disorder in Youths
Leibenluft E (NIMH, Bethesda, MD)
Am J Psychiatry 168:129-142, 2011

In recent years, increasing numbers of children have been diagnosed with bipolar disorder. In some cases, children with unstable mood clearly meet current diagnostic criteria for bipolar disorder, and in others, the diagnosis is unclear. Severe mood dysregulation is a syndrome defined to capture the symptomatology of children whose diagnostic status with respect to bipolar disorder is uncertain, that is, those who have severe, nonepisodic irritability and the hyperarousal symptoms characteristic of mania but who lack the well-demarcated periods of elevated or irritable mood characteristic of bipolar disorder. Levels of impairment are comparable between youths with bipolar disorder and those with severe mood dysregulation. An emerging literature compares children with severe mood dysregulation and those with bipolar disorder in longitudinal course, family history, and pathophysiology. Longitudinal data in both clinical and community samples indicate that nonepisodic irritability in youths is common and is associated with an elevated risk for anxiety and unipolar depressive disorders, but not bipolar disorder, in adulthood. Data also suggest that youths with severe mood dysregulation have lower familial rates of bipolar disorder than do those with bipolar disorder. While youths in both patient groups have deficits in face emotion labeling and experience more frustration than do normally developing children, the brain mechanisms mediating these pathophysiologic abnormalities appear to differ between the two patient groups. No specific treatment for severe mood dysregulation currently exists, but verification of its identity as a syndrome distinct from bipolar disorder by further research should include treatment trials.

▶ The differentiation of periods of severe mood dysregulation (SMD) from bipolar disorder marks a major advance for students of psychopathology as well as for the public health. The incredible overdiagnosis of bipolar disorder has occurred in adults, but more so in youth. Occasionally this has led to pathologization of behavior that may not be illness. This article is a compilation of information and data on SMD by its central figure. As one can see in Fig 1 in the original article, its criteria mark disturbance but exclude the "real" marks of mania or hypomania. The position of SMD does accept that these youth may have disturbance of the regulation of mood, particularly in terms of irritability, and calls for further research on this concept. These may be disorders on a continuum, but we have to get it straight in terms of definitions first. My own perspective is that although SMD is a valuable description of the impairment of many, I think we will still have excess diagnoses of bipolar disorder in youth in whom explosive and irritable behavior and reactivity are nonetheless interpreted as "special" to youth bipolar disorder, and the problem will persist to some degree.

A. H. Mack, MD

Stability of Autistic Traits in the General Population: Further Evidence for a Continuum of Impairment

Robinson EB, Munir K, Munafò MR, et al (Harvard School of Public Health, Boston, MA; Harvard Med School, Boston, MA; Univ of Bristol, UK)
J Am Acad Child Adolesc Psychiatry 50:376-384, 2011

Objective.—This study investigated the developmental course of autistic traits in a nationally representative sample of subjects 7 to 13 years of age.

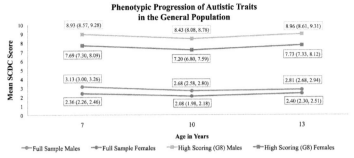

FIGURE 2.—Phenotypic progression of autistic traits in the general population. *Note:* Data labels indicate the predicted group mean and 95% confidence interval at each time point. (Reprinted from Journal of the American Academy of Child and Adolescent Psychiatry, Robinson EB, Munir K, Munafò MR, et al. Stability of autistic traits in the general population: further evidence for a continuum of impairment. *J Am Acad Child Adolesc Psychiatry.* 2011;50:376-384. Copyright 2011 with permission from Elsevier.)

Method.—The parents of 6,539 children in the Avon Longitudinal Study of Parents and Children completed the Social and Communication Disorders Checklist at ages 7, 10, and 13. The phenotypic progression of autistic traits was assessed in the full sample and in high-scoring individuals (e.g., top 10%, 5%). Gender, IQ, and overall behavior difficulties were examined as potentially relevant influences on autistic trait trajectories.

Results.—Autistic traits were highly stable in the general population overall and in the high-scoring groups. In the full sample, there was no change in mean Social and Communication Disorders Checklist scores for female subjects ages 7 to 13 ($p = .43$). Scores for male subjects decreased slightly, but significantly, on the order of 0.1 standard deviations ($p < .001$). There was no mean change in parent-rated autistic traits within any of the high-scoring groups. IQ was not related to phenotypic progression; high parent-rated behavior problems predicted slight improvement in Social and Communication Disorders Checklist scores over the course of the study period in high-scoring individuals ($p < .01$).

Conclusions.—These findings suggest that autistic traits are highly stable in the general population, even in individuals with the highest concentrations of autism-like behaviors. Phenotypic stability is consistent with expectations for individuals with autism spectrum disorders, providing further support for a phenomenologic continuum across the clinical threshold. Moreover, the gap between female and male risk for autistic symptomology is consistent over time.

▶ Here is an examination of the stability of autistic traits in the general population from 7 to 13 years; it is well documented in Fig 2. It is an important study, reviewing the phenotypic progression of autistic traits in a nationally representative sample of 6539 children. The population is key: a group of normal individuals as to their autistic traits (no disorder or illness). The main outcome measure was the Social Communication Disorders checklist. As seen in Fig 2, the rate of occurrence of these traits remained stable. There was a male to female ratio as documented in autism studies as well. The implication is that autistic traits as a disorder should be included in standard classifications of illnesses, that there is a subtle degree of autism in the community as well.

This study, as well done as it is, makes for concern and ideas at once. On one hand, maybe it is true that autism should be diagnosed on a spectrum. But even there, the spectrum has a limit. We must have cutoffs to state whether a person has an illness or not. This isn't just because of a clinging to our current system; it's just common sense. The documentation of autism traits in the population can lead to further understanding of the mechanisms of these specific traits.

A. H. Mack, MD

Trends in the Prevalence of Developmental Disabilities in US Children, 1997–2008
Boyle CA, Boulet S, Schieve LA, et al (Natl Ctr on Birth Defects and Developmental Disabilities, Atlanta, GA; et al)
Pediatrics 127:1034-1042, 2011

Objective.—To fill gaps in crucial data needed for health and educational planning, we determined the prevalence of developmental disabilities in US children and in selected populations for a recent 12-year period.

Participants and Methods.—We used data on children aged 3 to 17 years from the 1997–2008 National Health Interview Surveys, which are ongoing nationally representative samples of US households. Parent-reported diagnoses of the following were included: attention deficit hyperactivity disorder; intellectual disability; cerebral palsy; autism; seizures; stuttering or stammering; moderate to profound hearing loss; blindness; learning disorders; and/or other developmental delays.

Results.—Boys had a higher prevalence overall and for a number of select disabilities compared with girls. Hispanic children had the lowest prevalence for a number of disabilities compared with non-Hispanic white and black children. Low income and public health insurance were associated with a higher prevalence of many disabilities. Prevalence of any developmental disability increased from 12.84% to 15.04% over 12 years. Autism, attention deficit hyperactivity disorder, and other developmental delays increased, whereas hearing loss showed a significant decline. These trends were found in all of the sociodemographic subgroups, except for autism in non-Hispanic black children.

Conclusions.—Developmental disabilities are common and were reported in ~ 1 in 6 children in the United States in 2006–2008. The number of children with select developmental disabilities (autism, attention deficit hyperactivity disorder, and other developmental delays) has increased, requiring more health and education services. Additional study of the influence of risk-factor shifts, changes in acceptance, and benefits of early services is needed.

▶ Child and adolescent psychiatrists may or may not be well trained to elicit, assess, or diagnose the presence of developmental disorders. However, according to this report, there is an increasing likelihood that future patients will have some form of neurologic or developmental delay or deficit. As a result, there is, of course, a need for psychiatrists in this arena to improve their skills. This will not be easy, especially given other recent findings that there are insufficient numbers of screenings (by members of all professions). This is a major epidemiological study, but we do have to wonder how psychiatrists should change their practice: should all begin to do screening examinations? A generation (or 2) ago, becoming board certified required proficiency not only in psychiatry but in neurology as well. One might wonder whether our focus on just emotions, cognition, and behavior has led us to be too focused. It is hoped that the ongoing discussions on psychiatric workforce, which are especially important in child and adolescent psychiatry, will be revealing in this sense.

A. H. Mack, MD

Intervention Studies

Adolescent Substance Use: America's #1 Public Health Problem
The National Center on Addiction and Substance Abuse (Columbia Univ, NY)
1-406, 2011

Background.—Adolescence is the critical period when individuals begin to smoke, drink, or use other drugs and experience harmful consequences. Teens who use drugs are at greater risk for developing addiction, which is a complex brain disease that affects both the brain's structure and its functions. Nine of 10 persons who meet the clinical criteria for substance abuse began smoking, drinking, or using other drugs before age 18 years. One in four of those who begin substance use before age 18 years become addicted, whereas only one in 25 persons who begin substance abuse after age 21 years develops this problem. Factors contributing to the prevention of substance abuse in adolescents were evaluated. In addition, recommendations were offered to improve the prevention and treatment of substance abuse.

Method.—The information was taken from nationally representative online surveys of 1000 high school students, 1000 parents of high school students (75% of whom were from the same households as the high school student participants), and 500 school personnel. In addition, data came from extensive in-depth analyses of seven national data sets; interviews with about 50 experts in fields related to the report topic; five focus groups with students, parents, and school personnel; and a review of over 2000 scientific articles and reports.

Results.—The effects of substance use and addiction on the teen brain and its neurochemistry were noted. The teen brain was found to be more vulnerable to the effects of addictive substances than the adult brain because of its immaturity. Alcohol is the most preferred addictive substance for high school students. Adolescent substance abuse was also found to be a significant public health problem, presenting clear dangers to millions of teenagers but also dramatic consequences for the entire population. Among these consequences for the teen are injuries, unintended pregnancies, and medical conditions such as asthma, depression, anxiety, psychosis, and impaired brain function. Their academic performance and educational achievements are limited, and criminal behaviors can develop. Teens can also die. Consequences for others include the unhealthy smoke they breathe in, the assaults and other injuries or deaths caused by impaired teens, the contraction of sexually transmitted diseases, unplanned pregnancies, and the birth of children to teen mothers who abuse drugs during pregnancy.

Also noted were the broad factors in American culture that drive adolescent substance abuse. These include parental influences, school influences, community influences, medial influences, and the accessibility of addictive substances to adolescents. Individual factors can also contribute. Teens themselves view substance abuse differently depending on various factors, such as peer approval. There are also adverse effects contributed by genetic and family history influences, adverse childhood experiences, mental health disorders, the individual's temperament and self-esteem issues, peer victimization and bullying, academic performance, employment, parent's marital status, and risk-taking behaviors. Certain adolescents are at higher risk for abuse, including those in the child welfare system, high school dropouts, and those identified with the justice system, a minority sexual orientation, and athletics. The risks of teen substance abuse can be positively influenced by parental engagement; the presence of role models and other positive peer involvement; a focus on future personal goals; engagement in school, community, or athletic pursuits; and religious beliefs.

Recommendations.—Preventive approaches involve screening and interventions for adolescents as part of routine health care, governmental regulation of access to addictive substances, public awareness and education for parents and teens, school-based efforts, and community-based efforts. Barriers exist that hinder the ability of all these efforts to improve the substance abuse picture in teens. In addition, treatment efforts need to bridge the evidence-practice gap, but there are barriers to these efforts as well. All of the parties involved must actively engage in preventive and treatment efforts to achieve excellent results.

▶ This significant report by the National Center on Addiction and Substance Abuse (also known as CASA) again sets the bar on the degree of adolescent substance use that our society ought to accept: none. The report marshals data from several important sources and shows several points. One is the pervasive nature of substance use among adolescents in the United States today; the data show that there has been a slight decline over time. The second is the coalescing of data regarding the human, medical, and economic costs. Finally, the report emphasizes the need for prevention—as a need and as a consideration for society and policy makers. The basic perspective is that adolescent substance use is essentially the nation's primary public health problem and should be—and can be—tackled. This report is a primer on adolescent substance use, its risk factors, and its effects. It should be read by clinicians and patients alike.

A. H. Mack, MD

Children of Depressed Mothers 1 Year After Remission of Maternal Depression: Findings From the STAR*D-Child Study
Wickramaratne P, Gameroff MJ, Pilowsky DJ, et al (Columbia Univ and the New York State Psychiatric Inst; Univ of Texas Southwestern Med Ctr; Duke Univ-Natl Univ of Singapore; et al)
Am J Psychiatry 168:593-602, 2011

Objective.—Maternal major depressive disorder is an established risk factor for child psychopathology. The authors previously reported that 1 year after initiation of treatment for maternal depression, children of mothers whose depression remitted had significantly improved functioning and psychiatric symptoms. This study extends these findings by examining changes in psychiatric symptoms, behavioral problems, and functioning among children of depressed mothers during the first year after the mothers' remission from depression.

Method.—Children were assessed at baseline and at 3-month intervals with the Schedule for Affective Disorders and Schizophrenia for School-Age Children—Present and Lifetime Version, the Child Behavior Checklist, and the Children's Global Assessment Scale for 1 year after their mothers' remission or for 2 years if the mothers did not remit. The authors compared children of early remitters (0—3 months; N=36), late remitters (3—12 months; N=28), and nonremitters (N=16).

Results.—During the postremission year, children of early-remitting mothers showed significant improvement on all outcomes. Externalizing behavioral problems decreased in children of early- and late-remitting mothers but increased in children of nonremitting mothers. Psychiatric symptoms decreased significantly only in children of mothers who remitted, and functioning improved only in children of early-remitting mothers.

Conclusions.—Remission of mothers' depression, regardless of its timing, appears to be related to decreases in problem behaviors and symptoms in their children over the year after remission. The favorable effect of mothers' remission on children's functioning was observed only in children of early-remitting mothers.

▶ Children whose mothers are depressed have increased prevalence of psychiatric symptoms and behavioral dysfunction. One prior report from the Sequenced Treatment Alternatives to Relieve Depression (STAR*D) sample showed that after 3 months of antidepressant treatment, the mothers' remissions were significantly associated with reductions in the children's diagnoses and symptoms. However, children ages 7 to 17 years whose mothers' depression remitted in the course of the STAR*D studies showed substantial decrease in externalizing symptoms and improved psychosocial function in this study. Importantly, children who were asymptomatic at the initiation of treatment were significantly more likely to develop symptoms if their mothers did not remit. This report provides evidence that this finding extended over a longer period than previously reported.

What is of interest is considering why this is the case: It is easy to consider the possibility that maternal depression may be linked to a child's mood disorder or the child's functioning overall. However the effects of maternal depression have been shown to be more widespread, including effects on substance use and various externalizing conditions and anxiety. Nevertheless, attention to this component of the mother-child dyad should be taken into account by those who care about and care for both the mother and the child. Perhaps one set of future analyses will address the role and effect of the father as well or of the relationship of maternal depression to family size.

A. H. Mack, MD

Effects of a Brief Intervention for Reducing Violence and Alcohol Misuse Among Adolescents: A Randomized Controlled Trial

Walton MA, Chermack ST, Shope JT, et al (Univ of Michigan, Ann Arbor)
JAMA 304:527-535, 2010

Context.—Emergency department (ED) visits present an opportunity to deliver brief interventions to reduce violence and alcohol misuse among urban adolescents at risk of future injury.

Objective.—To determine the efficacy of brief interventions addressing violence and alcohol use among adolescents presenting to an urban ED.

Design, Setting, and Participants.—Between September 2006 and September 2009, 3338 patients aged 14 to 18 years presenting to a level I ED in Flint, Michigan, between 12 PM and 11 PM 7 days a week completed a computerized survey (43.5% male; 55.9% African American). Adolescents reporting past-year alcohol use and aggression were enrolled in a randomized controlled trial (SafERteens).

Intervention.—All patients underwent a computerized baseline assessment and were randomized to a control group that received a brochure (n = 235) or a 35-minute brief intervention delivered by either a computer (n = 237) or therapist (n = 254) in the ED, with follow-up assessments at 3 and 6 months. Combining motivational interviewing with skills training, the brief intervention for violence and alcohol included review of goals, tailored feedback, decisional balance exercise, role plays, and referrals.

Main Outcome Measures.—Self-report measures included peer aggression and violence, violence consequences, alcohol use, binge drinking, and alcohol consequences.

Results.—About 25% (n = 829) of screened patients had positive results for both alcohol and violence; 726 were randomized. Compared with controls, participants in the therapist intervention showed self-reported reductions in the occurrence of peer aggression (therapist, −34.3%; control, −16.4%; relative risk [RR], 0.74; 95% confidence interval [CI], 0.61-0.90), experience of peer violence (therapist, −10.4%; control, +4.7%; RR, 0.70; 95% CI, 0.52-0.95), and violence consequences (therapist, −30.4%; control, −13.0%; RR, 0.76; 95% CI, 0.64-0.90) at 3 months. At 6 months, participants in the therapist intervention showed self-reported reductions in alcohol

TABLE 1.—Baseline Background, Violence, and Substance Use Characteristics[a]

Characteristics	Computerized Brief Intervention (n = 237)	Therapist Brief Intervention (n = 254)	Control (n = 235)	Total (N = 726)
Demographics				
Male	100 (42.2)	114 (44.9)	102 (43.4)	316 (43.5)
Race				
African American	129 (54.4)	145 (57.1)	132 (56.2)	406 (55.9)
White	96 (40.4)	96 (37.8)	92 (39.2)	284 (39.1)
Other	12 (5.1)	13 (5.1)	11 (4.7)	36 (5.0)
Hispanic ethnicity	15 (6.3)	17 (6.7)	15 (6.4)	47 (6.5)
Age, mean (SD), y	16.7 (1.4)	16.8 (1.3)	16.8 (1.3)	16.8 (1.3)
Family receipt of public assistance	140 (59.1)	149 (58.7)	128 (54.5)	417 (57.4)
Failing grades (some Ds/Fs)[b]	83 (40.9)	104 (44.3)	101 (47.0)	288 (44.1)
Dropped out of school[c]	34 (14.4)	19 (7.5)	20 (8.5)	73 (10.1)
Live with parent	192 (81.0)	205 (80.7)	184 (78.3)	581 (80.0)
Gang involvement	18 (2.5)	21 (2.9)	14 (1.9)	53 (7.3)
Emergency department				
Chief concern injury	59 (24.9)	68 (26.9)	67 (28.6)	194 (26.8)
Chief concern intentional injury	12 (5.1)	25 (9.9)	17 (7.3)	54 (7.5)
Discharged from emergency department on day of recruitment	217 (91.6)	238 (93.7)	220 (93.6)	675 (93.0)
Past-year substance use				
Binge drinking (≥5 drinks)	115 (48.5)	134 (52.8)	127 (54.0)	376 (51.8)
Alcohol misuse on AUDIT-C	108 (45.6)	127 (50.0)	112 (47.7)	347 (47.8)
Alcohol consequences	102 (43.0)	122 (48.0)	102 (43.4)	326 (44.9)
Marijuana use	151 (63.7)	166 (65.4)	159 (67.7)	476 (65.6)
Past-year violence				
Severe peer aggression	179 (75.5)	210 (82.7)	183 (77.9)	572 (78.8)
Experienced peer violence	103 (43.5)	121 (47.6)	99 (42.1)	323 (44.5)
Violence consequences	183 (77.2)	213 (83.9)	195 (98.3)	591 (81.4)

Abbreviation: AUDIT-C, Alcohol Use Disorders Identification Test—Consumption.
[a]Data are expressed as No. (%) unless otherwise indicated.
[b]Among those in school (n=653 [89.9%]).
[c]*P*=.02.

consequences (therapist, -32.2%; control, -17.7%; odds ratio, 0.56; 95% CI, 0.34-0.91) compared with controls; participants in the computer intervention also showed self-reported reductions in alcohol consequences (computer, -29.1%; control, -17.7%; odds ratio, 0.57; 95% CI, 0.34-0.95).

Conclusion.—Among adolescents identified in the ED with self-reported alcohol use and aggression, a brief intervention resulted in a decrease in the prevalence of selfreported aggression and alcohol consequences.

Trial Registration.—clinicaltrials.gov Identifier: NCT00251212 (Table 1).

▶ Violence, which is often associated with substance use, is a pervasive problem in American society and with various prevention programs remaining unfunded, there is a need to intervene in as many moments as possible in adolescents' lives to prevent violence. Over the past several years, there have been a number of examples of brief therapies aimed at altering the behavior of teens. Here is one that is a randomized controlled trial, which gives it added weight. Of almost 4000 teens approached in this Flint, Michigan, urban emergency department, approximately one quarter agreed to participate in the study, with division into 3 parts, the prototype group that received a 35-minute intervention involving therapist counseling, versus computer-only and brochure-only interventions. It was found that the brief therapy intervention had the greatest effect at 3 and 6 months. This is an important outcome. The interventions were directed at a specific population, notwithstanding the exclusion criteria; Flint is a city with many needs. One must wonder why these youth even agreed to participate in the program (as seen in Table 1)—who they are, and in what degree of change they were already engaged—they are certainly ripe for change. This might be a good opportunity to study readiness for change as it pertains at least to alcohol use. Overall, however, this is a rigorous addition in the march toward addressing this problem—a problem that affects its perpetrators, its victims, and society generally.

A. H. Mack, MD

Preventing Children's Posttraumatic Stress After Disaster With Teacher-Based Intervention: A Controlled Study

Wolmer L, Hamiel D, Laor N (Tel Aviv-Brull Community Mental Health Ctr, Israel)

J Am Acad Child Adolesc Psychiatry 50:340-348, 2011

Objective.—The psychological outcomes that the exposure to mass trauma has on children have been amply documented in the past decades. The objective of this study is to describe the effects of a universal, teacher-based preventive intervention implemented with Israeli students before the rocket attacks that occurred during Operation Cast Lead, compared with a nonintervention but exposed control group.

Method.—The study sample consisted of 1,488 students studying in fourth and fifth grades in a city in southern Israel who were exposed to continuous rocket attacks during Operation Cast Lead. The intervention group included about half (53.5%) of the children who studied in six schools where the teacher-led intervention was implemented 3 months before the traumatic exposure. The control group (46.5% of the sample) included six schools matched by exposure in which the preventive intervention was not implemented. Children filled out the UCLA-PTSD Reaction Index and the Stress/Mood Scale 3 months after the end of the rocket attacks.

Results.—The intervention group displayed significantly lower symptoms of posttrauma and stress/mood than the control group ($p < .001$). Control children had 57% more detected cases of posttraumatic stress disorder (PTSD) than participant children. This difference was significantly more pronounced among boys (10.2% versus 4.4%) and less among girls (12.5% versus 10.1%).

Conclusions.—The teacher-based, resilience-focused intervention is a universal, cost-effective approach to enhance the preparedness of communities of children to mass trauma and to prevent the development of PTSD after exposure.

▶ This study provides another perspective on the care of children and adolescents exposed to trauma. When considering studies on posttraumatic stress and posttraumatic stress disorder, it is important to be able to generalize one's findings. This is simplest and most appropriate when using actual *Diagnostic and Statistical Manual of Mental Disorders* (4th ed.) criteria (albeit, this may change in the 5th edition). However, this goes for the definition of the traumatic event, the initial response, and the subsequent psychiatric symptoms and signs. All too often, those components are forgotten when this diagnosis is inappropriately made, and this serves to dilute the significance of the disorder among those who truly meet the diagnostic criteria. In Israel, ongoing fear of rockets comes alongside actual experience of rockets; one can go to Israel and see bomb shelters. This is an important study of an intervention with a group that has had exposure to traumatic events, and future studies should build on it.

A. H. Mack, MD

Policy Statement—Principles of Pediatric Patient Safety: Reducing Harm Due to Medical Care
Steering Committee on Quality Improvement and Management and Committee on Hospital Care
Pediatrics 127:1199-1210, 2011

Pediatricians are rendering care in an environment that is increasingly complex, which results in multiple opportunities to cause unintended harm. National awareness of patient safety risks has grown in the 10 years since the Institute of Medicine published its report *To Err Is Human*, and patients and society as a whole continue to challenge health care providers to examine their practices and implement safety solutions. The depth and breadth of harm incurred by the practice of medicine is still being defined as reports continue to uncover a variety of avoidable errors, from those that involve specific high-risk medications to those that are more generalizable, such as patient misidentification. Pediatricians in all venues must have a working knowledge of patient-safety language, advocate for best practices that attend to risks that are unique to children, identify and support a culture of safety, and lead efforts to eliminate avoidable harm in any setting in which medical care is rendered to children.

▶ Even if one disparages the estimate, as brought forward more than a decade ago,[1] that almost 100 000 US patients die each year because of errors in medical care, the movement toward the patient safety culture is forcefully driving institutions, accrediting bodies, and other components of the health care landscape. Because quality improvement is a component of the patient safety culture, almost all medical practitioners will be touched by this movement. Indeed, except perhaps for a small number of psychiatrists in private practice who are not in a group and who never prescribe medications or need laboratory studies, we all will function in some system of care. With the increasing complexity of our care and the machines, medications, or other interventions that we apply to patients, the risks for errors rise. This article, then, is important for pediatric psychiatrists to be aware at least where our pediatrician colleagues are. Of course, we have always considered safety in terms of violence to self and others; this is a slightly different paradigm, and its application to psychiatry continues to be contemplated and developed, but we all need to appreciate the culture of patient safety so that we accept, rather than resist, the practice changes that it will surely effect.

A. H. Mack, MD

Reference

1. Institute of Medicine. *To Err Is Human: Building a Safer Health System.* Washington, DC: National Academies Press; 2000.

Treatment Studies: Pharmacotherapy

A Double-Blind, Placebo-Controlled Study of Atomoxetine in Young Children With ADHD

Kratochvil CJ, Vaughan BS, Stoner JA, et al (Univ of Nebraska Med Ctr, Omaha; Univ of Oklahoma Health Sciences Ctr; et al)
Pediatrics 127:e862-e868, 2011

Objective.—To evaluate the efficacy and tolerability of atomoxetine for the treatment of attention-deficit/hyperactivity disorder (ADHD) in 5- and 6-year-old children.

Methods.—This was an 8-week, double-blind, placebo-controlled randomized clinical trial of atomoxetine in 101 children with ADHD. Atomoxetine or placebo was flexibly titrated to a maximum dose of 1.8 mg/kg per day. The pharmacotherapist reviewed psychoeducational material on ADHD and behavioral-management strategies with parents during each study visit.

Results.—Significant mean decreases in parent ($P = .009$) and teacher ($P = .02$) ADHD−IV Rating Scale scores were demonstrated with atomoxetine compared with placebo. A total of 40% of children treated with atomoxetine met response criteria (Clinical Global Impression−Improvement Scale indicating much or very much improved) compared with 22% of children on placebo, which was not significant ($P = .1$). Decreased appetite, gastrointestinal upset, and sedation were significantly more common with atomoxetine than placebo. Although some children demonstrated a robust response to atomoxetine, for others the response was more attenuated. Sixty-two percent of subjects who received atomoxetine were moderately, markedly, or severely ill according to the Clinical Global Impression−Severity Scale at study completion.

Conclusions.—To our knowledge, this is the first randomized controlled trial of atomoxetine in children as young as 5 years. Atomoxetine generally was well tolerated and reduced core ADHD symptoms in the children on the basis of parent and teacher reports. Reductions in the ADHD-IV Rating

Scale scores, however, did not necessarily translate to overall clinical and functional improvement, as demonstrated on the Clinical Global Impression—Severity Scale and the Clinical Global Impression—Improvement Scale. Despite benefits, the children in the atomoxetine group remained, on average, significantly impaired at the end of the study.

▶ Atomoxetine continues to be an alternative to the stimulant medications for the treatment of attention-deficit/hyperactivity disorder, and this study extends the literature's coverage of it down to age 5. Atomoxetine's efficacy continues to be moderate at best in whichever overall age group it is applied to—here, the rate of clinical improvement on this medication is not terrific and lags behind the standards set by the various stimulant medications. There is evidence here of the medication's tolerability, which may exceed that of the stimulants; perhaps clinicians should offer this choice to patients and their families—this is a medication that is better tolerated, although less effective than the stimulants. It is not clear that we are ready to say that in the absence of head-to-head trials. Clearly the effect size compared with placebo was low (not significant), but there may be further data that nonetheless provide support for the use of this nonstimulant medication in some clinical situations. One should stay tuned.

A. H. Mack, MD

Cardiovascular Events and Death in Children Exposed and Unexposed to ADHD Agents
Schelleman H, Bilker WB, Strom BL, et al (Univ of Pennsylvania School of Medicine, Philadelphia; et al)
Pediatrics 127:1102-1110, 2011

Objective.—The objective of this study was to compare the rate of severe cardiovascular events and death in children who use attention-deficit/hyperactivity disorder (ADHD) medications versus nonusers.

Patients and Methods.—We performed a large cohort study using data from 2 administrative databases. All children aged 3 to 17 years with a prescription for an amphetamine, atomoxetine, or methylphenidate were included and matched with up to 4 nonusers on the basis of data source, gender, state, and age. Cardiovascular events were validated using medical records. Proportional hazards regression was used to calculated hazard ratios.

Results.—We identified 241 417 incident users (primary cohort). No statistically significant difference between incident users and nonusers was observed in the rate of validated sudden death or ventricular arrhythmia (hazard ratio: 1.60 [95% confidence interval (CI): 0.19—13.60]) or all-cause death (hazard ratio: 0.76 [95% CI: 0.52—1.12]). None of the strokes identified during exposed time to ADHD medications were validated. No myocardial infarctions were identified in ADHD medication users. No statistically significant difference between prevalent users and nonusers (secondary cohort) was observed (hazard ratios for validated sudden death or ventricular arrhythmia: 1.43 [95% CI: 0.31−6.61]; stroke: 0.89 [95% CI: 0.11−7.11]; stroke/myocardial infarction: 0.72 [95% CI: 0.09−5.57]; and all-cause death: 0.77 [95% CI: 0.56−1.07).

Conclusions.—The rate of cardiovascular events in exposed children was very low and in general no higher than that in unexposed control subjects. Because of the low number of events, we have limited ability to rule out relative increases in rate.

▶ This article was selected because psychiatrists, pediatricians, and patients continue to have concerns about the cardiac safety profile of the stimulant medications that are used to treat attention-deficit/hyperactivity disorder (ADHD). Since the seminal article(s) from 3 to 4 years ago, which expressed grave concern about these medications and which advised the need for significant baseline cardiac testing on any candidate for these medications, there have been several studies to assess this concern. This review is made primarily by pediatricians who studied those who came for ADHD treatment and finds a very low incidence of such conditions. This highlights the need to understand as well as possible what effects stimulants do have on the body when taken in moderate doses and to understand what, if any, cardiac effects may be present. Clinicians should remain cautious and should always use excellent clinical judgment, but these findings provide increased perception about the safety of these medications.

A. H. Mack, MD

Clonidine Extended-Release Tablets for Pediatric Patients With Attention-Deficit/Hyperactivity Disorder

Jain R, Segal S, Kollins SH, et al (R/D Clinical Res, Inc, Lake Jackson, TX; Inst for Clinical Res, North Miami, FL; Duke Univ Med Ctr, Durham, NC; et al)
J Am Acad Child Adolesc Psychiatry 50:171-179, 2011

Objective.—This study examined the efficacy and safety of clonidine hydrochloride extended-release tablets (CLON-XR) in children and adolescents with attention-deficit/hyperactivity disorder (ADHD).

Method.—This 8-week, placebo-controlled, fixed-dose trial, including 3 weeks of dose escalation, of patients 6 to 17 years old with ADHD evaluated the efficacy and safety of CLON-XR 0.2 mg/day or CLON-XR 0.4 mg/day versus placebo in three separate treatment arms. Primary endpoint was mean change in ADHD Rating Scale−IV (ADHD-RS-IV) total score from baseline to week 5 versus placebo using a last observation carried forward method. Secondary endpoints were improvement in ADHD-RS-IV inattention and hyperactivity/impulsivity subscales, Conners Parent Rating Scale−Revised: Long Form, Clinical Global Impression of Severity, Clinical Global Impression of Improvement, and Parent Global Assessment from baseline to week 5.

Results.—Patients (N = 236) were randomized to receive placebo (n = 78), CLON-XR 0.2 mg/day (n = 78), or CLON-XR 0.4 mg/day (n = 80).

Improvement from baseline in ADHD-RS-IV total score was significantly greater in both CLON-XR groups versus placebo at week 5. A significant improvement in ADHD-RS-IV total score occurred between groups as soon as week 2 and was maintained throughout the treatment period. In addition, improvement in ADHD-RS-IV inattention and hyperactivity/impulsivity subscales, Conners Parent Rating Scale—Revised: Long Form, Clinical Global Impression of Improvement, Clinical Global Impression of Severity, and Parent Global Assessment, occurred in both treatment groups versus placebo. The most common treatment-emergent adverse event was mild-to-moderate somnolence. Changes on electrocardiogram were minor and reflected the known pharmacology of clonidine.

Conclusions.—Clonidine hydrochloride extended-release tablets were generally well tolerated by patients in the study and significantly improved ADHD symptoms in this pediatric population.

▶ The core basis for exploring alternatives to stimulants is the fact that some patients do not respond to stimulants. However, there are no alternatives that seem to come close to the stimulants in terms of efficacy. Many, if not all, alternatives, have fewer side effects, lesser risk for addiction, and require less attention in terms of their being a "controlled" substance. They may well have risks of their own, however, such as bupropion's seizure risk or anticholinergicity of tricyclic antidepressants. This study explores the risks of effects of clonidine, now in an extended pill package. The data provide interesting evidence as to the different time of action in this medication rather than the average 2 hours to peak concentration with the clonidine patch. The blood pressure and conduction issues of clonidine are raised here and deserve attention. Clinicians should read this review of safety, tolerability, and efficacy carefully as we likely will treat patients with this medication. One looks forward to additional research to demonstrate the conditions in which clonidine is the treatment of choice.

A. H. Mack, MD

Cognitive and behavioral complications of frontal lobe epilepsy in children: A review of the literature
Braakman HMH, Vaessen MJ, Hofman PAM, et al (Maastricht Univ Med Centre, The Netherlands; Epilepsy Centre Kempenhaeghe, Heeze, The Netherlands)
Epilepsia 52:849-856, 2011

Frontal lobe epilepsy (FLE) is considered the second most common type of the localization-related epilepsies of childhood. Still, the etiology of FLE in children, its impact on cognitive functioning and behavior, as well as the response to antiepileptic drug treatment in children has not been sufficiently studied. This review focuses on these aspects of FLE in childhood, and reveals that FLE in childhood is most often cryptogenic, and impacts on a broad range of cognitive functions. The nature and severity of cognitive deficits are highly variable, although impaired attention and executive functions are most frequent. Young age at seizure onset is the only potential risk factor for poor cognitive outcome that has been consistently reported. The behavioral disturbances associated with FLE are also highly variable, although attention deficit/hyperactivity disorder seems most frequent. In 40% of children with FLE satisfactory seizure control could not be achieved. This is a higher percentage than reported for the general population of children with epilepsy. Therefore, pediatric FLE, even if cryptogenic in nature, is frequently complicated by impairment of cognitive function, behavioral disturbances, and therapy-resistance. Given the impact of these complications, there is a need for studies of the etiology of frontal lobe epilepsy-associated cognitive and behavioral disturbances, as well as pharmacotherapy-resistance.

▶ We all are trained to consider temporal lobe epilepsy as a basis for certain abnormal behaviors, but seizures based around the frontal lobe are the second most common site-specific epilepsy disorders, and this review provides some assessment of them. It is of no surprise, however, that the more common findings are that youth affected by this type of neurologic syndrome are affected in terms of executive function and also impulsivity or attention. While the authors describe that they will explain a behavioral phenotype, it is less impressive as a type than for other disorders. What is of great interest is that these disorders are poorly amenable to treatment. As a result, children and youth who have disorders that will lead to frontal lobe epilepsy need close and ongoing attention and may well need trials of several medications before finding the correct one. This review is essentially a meta-analysis; further assessment is needed in order to further elucidate the findings in frontal lobe epilepsy and how to better treat it.

A. H. Mack, MD

Computer-Assisted Management of Attention-Deficit/Hyperactivity Disorder
Lavigne JV, Dulcan MK, LeBailly SA, et al (Children's Memorial Hosp, Chicago, IL; Northwestern Univ, Chicago, IL)
Pediatrics 128:e46-e53, 2011

Objectives.—Medication management of attention-deficit/hyperactivity disorder (ADHD) is often suboptimal. We examined whether (1) brief physician training plus computer-assisted medication management led to greater reduction in ADHD symptoms and (2) adherence to the recommended titration protocol produced greater symptomatic improvement.

Methods.—A randomized medication trial was conducted that included 24 pediatric practices. Children who met criteria for ADHD were randomly assigned by practice to treatment-as-usual or a specialized care group in which physicians received 2 hours of didactic training on medication management of ADHD plus training on a software program to assist in monitoring improvement. Parent and teacher reports were obtained before treatment and 4, 9, and 12 months after starting medication.

Results.—Children in both specialized care and treatment-as-usual groups improved on the ADHD Rating Scales and SNAP-IV, but there were no group differences in improvement rates. Brief physician training alone did not produce improvements. When recommended titration procedures were followed, however, outcomes were better for total and inattentive ADHD symptoms on both the ADHD Rating Scales and SNAP-IV parent and teacher scales. Results were not attributable to discontinuation because of adverse effects or failure to find an effective medication dose.

Conclusions.—Brief physician training alone did not lead to reductions in ADHD symptoms, but adherence to a protocol that involved titration until the child's symptoms were in the average range and had shown a reliable change led to better symptom reduction. Computer-assisted medication management can contribute to better treatment outcomes in primary care medication treatment of ADHD.

▶ The term "computer-assisted" can mean many things, but in this case, it relates to a system used to help promote regularized alterations in stimulant dose. The study demonstrated, as many others have, that improvement in the symptoms and signs of attention-deficit/hyperactivity disorder (ADHD) (as diagnosed by the Diagnostic Interview Schedule for Children, version IV) come as a result of stimulant use. Their other findings, such as that a specific training for pediatricians along with computer-programmed dosing changes were not helpful, suggests other issues. However, the intriguing finding of improvement simply related to an algorithm is important. Although there is no inherent defect in relying on instruments to determine dose, it is a system open to human fallibility and variation. Indeed, the authors have highlighted an issue that deserves further exploration as we continue to seek novel approaches to the treatment of this condition. A study like this, by the way, highlights how much more advanced the treatment of ADHD is for the child and adolescent population than for the adult population; clinicians dealing with patients claiming to have ADHD find themselves with insufficient data on which to make decisions, and further help is needed.

A. H. Mack, MD

Efficacy and Safety of Lisdexamfetamine Dimesylate in Adolescents With Attention-Deficit/Hyperactivity Disorder

Findling RL, Childress AC, Cutler AJ, et al (Case Western Reserve Univ, Cleveland, OH; Ctr for Psychiatry and Behavioral Medicine Inc, Las Vegas, NV; Florida Clinical Res Ctr, Bradenton; et al)
J Am Acad Child Adolesc Psychiatry 50:395-405, 2011

Objective.—To examine lisdexamfetamine dimesylate (LDX) efficacy and safety versus placebo in adolescents with attention-deficit/hyperactivity disorder (ADHD).

Method.—Adolescents (13 through 17) with at least moderately symptomatic ADHD (ADHD Rating Scale IV: Clinician Version [ADHD-RS-IV] score ≥28) were randomized to placebo or LDX (30, 50, or 70 mg/d) in a 4-week, forced-dose titration, double-blind study. Primary and secondary efficacy measures were the ADHD-RS-IV, Clinical Global Impressions—Improvement (CGI-I), and Youth QOL—Research Version (YQOL-R). Safety assessments included treatment-emergent adverse events (TEAEs), vital signs, laboratory findings, physical examinations, and ECG.

Results.—Overall, 314 participants were randomized; 309 were in efficacy analyses and 49 withdrew (11 due to TEAEs). Least squares mean (SE) change from baseline at endpoint in ADHD-RS-IV total scores were −18.3 (1.25), −21.1 (1.28), −20.7 (1.25) for 30, 50, and 70 mg/d LDX, respectively; −12.8 (1.25) for placebo ($p \leq .0056$ versus placebo for each). Differences in ADHD-RS-IV total scores favored all LDX doses versus placebo at all weeks ($p \leq .0076$). On the CGI-I, 69.1% of participants were rated very much/much improved at endpoint with LDX all doses versus placebo (39.5%) ($p < .0001$). YQOL-R changes at endpoint scores for LDX groups versus placebo were not significant. Commonly reported LDX (all doses combined) TEAEs (≥5%) were decreased appetite, headache, insomnia, decreased weight, and irritability. Small mean increases in pulse and blood pressure and no clinically meaningful trends in ECG changes were noted with LDX.

Conclusions.—LDX at all doses was effective versus placebo in treating adolescent ADHD and demonstrated a safety profile consistent with previous LDX studies.

Clinical Trials Registry Information.—Efficacy and Safety of Lisdexamfetamine Dimesylate (LDX) in Adolescents With Attention-Deficit/Hyperactivity Disorder (ADHD); http://www.clinicaltrials.gov; NCT00735371.

▶ A study on the safety and efficacy of lisdexamfetamine was expected, but the magnitude of this study is significant. The trial occurred in 45 sites around the United States among adolescents for whom attention-deficit/hyperactivity disorder (ADHD) was the primary diagnosis (although it is unclear whether ADHD not otherwise specified patients were included) and in whom the diagnosis was judged to be more than moderate in severity. Three efficacy measures were recorded as the forced titration occurred; safety was measured in terms of vital signs, electrocardiogram, and weight. The study compared exposure to lisdexamfetamine to placebo, and ratings were double blinded. Overall, the measures of efficacy and safety were within the range expected of d-amphetamine, which is the drug to which lisdexamfetamine is metabolized.

What, then, is the advantage of lisdexamfetamine over any other stimulant? The answer lies in pharmacokinetics—the prodrug feature of lisdexamfetamine makes for its period of action lasting up to 12 hours, with a 2-hour delay before onset of action. Furthermore, this compound is not easily snorted or injected, making it unwieldy as an abusable substance. These are important features indeed, although individual clinicians will need to weigh the benefits of this medication against its cost at the pharmacy and in its development.

A. H. Mack, MD

Evidence-Based Recommendations for Monitoring Safety of Second Generation Antipsychotics in Children and Youth

Pringsheim T, for the CAMESA guideline group (Univ of Calgary, Canada; et al)
J Can Acad Child Adolesc Psychiatry 20:218-233, 2011

Background.—The use of antipsychotics, especially second generation antipsychotics (SGAs), for children with mental health disorders in Canada has increased dramatically over the past five years. These medications have the potential to cause major metabolic and neurological complications with chronic use.

Objective.—Our objective was to synthesize the evidence for specific metabolic and neurological side effects associated with the use of SGAs in children and make evidence-based recommendations for the monitoring of these side effects.

Methods.—We performed a systematic review of controlled clinical trials of SGAs in children. Recommendations for monitoring SGA safety were made according to a classification scheme based on the GRADE system. When there was inadequate evidence to make recommendations, recommendations were based on consensus and expert opinion. A multidisciplinary consensus group reviewed all relevant evidence and came to consensus on recommendations.

Results.—Evidence-based recommendations for monitoring SGA safety are provided in the guideline. The strength of recommendations for specific physical examination maneuvers and laboratory tests are provided for each SGA medication at specific time points.

Conclusion.—Multiple randomized controlled trials (RCTs) have established the efficacy of many of the SGAs in pediatric mental health disorders. These benefits however do not come without risk; both metabolic and neurological side effects occur in children treated with these SGAs. The risk of weight gain, increased BMI and abnormal lipids appears greatest with olanzapine, followed by clozapine and quetiapine. The risk of neurological side effects of treatment appears greatest with risperidone, olanzapine and aripiprazole. Appropriate monitoring procedures for adverse effects will improve the quality of care of children treated with these medications.

▶ This is an invaluable article; one can understand why it was published in a Canadian-based journal, but hopefully it will be disseminated to a broader audience. It provides a review of the evidence of each of the second-generation antipsychotics in terms of safety profile and experience with adverse reactions and side effects, and it utilizes a systematic review approach to provide recommendations on several forms of monitoring for these medications in children.

This is not simply laboratory values but other somatic measurements as well. The systematic approach provides levels of support for each of the types of monitoring. One reason that this article is so well made is that it is the product of a multidisciplinary work group, of experts in family medicine, neurology, as well as psychiatry, all interested in the safest manner of monitoring these medications. While they may not all be on-label for any child, their use is pervasive, especially in the pervasive developmental disorders, and so this article should protect the health and safety of children with psychiatric problems.

A. H. Mack, MD

Pharmacokinetically and Clinician-Determined Adherence to an Antidepressant Regimen and Clinical Outcome in the TORDIA Trial
Woldu H, Porta G, Goldstein T, et al (Mt. Sinai School of Medicine, NY; Univ of Pittsburgh, PA; et al)
J Am Acad Child Adolesc Psychiatry 50:490-498, 2011

Objective.—Nonadherence to antidepressant treatment may contribute to poor outcome and to suicidal adverse events in adolescent depression. We examine the relationship between adherence and both clinical response and suicidal events in participants in the Treatment of Resistant Depression in Adolescents (TORDIA) study.

Method.—The relationship between adherence to medication and clinical outcome was assessed in 190 treatment-resistant depressed adolescents who were randomized to one of four cells: switch to another selective serotonin reuptake inhibitor (SSRI), switch to venlafaxine, or either of these two medication switches plus cognitive behavioral therapy. Plasma levels of antidepressant drug and metabolites were determined after 6 and 12 weeks of treatment. A twofold or greater variation in the dose-adjusted concentration of drug plus metabolites (level/dose ratio [LDR]) was defined as nonadherence. Nonadherence was also determined by clinician pill counts (CPC) of the proportion of prescribed pills that were unused and was defined as having greater than 30% of the prescribed pills remaining.

Results.—LDR and CPC showed low concordance. LDR was unrelated to clinical response. CPC adherence was related to a higher response rate overall (adherent, 63.0% versus nonadherent, 47.2%, $p = .03$). Approximately half (50.8%) of the sample surveyed showed evidence of nonadherence by CPC. Neither measure of adherence was related to the occurrence of suicidal events or to the pace of decline in suicidal ideation.

Conclusions.—Clinician pill counts may be a relevant measure of adherence that is related to outcome under formal clinical trial conditions in depressed adolescents. Nonadherence appears to be a common and significant source of treatment nonresponse. Clinical Trial Registration

Information—Treatment of SSRI-Resistant Depression in Adolescents (TORDIA); http://www.clinicaltrials.gov; NCT00018902.

▶ There are 2 concurrent themes to this report that use the data from the Treatment of Resistant Depression in Adolescents study. The first is the question of noncompliance, which is certainly an important consideration in any psychiatric treatment, and it is all the more common in the medication treatment of adolescents. Indeed, the report documents a high rate of medication noncompliance. This is a major concern in that the focus of the study is the treatment-resistant depressed patient. But a second theme is the fact that the forms of physician assessment of noncompliance were not reliable. They did not necessarily provide consistent counts of the degree of noncompliance. This is a further frontier in the understanding of treatment-resistant depression, but it will be necessary to move ahead to elucidate this phenomenon to better treat depression in this population. It may be difficult to contemplate the use of plasma draws in everyday outpatient child psychiatric practice. Yet it does fall into the emerging concept that all care will be delivered in systems of care, which have patients as a part of the team, and perhaps this will provide benefits in several realms of care.

A. H. Mack, MD

Treatment Studies: Psychotherapies

A New Parenting-Based Group Intervention for Young Anxious Children: Results of a Randomized Controlled Trial

Cartwright-Hatton S, McNally D, Field AP, et al (Univ of Manchester, UK; Central Manchester Foundation Trust, UK; Univ of Sussex, UK)
J Am Acad Child Adolesc Psychiatry 50:242-251, 2011

Objective.—Despite recent advances, there are still no interventions that have been developed for the specific treatment of young children who have anxiety disorders. This study examined the impact of a new, cognitive—behaviorally based parenting intervention on anxiety symptoms.

Method.—Families of 74 anxious children (aged 9 years or less) took part in a randomized controlled trial, which compared the new 10-session, group-format intervention with a wait-list control condition. Outcome measures included blinded diagnostic interview and self-reports from parents and children.

Results.—Intention-to-treat analyses indicated that children whose parent(s) received the intervention were significantly less anxious at the end of the study than those in the control condition. Specifically, 57% of those receiving the new intervention were free of their primary disorder, compared with 15% in the control condition. Moreover, 32% of treated children were free of any anxiety diagnosis at the end of the treatment period, compared with 6% of those in the control group. Treatment gains were maintained at 12-month follow-up.

Conclusions.—This new parenting-based intervention may represent an advance in the treatment of this previously neglected group. Clinical trial registration information: Anxiety in Young Children: A Randomized Controlled Trial of a New Cognitive-Behaviourally Based Parenting Intervention; http://www.isrctn.org/; ISRCTN12166762.

▶ A search for new modalities for anxiety in children begins with the interpretation that the extant forms of treatment are insufficient but that focus on cognitive models is central to understanding anxiety, as is the perspective of parental influences promoting anxiety among children. As some groups have indicated, providing attention, education, or training to parents of diagnosed children can be effective, just as cognitive-behavioral therapy has been for children with obsessive-compulsive disorder. This study includes a wider group of anxiety disorders, and its modality is structured and manualized. Here the intervention was compared to control cases, so ultimately head-to-head comparisons will be effective not only for differentiating among treatments but also for understanding the development and pathophysiology of anxiety in this age group. If it is not purely cognitive-behavioral, then what is it? How is this affecting the child's reaction? We shall learn.

A. H. Mack, MD

Altering the Trajectory of Anxiety in At-Risk Young Children
Rapee RM, Kennedy SJ, Ingram M, et al (Macquarie Univ, Sydney, New South Wales, Australia)
Am J Psychiatry 167:1518-1525, 2010

Objective.—Increasing evidence for the importance of several risk factors for anxiety disorders is beginning to point to the possibility of prevention. Early interventions targeting known risk for anxiety have rarely been evaluated. The authors evaluated the medium-term (3-year) effects of a parent-focused intervention for anxiety in inhibited preschool-age children.

Method.—The study was a randomized controlled trial of a brief intervention program provided to parents compared with a monitoring-only condition. Participants were 146 inhibited preschool-age children and their parents; data from two or more assessment points were available at 3 years for 121 children. Study inclusion was based on parent-reported screening plus laboratory-observed inhibition. The six-session group-based intervention included parenting skills, cognitive restructuring, and in vivo exposure. The main outcome measures were number and severity of anxiety disorders, anxiety symptoms, and extent of inhibition.

Results.—Children whose parents received the intervention showed lower frequency and severity of anxiety disorders and lower levels of anxiety symptoms according to maternal, paternal, and child report. Levels of inhibition did not differ significantly based on either parent report or laboratory observation.

Conclusions.—This brief, inexpensive intervention shows promise in potentially altering the trajectory of anxiety and related disorders in young inhibited children.

▶ Anxiety disorders and subdiagnostic anxiety symptomatology are indeed disabling and highly prevalent forms of childhood psychopathology. Many children suffer from anxiety, so the need to effect a change in this large scale problem looms large. This study extends previous findings on a specific preventative intervention in at-risk children while addressing developmental progress, some environmental factors, and outcome goals. Their study was able to review progress for young children (age < 4 years on average) and the lasting effect of this intervention, which was psycho-education to the parents only. A control group was used as well. No analysis was made as to gender, and some could quibble with the ethnic composition of the study group. Nevertheless, this is a very promising form of intervention for many reasons—its brevity, focus on parental contact, empirical analyzability, and lack of theoretical bias. While further follow-up will be necessary, this study provides justification for further investigation into this form of intervention.

A. H. Mack, MD

Prolonged Exposure Versus Dynamic Therapy for Adolescent PTSD: A Pilot Randomized Controlled Trial
Gilboa-Schechtman E, Foa EB, Shafran N, et al (Bar-Ilan Univ, Ramat-Gan, Israel; Univ of Pennsylvania, Philadelphia; et al)
J Am Acad Child Adolesc Psychiatry 49:1034-1042, 2010

Objective.—To examine the efficacy and maintenance of developmentally adapted prolonged exposure therapy for adolescents (PE-A) compared with active control time-limited dynamic therapy (TLDP-A) for decreasing posttraumatic and depressive symptoms in adolescent victims of single-event traumas.

Method.—Thirty-eight adolescents (12 to 18 years old) were randomly assigned to receive PE-A or TLDP-A.

Results.—Both treatments resulted in decreased posttraumatic stress disorder and depression and increased functioning. PE-A exhibited a greater decrease of posttraumatic stress disorder and depression symptom severity and a greater increase in global functioning than did TDLP-A. After treatment, 68.4% of adolescents beginning treatment with PE-A and 36.8% of those beginning treatment with TLDP-A no longer met diagnostic criteria for posttraumatic stress disorder. Treatment gains were maintained at 6- and 17-month follow-ups.

Conclusions.—Brief individual therapy is effective in decreasing posttraumatic distress and behavioral trauma-focused components enhance efficacy.

Clinical Trial Registry Information.—Prolonged Exposure Therapy Versus Active Psychotherapy in Treating Post-Traumatic Stress Disorder in Adolescents, URL: http://clinicaltrials.gov, unique identifier: NCT00183690.

▶ This is an attempt to examine the efficacy and maintenance of developmentally adapted prolonged exposure therapy (PE-A) for adolescents compared with active control time-limited dynamic therapy (TLDP). The subjects had experienced single-event traumas. The authors cite a study to suggest that "adolescents exhibit a unique clinical expression of posttraumatic distress characterized by significant emotional and behavioral dysregulation" and use that as the basis of the investigation. One should keep in mind that these may be different from sexual abuse trauma, which often seems to be the main content of child literature on trauma. Here the comparison therapy, (PE-A), has been adapted for adolescents. Various measures were assessed, such as K-SADS-PL (Schedule of Affective Disorders and Schizophrenia for School-Age Children—Revised for DSM-IV), CGAS (Children's Global Assessment Scale), Child PTSD Symptom Scale, and others, including the Beck Depression Inventory. Both forms of treatment were successful at 6 and 17 months; the PE-A was superior to TLDP-A (time-limited dynamic psychotherapy) at 6 but not 17 months. Overall this is a good study, but its main limitation is its small size of 38.

A. H. Mack, MD

Computer-Assisted Cognitive Behavioral Therapy for Child Anxiety: Results of a Randomized Clinical Trial
Khanna MS, Kendall PC (Univ of Pennsylvania, Philadelphia; Temple Univ, Japan)
J Consult Clin Psychol 78:737-745, 2010

Objective.—This study examined the feasibility, acceptability, and effects of Camp Cope-A-Lot (CCAL), a computer-assisted cognitive behavioral therapy (CBT) for anxiety in youth.

Method.—Children (49; 33 males) ages 7–13 ($M = 10.1 \pm 1.6$; 83.7% Caucasian, 14.2% African American, 2% Hispanic) with a principal anxiety disorder were randomly assigned to (a) CCAL, (b) individual CBT (ICBT), or (c) a computer-assisted education, support, and attention (CESA) condition. All therapists were from the community (school or counseling psychologists, clinical psychologist) or were PsyD or PhD trainees with no experience or training in CBT for child anxiety. Independent diagnostic interviews and self-report measures were completed at pre- and posttreatment and 3-month follow-up.

Results.—At posttreatment, ICBT or CCAL children showed significantly better gains than CESA children; 70%, 81%, and 19%, respectively, no longer met criteria for their principal anxiety diagnosis. Gains were maintained at follow-up, with no significant differences between ICBT and CCAL. Parents and children rated all treatments acceptable,

TABLE 1.—Means, Standard Deviations, and Group Differences for Measures of Disorder at Pretreatment, Posttreatment, and 3-Month Follow-Up Across Conditions

Measure	Pretreatment			Posttreatment			3-Month Follow-Up	
	ICBT ($N=17$)	CCAL ($N=16$)	CESA ($N=16$)	ICBT ($N=17$)	CCAL ($N=16$)	CESA ($N=16$)	ICBT ($N=14$)	CCAL ($N=12$)
CSR (95% CI)								
M	5.8	5.7	5.2	3.1	2.9	4.2**	3.3	2.4
SD	1.2	.87	1.2	1.6	1.0	1.3	1.0	1.0
CGAS rating (95% CI)								
M	54.1	53.8	60.5	69.9	68.2	63.8**	76.7	75.1
SD	12.1	7.5	13.7	7.7	7.0	10.5	8.7	7.1
MASC total score (95% CI)								
M	48.9	50.5	48.2	35.8	35.2	39**	32.4	31.5
SD	14.5	12.8	15.0	13.1	12.3	16.1	12.4	12.7
CDI total score (95% CI)								
M	25.2	27.2	23.2	22.7	21.3	21.8*	20.3	19.4
SD	8.3	4.4	7.6	9.1	10.7	9.2	9.5	8.7

Note. ICBT = individual cognitive behavioral therapy; CCAL = Camp Cope-A-Lot (computer-assisted therapy); CESA = computer-assisted education, support, and attention control; CSR = Clinical Severity Rating (based on ADIS-C/P); CGAS = Clinical Global Assessment Scale; MASC = Multidimensional Anxiety Scale for Children; CDI = Children's Depression Inventory.
*$p<.05$.
**$p<.01$.

with CCAL and ICBT children rating higher satisfaction than CESA children.

Conclusions.—Findings support the feasibility, acceptability and beneficial effects of CCAL for anxious youth. Discussion considers the potential of computer-assisted treatments in the dissemination of empirically supported treatments (Table 1).

▶ As the authors point out, there is considerable evidence that cognitive behavioral therapy (CBT) is effective for anxiety disorders in children, yet this approach is not practiced by many child therapists. Thus, there is a need to disseminate this method.

Also, most children these days are glued to their computers or smartphones, so the idea of a computer-based treatment makes a lot of sense.

This study compared the effectiveness of a computer-based anxiety treatment, based on their own empirically validated CBT intervention, with individual face-to-face CBT, and a computer-based attentional control. These were definitely the appropriate comparison groups, as one provides CBT and the other provides interaction with a computer. This is just a preliminary study, but it does suggest that this method of intervening with anxious children holds potential.

Of course, the main question that arises in comparing a computer-based treatment with the more traditional method of psychotherapy pertains to the issue of the therapeutic relationship. Since most studies indicate the importance of the therapy relationship, is it as strong an attachment when in the computer-based treatment the child has only a coach who is not there in person? The authors, anticipating this question, address it and report that the rating of the therapy relationship was comparable to that in the face-to-face therapy.

One question I had was why such a large proportion of the subjects were male, that is, 33 of 49. This issue was not addressed in the article, but it is difficult to imagine that the prevalence of anxiety disorders is so much higher in males than in females.

It was nice to see examples of the type of cartoons and interactive exercises they used. Clearly, the language and cognitive ability of the age group was considered, and it's easy to see why children might have found the program appealing. It would have been useful to hear how the researchers coped with people forgetting to log onto the program. At any rate, this new method offers promise (Table 1), particularly in cases where parents find it difficult to get their children to a clinic office and in communities where evidence-based treatments are not being offered.

J. L. Krupnick, PhD

Does Cognitive Behavioral Therapy for Youth Anxiety Outperform Usual Care in Community Clinics? An Initial Effectiveness Test

Southam-Gerow MA, Weisz JR, Chu BC, et al (Virginia Commonwealth Univ, Richmond; Harvard Univ and the Judge Baker Children's Ctr, MA; State Univ of New Jersey, Newark; et al)
J Am Acad Child Adolesc Psychiatry 49:1043-1052, 2010

Objective.—Most tests of cognitive behavioral therapy (CBT) for youth anxiety disorders have shown beneficial effects, but these have been efficacy trials with recruited youths treated by researcher-employed therapists. One previous (nonrandomized) trial in community clinics found that CBT did not outperform usual care (UC). The present study used a more stringent effectiveness design to test CBT versus UC in youths referred to community clinics, with all treatment provided by therapists employed in the clinics.

Method.—A randomized controlled trial methodology was used. Therapists were randomized to training and supervision in the Coping Cat CBT program or UC. Forty-eight youths (56% girls, 8 to 15 years of age, 38% Caucasian, 33% Latino, 15% African-American) diagnosed with *DSM-IV* anxiety disorders were randomized to CBT or UC.

Results.—At the end of treatment more than half the youths no longer met criteria for their primary anxiety disorder, but the groups did not differ significantly on symptom (e.g., parent report, eta-square $= 0.0001$; child report, eta-square $= 0.09$; both differences favoring UC) or diagnostic (CBT, 66.7% without primary diagnosis; UC, 73.7%; odds ratio 0.71) outcomes. No differences were found with regard to outcomes of comorbid conditions, treatment duration, or costs. However, youths receiving CBT used fewer additional services than UC youths ($\chi_1^2 = 8.82$, $p = .006$).

Conclusions.—CBT did not produce better clinical outcomes than usual community clinic care. This initial test involved a relatively modest sample size; more research is needed to clarify whether there are conditions under which CBT can produce better clinical outcomes than usual clinical care.

TABLE 1.—Descriptive Data Before and After Treatment, by Treatment Group

| | Before Treatment | | | | | | After Treatment | | | | | |
| | UC | | | CBT | | | UC | | | CBT | | |
	Mean	SD	n	Mean	SD	n	Mean	SD	n	Mean	SD	n
Child self-report												
STAIC-Trait	35.75	7.25	24	34.33	6.12	24	29.68	6.81	19	36.53	9.86	17
DISC-C Anx sx count	17.19	8.33	24	19.42	7.88	24	6.21	6.97	14	11.15	7.66	17
Child Anxiety Factor	−0.02	0.97	24	0.02	0.81	24	−1.01	0.98	19	−0.29	1.07	18
Parent report												
STAIC-P-Trait	45.21	8.22	24	46.52	7.91	21	41.80	7.88	19	42.75	8.89	16
CBCL Anx/Dep	68.65	8.61	20	67.65	9.09	23	58.94	9.04	17	60.19	8.46	16
CBCL Internalizing	66.30	8.23	20	66.52	9.23	23	56.12	10.36	17	58.87	9.03	15
DISC-P Anx sx count	20.75	7.45	24	19.17	8.80	24	9.08	7.97	19	10.77	8.11	17
Parent Anxiety Factor	−0.002	0.81	24	0.03	0.90	24	−0.94	0.84	19	−0.82	0.80	18
DISC-P DBD diagnoses	1.00	0.78	24	0.75	0.79	24	1.00	1.00	19	0.39	0.61	18
Combined report												
DISC-Anx diagnoses	2.28	1.22	24	2.17	1.31	24	1.21	1.62	19	1.44	1.15	18
DISC-Dep diagnoses	0.04	0.20	24	0.25	0.54	24	0.11	0.32	19	0.11	0.32	18
DISC-Total diagnoses	3.25	1.60	24	3.17	1.93	24	2.32	2.00	19	1.94	1.55	18
Other variables												
Estimated cost (US$)							3055.76	1301.94	24	2543.29	1740.37	24
Treatment duration (sessions)							14.00	5.92	24	13.96	8.15	24
Treatment duration (wk)							27.68	18.77	24	21.542	13.971	24

Note: CBCL Anx/Dep = Child Behavior Checklist—Anxiety/Depression Scale; CBCL Internalizing = Child Behavior Checklist—Internalizing Behavior Scale; CBT = cognitive-behavioral therapy group; DISC-Anx diagnoses = total number of comorbid (nonprimary) anxiety diagnoses on Diagnostic Interview Schedule for Children, composite report; DISC-Dep diagnoses = total number of comorbid depressive disorder diagnoses on Diagnostic Interview Schedule for Children, composite report; DISC-C anx sx count = number of anxiety disorder symptoms (social phobia, separation anxiety disorder, generalized anxiety disorder, and specific phobia only) on child-report Diagnostic Interview Schedule for Children; DISC-P anx sx count = number of anxiety disorder symptoms (social phobia, separation anxiety disorder, generalized anxiety disorder, and specific phobia only) on parent-report Diagnostic Interview Schedule for Children; DISC-P DBD Diagnoses = number of disruptive behavior disorder diagnoses on Diagnostic Interview Schedule for Children—Parent Report; DISC-Total diagnoses = total number of diagnoses on Diagnostic Interview Schedule for Children, composite report; STAIC-P-Trait = State-Trait Anxiety Inventory for Children, Trait Version, parent report; STAIC-Trait = State-Trait Anxiety Inventory for Children, Trait Version; UC = usual care group.

Clinical Trial Registry Information.—Community Clinic Test of Youth Anxiety and Depression Study, URL: http://clinicaltrials.gov, unique identifier: NCT01005836 (Table 1).

▶ This study produced an unexpected finding, that is, that cognitive behavioral therapy (CBT), an evidence-based treatment for youth anxiety disorders, did not produce better clinical outcomes than usual community clinic care. This flies in the face of the usual assumption that evidence-based care is more effective and should be disseminated as much as possible into the community. At the same time, it follows the usual pattern of showing that when treatments that are found efficacious (tested in university-based settings with carefully selected patients, extensive supervision, etc) in carefully controlled circumstances are moved into community settings, they typically do not fare as well. Table 1 shows the pre-post statistics for each group.

This study incorporated a number of design features that make it compelling; for example, it is the first randomized controlled trial focusing on childhood anxiety disorders in which treatment was delivered within public mental health clinics, to clinically referred youths, by providers who were employees of the clinics. This makes it an excellent test of how the treatment method works in a less rarified atmosphere than one finds in efficacy studies. It seems likely that the socioeconomic status of the patients in this study was considerably lower than those seen at university-based clinics, the clinicians were probably less well trained, and the families from which the children came probably were more likely multiproblem families. Thus, this was truly a test of how well the method might perform under the toughest of circumstances.

The authors make some interesting points in speculating about why CBT was not significantly more effective then usual care. Among these is the idea that CBT therapists maintained a focus on anxiety, whereas the usual care therapists were free to attend to and address nonanxiety problems. In a population with a high rate of comorbid disorders, this may have provided flexibility that was important for this population. However, these are the patients that clinicians are likely to encounter in lower income samples. These results serve as a reminder that an intervention with a more carefully screened sample may not carry the same power with patients with more complex clinical profiles.

J. L. Krupnick, PhD

Preventing Substance Use Among Early Asian—American Adolescent Girls: Initial Evaluation of a Web-Based, Mother—Daughter Program
Fang L, Schinke SP, Cole KCA (Univ of Toronto, Ontario, Canada; Columbia Univ, NY)
J Adolesc Health 47:529-532, 2010

Purpose.—This study examined the efficacy and generalizability of a family-oriented, web-based substance use prevention program to young Asian—American adolescent girls.

Methods.—Between September and December 2007, a total of 108 Asian—American girls aged 10—14 years and their mothers were recruited through online advertisements and from community service agencies. Mother—daughter dyads were randomly assigned to an intervention arm or to a test-only control arm. After pretest measurement, intervention-arm dyads completed a 9-session web-based substance use prevention program. Guided by family interaction theory, the program aimed to improve girls' psychological states, strengthen substance use prevention skills, increase mother—daughter interactions, enhance maternal monitoring, and prevent girls' substance use. Study outcomes were assessed using generalized estimating equations.

Results.—At posttest, relative to control-arm girls, intervention-arm girls showed less depressed mood; reported improved self-efficacy and refusal skills; had higher levels of mother—daughter closeness, mother—daughter communication, and maternal monitoring; and reported more family rules against substance use. Intervention-arm girls also reported fewer instances of alcohol, marijuana, and illicit prescription drug use, and expressed lower intentions to use substances in the future.

Conclusions.—A family-oriented, web-based substance use prevention program was efficacious in preventing substance use behavior among early Asian-American adolescent girls.

▶ What is most intriguing about this study is the sample. One does not typically think about Asian American adolescents as being at high risk for substance abuse since, as the authors point out, the popular image of Asian Americans is one of being a model minority group. Given this, it is not surprising to read that little research has been done in terms of developing or testing prevention programs for this population. This study begins to address this omission.

A strength of the study is its grounding in theory, in this case, family interaction theory. It also reflects use of modern technology in that it is a Web-based approach. Given the degree to which young adolescents are invested in Internet activities, this approach probably increases their level of interest in participation. The methods in the approach, ie, use of animated graphics and games and interactive exercises, also seem like good choices to keep participants motivated.

A couple of concerns about the study include the following: (1) despite the finding that the girls who participated in the intervention arm expressed lower intentions to use substances in the future, intentions don't necessarily translate into behavior, making it important to follow up to see if these intentions do translate into less substance use and (2) since mothers had to actively participate, the sample probably skewed toward girls who had more involved families, ie, those who would likely be at lower risk for substance abuse in the future.

J. L. Krupnick, PhD

Services and Outcomes

Brief Rating of Aggression by Children and Adolescents (BRACHA): Development of a Tool for Assessing Risk of Inpatients' Aggressive Behavior
Barzman DH, Brackenbury L, Sonnier L, et al (Cincinnati Children's Hosp Med Ctr, OH; Reed College, Portland, OR; et al)
J Am Acad Psychiatry Law 39:170-179, 2011

This study evaluated the Brief Rating of Aggression by Children and Adolescents—Preliminary Version (BRACHA 0.8), an actuarial method of assessing the risk of aggressive behavior by hospitalized children and adolescents. Licensed psychiatric social workers used a 16-item questionnaire to assess all patients seen in the emergency department (ED) of a major urban children's hospital. Over a six-month period, 418 patients

TABLE 1.—Sixteen Questionnaire Items and Their Associations With Aggression

Item	Response	Without Aggression ($n = 298$)	With Aggression ($n = 120$)	χ^2 ($df = 1$)	p
1. Does the patient have a history of psychiatric hospitalization?	Yes	117	75	18.6	<.0001
	No	181	45		
2. Does the patient have a history of suspensions or expulsions?	Yes	140	83	16.9	<.0001
	No	158	37		
3. Does the patient have trouble accepting adult authority?	Yes	197	104	17.9	<.0001
	No	101	16		
4. Has the patient ever been physically abused?	Yes	68	25	0.195	.659
	No	230	95		
5. Has the patient ever been sexually abused?	Yes	68	28	0.013	.9100
	No	230	92		
6. Has the patient ever physically assaulted others?	Yes	176	97	17.9	<.0001
	No	122	23		
7. Has the patient exhibited impulsivity while in the ED (e.g., needs redirection)?	Yes	58	51	23.6	<.0001
	No	240	69		
8. Has the patient been intrusive to others while in the ED?	Yes	28	34	24.3	<.0001
	No	270	86		
9. Has the patient attempted or committed acts of violence more than 7 days ago?	Yes	134	82	18.7	<.0001
	No	164	38		
10. Does the patient have past violent ideation?	Yes	138	83	17.9	<.0001
	No	160	37		
11. Does the patient have past violent intent or plan?	Yes	122	76	17.2	<.0001
	No	176	44		
12. Has the patient ever destroyed property (e.g., broken a vase or vandalism)?	Yes	183	95	12.1	.0005
	No	115	25		
13. Has the patient been aggressive towards self or others in the last 24 hours?	Yes	182	90	7.30	.0068
	No	116	30		
14. Has the patient ever displayed a pattern of either verbal or physical aggression against self or others, either as a delayed or immediate emotional reaction to a trigger (e.g., threatening a peer who accidentally bumps into him/her in the hall or impulsively cutting self when angry)?	Yes	230	107	7.87	.0050
	No	68	13		
15. Has the patient exhibited aggression or antisocial behaviors prior to age 10 (e.g., fire-setting, destruction of property, stealing, or trying to injure a person or animal)?	Yes	102	68	17.9	<.0001
	No	196	52		
16. Does the patient appear to lack remorse, shame, or guilt in the past or present?	Yes	86	54	10.0	.0015
	No	212	66		

(age range, 3.5–19.0 years) underwent psychiatric hospitalization after ED evaluation. The hospital nursing staff recorded the inpatients' behavior, with the Overt Aggression Scale (OAS). Inpatients were deemed aggressive if, during the first six days of their hospital stay, they scored one or higher on any OAS subscale. We evaluated questionnaire properties, items, and demographic covariates (e.g., age, sex, and living situation) by using factor analyses, logistic regression models, and receiver operating characteristic (ROC) methods. A total of 292 aggressive acts were committed by 120 (29% of 418) patients. Fourteen of the 16 items predicted ($p < .007$) inpatient aggression and showed good internal consistency (Cronbach's $\alpha = 0.837$). Age was inversely related to probability of aggression and was incorporated into the final assessment instrument. Predictive power was comparable with other published risk assessment instruments (ROC areas of .75 for any aggression and .82 for aggression toward others). BRACHA 0.8 shows promise in rapidly assessing risk of inpatient aggression, but further studies are needed to establish the reliability and validity of the instrument (Table 1).

▶ Students of violence and aggression among adults will recognize the value of this study, which presents the development of the Brief Rating of Aggression by Children and Adolescents (BRACHA), an actuarial rating scale intended to assess risk of aggressive behavior among the population of youths who are hospitalized as inpatients. This phase of the study compared initial findings on the BRACHA with outcomes, measured by the Overt Aggression Scale (which has been validated for use on child psychiatry units). Here is an important pathway toward an improved analysis of violence in children and adolescents. This assessment is sorely needed given that violence or aggression in this population can be quite damaging. A second point is to recall that aggression may include verbal threats (and the law includes verbal threats as a type of assault). The findings of increased violence following a higher BRACHA score (see Table 1 for the 16 BRACHA questions and their relationship to outcomes) may provide us with important tools for safety and patient placement in the future.

A. H. Mack, MD

Patterns and Correlates of Tic Disorder Diagnoses in Privately and Publicly Insured Youth
Olfson M, Crystal S, Gerhard T, et al (New York State Psychiatric Inst; Rutgers Univ, New Brunswick, NJ; et al)
J Am Acad Child Adolesc Psychiatry 50:119-131, 2011

Objective.—This study examined the prevalence and demographic and clinical correlates of children diagnosed with Tourette disorder, chronic motor or vocal tic disorder, and other tic disorders in public and private insurance plans over the course of a 1-year period.

Method.—Claims were reviewed of Medicaid (n = 10,247,827) and privately (n = 16,128,828) insured youth (4-18 years old) focusing on tic disorder diagnoses during a 1-year period. Rates are presented for children with each tic disorder diagnosis overall and stratified by demographic characteristics and co-identified mental disorders. Mental health service use, including medications prescribed, and co-existing psychiatric disorders were also examined.

Results.—In Medicaid-insured children, rates of diagnosis per 1,000 were 0.53 (95% confidence interval [CI] 0.51-0.55) for Tourette disorder, 0.08 (95% CI 0.07-0.08) for chronic motor or vocal tic disorder, and 0.43 (95% CI 0.41-0.44) for other tic disorders. In privately insured children, comparable rates were 0.50 (95% CI 0.49-0.52), 0.10 (95% CI 0.10-0.11), and 0.59 (95% CI 0.58-0.61). In 1 year, children diagnosed with tic disorders also frequently received other psychiatric disorder diagnoses.

Compared with privately insured youth, children under Medicaid diagnosed with Tourette disorder had higher rates of attention-deficit/hyperactivity disorder (50.2% versus 25.9%), other disruptive behavior (20.6% versus 5.6%), and depression (14.6% versus 9.8%) diagnoses and higher rates of antipsychotic medication use (53.6% versus 33.2%).

Conclusions.—Despite similarities in annual rates of tic disorder diagnoses in publicly and privately insured children, important differences exist in patient characteristics and service use of publicly and privately insured youth who are diagnosed with tic disorders.

▶ The position of this study is that too few tic disorders, of any severity or duration, are being diagnosed. A major consideration is that there are many individuals with tic disorders, particularly children, but they do not seek treatment. Their initial premise is that the real rate must be someplace between then 0.5 per 1000 and the 10 per 1000, the prevalence figures that have been used or in the literature, respectively. One initial question is whether there is a difference in diagnosis rate among publicly and privately funded groups. Indeed, the authors use a large grouping of clinical data. They provide characteristics of those who have been diagnosed or treated for tic disorders. Generally speaking, they conclude that the various other prevalence studies should be taken in comparison with this one to suggest that in Medicaid and privately insured cases, there is an insufficient degree of closeness between the prevalence rates and the rate of real diagnosis rate, but they should approach each other. Clinicians should be aware of the need to recognize and possibly treat tic disorders when they are found.

A. H. Mack, MD

Recovery and Recurrence Following Treatment for Adolescent Major Depression
Curry J, Silva S, Rohde P, et al (Duke Univ Med Ctr, Durham, NC; Oregon Res Inst, Eugene; et al)
Arch Gen Psychiatry 68:263-269, 2011

Context.—Major depressive disorder in adolescents is common and impairing. Efficacious treatments have been developed, but little is known about longer-term outcomes, including recurrence.

Objectives.—To determine whether adolescents who responded to short-term treatments or who received the most efficacious short-term treatment would have lower recurrence rates, and to identify predictors of recovery and recurrence.

Design.—Naturalistic follow-up study.

Setting.—Twelve academic sites in the United States.

Participants.—One hundred ninety-six adolescents (86 males and 110 females) randomized to 1 of 4 short-term interventions (fluoxetine hydrochloride treatment, cognitive behavioral therapy, their combination, or placebo) in the Treatment for Adolescents With Depression Study were followed up for 5 years after study entry (44.6% of the original Treatment for Adolescents With Depression Study sample).

Main Outcome Measures.—Recovery was defined as absence of clinically significant major depressive disorder symptoms on the Schedule for Affective Disorders and Schizophrenia for School-Age Children—Present and Lifetime Version interview for at least 8 weeks, and recurrence was defined as a new episode of major depressive disorder following recovery.

Results.—Almost all participants (96.4%) recovered from their index episode of major depressive disorder during the follow-up period. Recovery by 2 years was significantly more likely for short-term treatment responders (96.2%) than for partial responders or nonresponders (79.1%) ($P < .001$) but was not associated with having received the most efficacious short-term treatment (the combination of fluoxetine and cognitive behavioral therapy). Of the 189 participants who recovered, 88 (46.6%) had a recurrence. Recurrence was not predicted by full short-term treatment response or by original treatment. However, full or partial responders were less likely to have a recurrence (42.9%) than were nonresponders (67.6%) ($P = .03$). Sex predicted recurrence (57.0% among females vs 32.9% among males; $P = .02$).

Conclusions.—Almost all depressed adolescents recovered. However, recurrence occurs in almost half of recovered adolescents, with higher probability in females in this age range. Further research should identify and address the vulnerabilities to recurrence that are more common among young women.

▶ This report provides evidence as to the long-term course of major depressive disorder in adolescents. It used data from the care of 196 adolescents with a major depressive episode in the Treatment for Adolescents With Depression Study and found that girls were more likely than boys to have a recurrence, that initial remission was the norm by far when treated with either cognitive behavioral therapy or fluoxetine or both, and that recurrence occurred within 5 years in nearly half. This is important for several reasons. As we continue to probe more into the nature of depressive disorders in the adolescent population, we are seeing the ways in which the disorder resembles or contrasts with major depressive disorder in adults. That women with major depressive disorder outnumber adult men has been found over many years, but here are findings of this extending into adolescence. Future studies could work off this interesting finding to determine whether this applied to younger girls in the study—if it was age dependent. But the main finding is the reification of the serious nature of the depressive episodes experienced by this population, the hope that there are effective treatments for it, and that there is a need for future vigilance for recurrence.

A. H. Mack, MD

Miscellaneous

Latent Classes of Adolescent Posttraumatic Stress Disorder Predict Functioning and Disorder After 1 Year

Ayer L, Danielson CK, Amstadter AB, et al (Univ of Vermont, Burlington; Med Univ of South Carolina, Charleston; Virginia Commonwealth Univ, Richmond)
J Am Acad Child Adolesc Psychiatry 50:364-375, 2011

Objective.—To identify latent classes of posttraumatic stress disorder (PTSD) symptoms in a national sample of adolescents, and to test their associations with PTSD and functional impairment 1 year later.

Method.—A total of 1,119 trauma-exposed youth aged 12 through 17 years (mean = 14.99 years, 51% female and 49% male) participating in the National Survey of Adolescents—Replication were included in this study. Telephone interviews were conducted to assess PTSD symptoms and functional impairment at Waves 1 and 2.

Results.—Latent Class Analysis revealed three classes of adolescent PTSD at each time point: pervasive disturbance, intermediate disturbance, and no disturbance. Three numbing and two hyperarousal symptoms best distinguished the pervasive and intermediate disturbance classes at Wave 1. Three re-experiencing, one avoidance, and one hyperarousal symptom best distinguished these classes at Wave 2. The Wave 1 intermediate disturbance class was less likely to have a PTSD diagnosis, belong to the Wave 2 pervasive disturbance class, and report functional impairment 1 year later compared with the Wave 1 pervasive disturbance class. The Wave 1 no disturbance class was least likely to have PTSD, belong to the pervasive disturbance class, and report functional impairment at Wave 2.

Conclusions.—This study suggests that PTSD severity—distinguishing symptoms change substantially in adolescence and are not characterized by the numbing cluster, contrary to studies in adult samples. These results may help to explain inconsistent factor analytic findings on the structure and diagnosis of PTSD, and emphasize that developmental context is critical to consider in both research and clinical work in PTSD assessment and diagnosis.

▶ This article was selected because it highlights the need for further attention to the presentation of posttraumatic stress disorder (PTSD) in children and adolescents, particularly the possibility that the caseness differs from that in adults or that there should be a different mode of diagnosis. However, this report, which comes from an institution well known for its study of PTSD, has various flaws that make its findings inapplicable to action on PTSD itself. First, it does not necessarily include subjects who have PTSD. This begins with overly vague reporting as to whether the subject truly meets criterion A, by reducing A2 (that the individual experienced "helplessness or horror" during the trauma) to a more vague question. Furthermore, this was not a clinical sample. The report also indicates that the team assessed for whether the subject met any criteria in the PTSD B, C, or D sections. Also, in diagnosing subjects with PTSD, the study did not require that any B-, C,- or D-like symptoms be related to the traumatic event itself. The authors seem focused on the trauma of interpersonal situations rather than being open to that of disasters or war. They assert that PTSD should be a dimensional disorder as well. As a result, it is important to be aware of this report while continuing to search for other means of describing this condition.

A. H. Mack, MD

Prevalence and correlates of auditory vocal hallucinations in middle childhood

Bartels-Velthuis AA, Jenner JA, van de Willige G, et al (Univ of Groningen, The Netherlands; et al)
Br J Psychiatry 196:41-46, 2010

Background.—Hearing voices occurs in middle childhood, but little is known about prevalence, aetiology and immediate consequences.

Aims.—To investigate prevalence, developmental risk factors and behavioural correlates of auditory vocal hallucinations in 7- and 8-year-olds.

Method.—Auditory vocal hallucinations were assessed with the Auditory Vocal Hallucination Rating Scale in 3870 children. Prospectively recorded data on pre- and perinatal complications, early development and current problem behaviour were analysed in children with auditory vocal hallucinations and matched controls.

Results.—The 1-year prevalence of auditory vocal hallucinations was 9%, with substantial suffering and problem behaviour reported in 15% of those affected. Prevalence was higher in rural areas but auditory vocal hallucinations were more severe and had greater functional impact in the urban environment. There was little evidence for associations with developmental variables.

Conclusions.—Auditory vocal hallucinations in 7- and 8-year-olds are prevalent but mostly of limited functional impact. Nevertheless, there may be continuity with more severe psychotic outcomes given the serious suffering in a subgroup of children and there is evidence for a poorer prognosis in an urban environment.

▶ Despite the rarity of schizophrenia in childhood and early adolescence, psychotic symptoms are present in this age group. Among those with intact reality testing, abnormal auditory experiences may include either eidetic imagery or hallucinations, and in both children and adults, the presence of auditory hallucinations may occur among populations without psychiatric conditions.[1,2] This review is a cross-sectional assessment of 7- and 8-year-olds, and the prevalence of auditory hallucinations was around 9% in a sample of school population in the Netherlands. Further analysis of the group with psychosis found no difference on the Child Behavior Checklist compared with those without psychosis nor were there differences in analyses in terms of lower socioeconomic status or immigration. This remains a condition of great interest, and further reflection is deserved in our analysis of the causes of psychosis.

A. H. Mack, MD

References

1. Olfson M, Lewis-Fernández R, Weissman MM, et al. Psychotic symptoms in an urban general medicine practice. *Am J Psychiatry.* 2002;159:1412-1419.
2. Edelsohn GA, Rabinovich H, Portnoy R. Hallucinations in nonpsychotic children: findings from a psychiatric emergency service. *Ann N Y Acad Sci.* 2003;1008: 261-264.

Sexual Identity, Sex of Sexual Contacts, and Health-Risk Behaviors Among Students in Grades 9–12 — Youth Risk Behavior Surveillance, Selected Sites, United States, 2001–2009
Kann L, Olsen EO, McManus T, et al (Natl Ctr for Chronic Disease Prevention and Health Promotion, Atlanta, GA)
MMWR Surveill Summ 60:1-133, 2011

Problem.—Sexual minority youths are youths who identify themselves as gay or lesbian, bisexual, or unsure of their sexual identity or youths who have only had sexual contact with persons of the same sex or with both sexes. Population-based data on the health-risk behaviors practiced by sexual minority youths are needed at the state and local levels to most effectively monitor and ensure the effectiveness of public health interventions designed to address the needs of this population.

Reporting Period Covered.—January 2001–June 2009.

Description of the System.—The Youth Risk Behavior Surveillance System (YRBSS) monitors priority health-risk behaviors (behaviors that contribute to unintentional injuries, behaviors that contribute to violence, behaviors related to attempted suicide, tobacco use, alcohol use, other drug use, sexual behaviors, dietary behaviors, physical activity and sedentary behaviors, and weight management) and the prevalence of obesity and asthma among youths and young adults. YRBSS includes state and local school-based Youth Risk Behavior Surveys (YRBSs) conducted by state and local education and health agencies. This report summarizes results from YRBSs conducted during 2001–2009 in seven states and six large urban school districts that included questions on sexual identity (i.e., heterosexual, gay or lesbian, bisexual, or unsure), sex of sexual contacts (i.e., same sex only, opposite sex only, or both sexes), or both of these variables. The surveys were conducted among large population-based samples of public school students in grades 9–12.

Across the nine sites that assessed sexual identity, the prevalence among gay or lesbian students was higher than the prevalence among heterosexual students for a median of 63.8% of all the risk behaviors measured, and the prevalence among bisexual students was higher than the prevalence among heterosexual students for a median of 76.0% of all the risk behaviors measured. In addition, the prevalence among gay or lesbian students was more likely to be higher than (rather than equal to or lower than) the prevalence among heterosexual students for behaviors in seven of the 10 risk behavior categories (behaviors that contribute to violence, behaviors related to attempted suicide, tobacco use, alcohol use, other drug use, sexual behaviors, and weight management). Similarly, the prevalence among bisexual students was more likely to be higher than (rather than equal to or lower than) the prevalence among heterosexual students for behaviors in eight of the 10 risk behavior categories (behaviors that contribute to unintentional injuries, behaviors that contribute to violence, behaviors related to attempted suicide, tobacco use, alcohol use, other drug use, sexual behaviors, and weight management).

Across the 12 sites that assessed sex of sexual contacts, the prevalence among students who had sexual contact with both sexes was higher than the prevalence among students who only had sexual contact with the opposite sex for a median of 71.1% of all the risk behaviors measured, and the prevalence among students who only had sexual contact with the same sex was higher than the prevalence among students who only had sexual contact with the opposite sex for a median of 29.7% of all the risk behaviors measured. Furthermore, the prevalence among students who had sexual contact with both sexes was more likely to be higher than (rather than equal to or lower than) the prevalence among students who only had sexual contact with the opposite sex for behaviors in six of the 10 risk behavior categories (behaviors that contribute to violence, behaviors related to attempted suicide, tobacco use, alcohol use, other drug use, and weight management). The prevalence among students who only had sexual contact with the same sex was more likely to be higher than (rather than equal to or lower than) the prevalence among students who only had sexual contact with the opposite sex for behaviors in two risk behavior categories (behaviors related to attempted suicide and weight management).

Interpretation.—Sexual minority students, particularly gay, lesbian, and bisexual students and students who had sexual contact with both sexes, are more likely to engage in health-risk behaviors than other students.

Public Health Action.—Effective state and local public health and school health policies and practices should be developed to help reduce the prevalence of health-risk behaviors and improve health outcomes among sexual minority youths. In addition, more state and local surveys designed to monitor health-risk behaviors and selected health outcomes among population-based samples of students in grades 9—12 should include questions on sexual identity and sex of sexual contacts.

▶ At the outset, there is not any basis to explain these findings, but they are based on a survey performed on a wide range of youth in varied parts of the nation, spanning from 9th to 12th grade, and involving a large number of subjects. The findings are that those youth who identify themselves as gay or bisexual or whose sexual contacts are same-sex tend to engage in riskier behaviors. The domains ranged from safe-sex practices to unintentional injuries to diet to physical activity to substance use to driving practices, among others. The distinctions were, in most cases, significant. For example, whereas 8% to 19% of straight teens reported smoking cigarettes, about 20% to 48% of gay teens reported the same. Bisexual teens reported the highest rates of many risky behaviors, even higher than gay and lesbian students; 33% to 63% of bisexual students reported binge drinking, for instance, compared with up to 16% to 44% of straight students and 17% to 44% of gay students. So this report provides important new information, but further elucidation of these behaviors and their basis is needed.

A. H. Mack, MD

Sleep Items in the Child Behavior Checklist: A Comparison With Sleep Diaries, Actigraphy, and Polysomnography
Gregory AM, Cousins JC, Forbes EE, et al (Univ of London, UK; Univ of Pittsburgh School of Medicine, PA; Univ of Pittsburgh, PA; et al)
J Am Acad Child Adolesc Psychiatry 50:499-507, 2011

Objective.—The Child Behavior Checklist is sometimes used to assess sleep disturbance despite not having been validated for this purpose. This study examined associations between the Child Behavior Checklist sleep items and other measures of sleep.

Method.—Participants were 122 youth (61% female, aged 7 through 17 years) with anxiety disorders (19%), major depressive disorder (9%), both anxiety and depression (26%), or a negative history of any psychiatric disorder (46%). Parents completed the Child Behavior Checklist and children completed a sleep diary, wore actigraphs for multiple nights, and spent 2 nights in the sleep laboratory. Partial correlations ([pr], controlling for age, gender and diagnostic status) were used to examine associations.

Results.—Child Behavior Checklist sleep items were associated with several other sleep variables. For example, "trouble sleeping" correlated significantly with sleep latency assessed by both diary ($pr(113) = 0.25$, $p = .008$) and actigraphy ($pr(105) = 0.21$, $p = .029$). Other expected associations were not found (e.g., "sleeps more than most kids" was not significantly correlated with EEG-assessed total sleep time: $pr(84) = 0.12$, $p = .258$).

Conclusions.—Assessing sleep using the Child Behavior Checklist exclusively is not ideal. Nonetheless, certain Child Behavior Checklist items (e.g., "trouble sleeping") may be valuable. Although the Child Behavior Checklist may provide a means of examining some aspects of sleep from existing datasets that do not include other measures of sleep, hypotheses generated from such analyses need to be tested using more rigorous measures of sleep.

▶ "Everybody sleeps ..." goes the old Sesame Street song, and yet adolescents, along with children, tend to receive insufficient clinical attention to their sleep. This is mainly in terms of early insomnia, but other phenomena, such as night terrors, enuresis, sleepwalking, or even narcolepsy, are important consider-ations. Furthermore, the normal delay in circadian rhythm is essential informa-tion for any parent or teacher or clinician. As in other selections this year and in the past, there has been an interest in challenging inappropriate extensions of clinical instruments. Here, it is the discrepancy between parent report and reality that is being addressed. This is similar to the problems in parental reporting of internalizing disorders. Should not we consider sleep to be an "internalizing" mental phenomenon? The Child Behavior Checklist has been an invaluable resource in child and adolescent psychiatry, but it cannot do everything, and we need sometimes to have evidence that demands that we use the most reli-able instruments rather than idealized ones.

A. H. Mack, MD

2 Psychotherapy

Introduction

This year's selection of articles reflects a mix of research and statistical techniques as well as assessments of different types of theoretical approaches. The section begins with 3 meta-analyses: on cognitive remediation in schizophrenia, on dialectical behavior therapy for research participants with borderline personality, and on long-term psychodynamic psychotherapy. There is also a review of randomized clinical trials in psychodynamic psychotherapy as well as a range of randomized clinical trials covering various demographic groups and psychiatric diagnoses. Among the approaches explored are cognitive therapy, interpersonal therapy, prolonged exposure, dialectical behavior therapy, parenting interventions, and others. As in other years, the diagnoses addressed include major depressive disorder, bipolar disorder, eating disorders, obsessive-compulsive disorder, and fibromyalgia. Other problems addressed include self-injury, suicidality, attachment problems, and bereavement. In summary, there is likely to be some area of inquiry into something relevant for each reader.

Janice L. Krupnick, PhD

Outcome Studies

A Meta-Analysis of Cognitive Remediation for Schizophrenia: Methodology and Effect Sizes

Wykes T, Huddy V, Cellard C, et al (King's College London, UK; Université Laval Robert-Giffard, Quebec City, Canada; Dartmouth Med School, Concord, NH; et al)
Am J Psychiatry 168:472-485, 2011

Objective.—Cognitive remediation therapy for schizophrenia was developed to treat cognitive problems that affect functioning, but the treatment effects may depend on the type of trial methodology adopted. The present meta-analysis will determine the effects of treatment and whether study method or potential moderators influence the estimates.

Method.—Electronic databases were searched up to June 2009 using variants of the key words "cognitive," "training," "remediation," "clinical trial," and "schizophrenia." Key researchers were contacted to ensure that all studies meeting the criteria were included. This produced 109 reports of 40 studies in which ≥70% of participants had a diagnosis of schizophrenia, all of whom received standard care. There was a comparison group and allocation procedure in these studies. Data were available to calculate effect sizes on cognition and/or functioning. Data were independently extracted by two reviewers with excellent reliability. Methodological moderators were extracted through the Clinical Trials Assessment Measure and verified by authors in 94% of cases.

Results.—The meta-analysis (2,104 participants) yielded durable effects on global cognition and functioning. The symptom effect was small and disappeared at follow-up assessment. No treatment element (remediation approach, duration, computer use, etc.) was associated with cognitive outcome. Cognitive remediation therapy was more effective when patients were clinically stable. Significantly stronger effects on functioning were found when cognitive remediation therapy was provided together with other psychiatric rehabilitation, and a much larger effect was present when a strategic approach was adopted together with adjunctive rehabilitation. Despite variability in methodological rigor, this did not moderate any of the therapy effects, and even in the most rigorous studies there were similar small-to-moderate effects.

Conclusions.—Cognitive remediation benefits people with schizophrenia, and when combined with psychiatric rehabilitation, this benefit generalizes to functioning, relative to rehabilitation alone. These benefits cannot be attributed to poor study methods.

▶ This is an important article to read for any clinician or researcher who is working in the area of treatments for schizophrenia. As the title indicates, it is a meta-analysis of cognitive remediation for schizophrenia, an intervention that targets various aspects of cognitive functioning that are affected by this illness. The article indicates that previous meta-analyses have been conducted with regard to this intervention, but this one offers a number of features that seem to make this the most comprehensive assessment of the intervention to date. For example, they note that this meta-analysis assesses treatment effects using "double the number of studies included in the most recent analysis." Their study included a very large number, ie, 2104 participants, including only studies in which at least 70% of the participants had a diagnosis of schizophrenia. They used a standardized measure, the Clinical Trials Assessment measure, to extract methodologic moderators. Also, they calculated the effect sizes of the intervention on cognition or functioning. Based on their methodology, they were able to answer some of the questions that had apparently dogged researchers of this type of treatment. For example, there were questions about whether the methodology used in some studies might have inflated effect sizes. This is a comprehensive, carefully conducted study that ultimately yields important clinical evidence about the place and role of cognitive remediation for a population much in need of effective interventions.

J. L. Krupnick, PhD

Dialectical Behavior Therapy for Borderline Personality Disorder: A Meta-Analysis Using Mixed-Effects Modeling

Kliem S, Kröger C, Kosfelder J (Technical Univ of Braunschweig, Germany; Univ of Applied Sciences Düsseldorf, Germany)
J Consult Clin Psychol 78:936-951, 2010

Objective.—At present, the most frequently investigated psychosocial intervention for borderline personality disorder (BPD) is dialectical behavior therapy (DBT). We conducted a meta-analysis to examine the efficacy and long-term effectiveness of DBT.

Method.—Systematic bibliographic research was undertaken to find relevant literature from online databases (PubMed, PsycINFO, PsychSpider, Medline). We excluded studies in which patients with diagnoses other than BPD were treated, the treatment did not comprise all components specified in the DBT manual or in the suggestions for inpatient DBT programs, patients failed to be diagnosed according to the *Diagnostic and Statistical Manual of Mental Disorders*, and the intervention group comprised fewer than 10 patients. Using a mixed-effect hierarchical modeling approach, we calculated global effect sizes and effect sizes for suicidal and self-injurious behaviors.

Results.—Calculations of postintervention global effect sizes were based on 16 studies. Of these, 8 were randomized controlled trials (RCTs), and 8 were neither randomized nor controlled (nRCT). The dropout rate was 27.3 pre- to posttreatment. A moderate global effect and a moderate effect size for suicidal and self-injurious behaviors were found, when including a moderator for RCTs with borderline-specific treatments. There was no evidence for the influence of other moderators (e.g., quality of studies, setting, duration of intervention). A small impairment was shown from posttreatment to follow-up, including 5 RCTs only.

Conclusions.—Future research should compare DBT with other active borderline-specific treatments that have also demonstrated their efficacy using several long-term follow-up assessment points (Table 1).

▶ Dialectical behavior therapy (DBT) has become a widely disseminated and widely used method in the treatment of borderline personality disorder (BPD). For this reason, a meta-analysis to determine its efficacy across studies is certainly warranted, and this meta-analysis is one that reflects state-of-the-art methodology. It is interesting that of the 16 studies that were included in this review, 3, including this meta-analysis, were conducted by researchers from Germany.

What I particularly appreciated about the approach used in this study was their inclusion criteria (ie, the focus on studies that included only patients with a borderline personality diagnosis, only studies that comprised all components of DBT, and studies with a total sample size of at least 10 in the intervention group). This was also the first time that a meta-analysis of this type of treatment included data on the long-term effectiveness of DBT for posttraumatic stress

TABLE 1.—Studies Included in a Meta-Analysis of Dialectical Behavior Therapy (DBT) for Borderline Personality Disorders (BPDs)

Study	Design	Sample Size	Assessment Points	Mean age (SD), Gender	Exclusion Criteria	Inclusion Criteria	Dropout	Method	Setting
Bohus et al., 2004, 2000; Kleindienst et al., 2008	nRCT	DBT = 31	0, 4 (post), 12, 24 (FU) month	29.6 (7.5), 100% female	Axis I: schizophrenia, bipolar I disorder, substance abuse; Axis II: mental retardation	BPD, female, one suicide attempt or a minimum of two non-suicidal self-injuries within the last 2 years	Post = 25.8%, FU = 29%	ITT-LOCF	In
Clarkin et al., 2004, 2007	RCT	DBT = 30, ST = 30, TFP = 30	0, 4, 8, 12 (post) month	30.9 (7.85), ?% female	Axis I: psychotic disorder, bipolar I disorder; substance dependence, delirium, dementia, amnestic disorder, other cognitive disorders; Axis II: mental retardation	BPD	Post = 31.1%, post-DBT = 43.3%	ITT-LOCF	Out
Comtois et al., 2007	nRCT	DBT = 38	0, 12 (post) month	34 (range: 19–54), 96% female	Axis I: substance dependence; Axis II: mental retardation	BPD, extensive suicide attempts, crisis service history	Post = 37%	Completers	Out
Fassbinder et al., 2007; Kröger et al., 2006	nRCT	DBT = 50	0, 3 (post), 15, 30 (FU) month	30.5 (7.7), 88% female	Axis I: schizophrenia, bipolar I disorder, substance abuse; substance dependence, dementia; Axis II: mental retardation; Axis III: current symptoms	BPD, age > 18	Post = 12%, FU = 40%	ITT-LOCF	In
Friedrich et al., 2003	nRCT	DBT = 33	0, 3, 6, 9, 12 (post) month	33.4 (8.8), 91% female	Axis I: acute psychosis	BPD	Post = 8%	Completers	Out
Harned et al., 2008; Linehan, Comtois, Murray, et al., 2006	RCT	DBT = 52, CTBE = 49	0, 12 (post), 24 (FU) month	29.3 (7.5), 100% female	Axis I: schizophrenia, schizoaffective disorder, psychotic disorder not otherwise specified, bipolar disorder; Axis II: mental retardation; Axis III: seizure disorder; Other: requiring medication, a mandate to treatment	BPD, female, recent and recurrent self-injury	Post = 11.8%, FU = 19.8%, post-DBT = 3.8%, FU-DBT = 11.5%	ITT-RRM	Out

Study	Design	Time points	Groups	Age (SD), % female	Diagnostic criteria	Sample	Dropout	Analysis	In/Out
Höschel, 2006	nRCT	0, 2, 8, 12 (post) weeks	DBT = 24	28.3 (6.86), 87.5% female	Axis I: schizophrenic disorder, substance dependence; Axis II: mental retardation, antisocial personality disorder	BPD	Post = 4.2%	Completers	In
Koons et al., 2001	RCT	0, 3, 6 (post) month	DBT = 14, TAU = 14	34.5 (7.5), 100% female	Axis I: schizophrenic disorder, bipolar disorder, substance dependence; Axis II: mental retardation, antisocial personality disorder	BPD, female veterans	Post = 28.8%, post-DBT = 28.8%	Completers	Out
Linehan et al., 1991, 1993, 1994	RCT	0, 4, 8, 12 (post), 18, 24 (FU) month	DBT = 22, TAU = 22	26.7 (7.8), 100% female	Axis I: Schizophrenic disorder, bipolar disorder, substance dependence; Axis II: mental retardation	BPD, female 18 < age < 45, suicide attempt in the past 8 weeks, one other in the past 5 years	Post = 6.8%, FU = 18.2%, post-DBT = 9.1%, FU-DBT = 18.2%	ITT-LOCF	Out
Linehan et al., 2002	RCT	0, 4, 8, 12 (post), 16 (FU) month	DBT = 11, CVT + 12 = 12	36.1 (7.3), 100% female	Axis I: psychotic disorder, bipolar disorder; Axis II: mental retardation; Axis III: seizure disorder	BPD, female, current opiate dependence	Post = 20.8%, FU = 20.8%, post-DBT = 36.4%, FU-DBT = 36.4%	ITT-LOCF	Out
Linehan et al., 2008	nRCT	0, 7, 12, 21 (post) weeks	DBT = 24	26.8 (9,0), 100% female	Axis I: psychotic disorder, major depressive disorder with psychotic features, substance dependence; Axis II: mental retardation; Axis III: seizure disorder, pregnant, breastfeeding, planning to become pregnant; Other: episode of self-inflicted injury in the 8 weeks prior to the screening interview	BPD, female, OAS-M ≤ 6	Post = 33%	ITT-RRM	Out
Linehan et al., 1999	RCT	0, 4, 8, 12 (post), 16 (FU) month	DBT = 12, TAU = 16	30.4 (6.6), 100% female	Axis I: psychotic disorder, bipolar disorder; Axis II: mental retardation	BPD female, current drug dependence	Post = 61.1%, FU = 64.3%, FU-DBT = 33.3%, post-DBT = 41.7%	ITT-LOCF	Out

(Continued)

Table 1.—(*Continued*)

Study	Design	Assessment Points	Sample Size	Mean age (SD), Gender	Exclusion Criteria	Inclusion Criteria	Dropout	Method	Setting
McMain et al., 2009	RCT	0, 4, 8, 12 (post) month	DBT = 90, GPM = 90	29.4 (9.1), 90% female	Axis I: psychotic disorder, bipolar I disorder, delirium, dementia; Axis II: mental retardation; Other: a diagnosis of substance dependence in the preceding 30 days, having a medical condition that precluded psychiatric medications	BPD, 18 < age < 60, at least two episodes of suicidal or non-suicidal self-injurious episodes in the past 5 years, at least one of which was in the 3 months preceding enrollment	Post = 38.3%, post-DBT = 38.9%	ITT-LOCF	Out
Prendergast &McCausland, 2007	nRCT	0, 6 (post) month	DBT = 16	36.35 (7.42), 100% female	Axis I: psychotic disorder, substance dependence	BPD, female	Post = 31%	SC	Out
Simpson et al., 2004	nRCT	0, 12 (post) weeks	DBT = 25	35.3 (10.1), 100% female	Axis I: schizophrenia, bipolar 1 disorder, substance dependence; Axis III: seizure disorder, pregnant, lactating; Other: unwilling to use effective birth control, unstable medical conditions, monoamine oxidase inhibitor treatment in the last 2 weeks, a previous adequate trial of fluoxetine	BPD	Post = 20%	SC	In
van den Bosch et al., 2005, 2002, 2001; Verheul et al., 2003	RCT	Baseline, 0, 52 (post), 78 (FU) weeks	DBT = 27, TAU = 31	34.9 (7.7), 100% female	Axis I: psychotic disorder, bipolar disorder; Axis II: mental retardation	BPD, female	Post = 17.2%, FU = 24.1%, post-DBT = 14.6%, FU-DBT = 25.9%	ITT-RRM	Out

Note. nRCT = nonrandomized and noncontrolled trial; RCT = randomized controlled trial; post = postintervention; FU = follow-up; ITT = intention to treat; LOCF = last observation carried forward; In = inpatient setting; Out = outpatient setting; ? = no information available; ST = supportive treatment; TFP = transference-focused psychotherapy; SC = statistical control; TAU = therapy as usual; CTBE = community therapy by experts; RRM = random-effects regression model; CVT +12 = comprehensive validation plus 12-step therapy; OAS-M = Overt Aggression Scale–Modified; GPM = general psychiatric management.
Editor's Note: Please refer to original journal article for full references.

disorder, an important measure of any treatment's effectiveness and particularly for a condition that typically lasts for many years.

Table 1 nicely describes the primary features of the studies that were included in the meta-analysis. It is worth noting that 4 of these included only completers of treatment. In recent years, it is expected that researchers will use intent-to-treat samples.

The most interesting finding (I thought) was the one that found that different types of treatments had different impacts on the symptoms of BPD. Specifically, they found that transference-focused psychotherapy (along the lines of the approach developed by Kernberg for patients with BPD) was consistently related to the reduction in aggression compared with DBT. It was also found that effect sizes were small when DBT was compared with borderline-specific treatments, such as transference-focused treatment.

It is important to have treatments studied by researchers other than those who develop a method, making this a more objective view of the treatment under review.

J. L. Krupnick, PhD

Long-term psychodynamic psychotherapy in complex mental disorders: update of a meta-analysis
Leichsenring F, Rabung S (Univ of Giessen, Germany; Univ Med Centre Hamburg-Eppendorf, Germany)
Br J Psychiatry 199:15-22, 2011

Background.—Dose—effect relationship data suggest that short-term psychotherapy is insufficient for many patients with chronic distress or personality disorders (complex mental disorders).

Aims.—To examine the comparative efficacy of long-term psychodynamic psychotherapy (LTPP) in complex mental disorders.

Method.—We conducted a meta-analysis of controlled trials of LTPP fulfilling the following inclusion criteria: therapy lasting for at least a year or 50 sessions; active comparison conditions; prospective design; reliable and valid outcome measures; treatments terminated. Ten studies with 971 patients were included.

Results.—Between-group effect sizes in favour of LTPP compared with less intensive (lower dose) forms of psychotherapy ranged between 0.44 and 0.68.

Conclusions.—Results suggest that LTPP is superior to less intensive forms of psychotherapy in complex mental disorders. Further research on long-term psychotherapy is needed, not only for psychodynamic psychotherapy, but also for other therapies (Table 1).

▶ As anyone who practices short-term psychotherapy knows from clinical experience, there are some individuals for whom short-term treatment is inadequate. There is a good deal of clinical agreement that this applies to patients with personality disorders, as this article points out, as well as patients who

TABLE 1.—Comparison of Long-Term Psychodynamic Psychotherapy With Other Forms of Psychotherapy: Between-Group Effect Sizes

Outcome Domain	Number of Comparisons	Hedges' d		Q	I^2, %
		d^a	95% CI^b		
Overall effectiveness	10	0.54 (0.52)	0.26–0.83	11.72	23
Target problems	9	0.49 (0.48)	0.27–0.71	9.12	12
Psychiatric symptoms	9	0.44 (0.41)	0.15–0.73	11.52	31
Personality functioning	7	0.68 (0.63)	0.31–1.04	5.97	0
Social functioning	8	0.62 (0.59)	0.18–1.06	12.44	44

ITT, intention to treat.
[a]Adjusted for ITT sample.
[b]Unadjusted d.

have more complex issues. Given that, it is important to have empirical evidence to substantiate this clinical observation, and this study achieves that goal. It is a carefully conducted study, using solid methodology, so the results can be trusted. I was also pleased to see that they were looking at outcome in a comprehensive way, assessing a number of domains. A useful contribution of the study was also that they looked at the potential for publication bias, identifying and assessing the results of unpublished studies. It was disappointing to see that so few studies had been conducted of long-term psychotherapy and that so few had follow-up results to determine if gains in treatment had been maintained. In some domains, such as social functioning, only 8 comparisons were possible, and for personality functioning, only 7 comparisons were possible (Table 1). This constitutes fairly limited data. Also, half of the studies were of patients with borderline personality so there was not a lot of variation in the types of patients who were studied.

J. L. Krupnick, PhD

A Quality-Based Review of Randomized Controlled Trials of Psychodynamic Psychotherapy

Gerber AJ, Kocsis JH, Milrod BL, et al (Columbia College of Physicians and Surgeons and the New York State Psychiatric Inst; Weill Cornell Med College, NY; Univ of Pennsylvania, Philadelphia; et al)
Am J Psychiatry 168:19-28, 2011

Objective.—The Ad Hoc Subcommittee for Evaluation of the Evidence Base for Psychodynamic Psychotherapy of the APA Committee on Research on Psychiatric Treatments developed the Randomized Controlled Trial Psychotherapy Quality Rating Scale (RCT-PQRS). The authors report results from application of the RCT-PQRS to 94 randomized controlled trials of psychodynamic psychotherapy published between 1974 and May 2010.

Method.—Five psychotherapy researchers from a range of therapeutic orientations rated a single published paper from each study.

Results.—The RCT-PQRS had good interrater reliability and internal consistency. The mean total quality score was 25.1 (SD=8.8). More recent studies had higher total quality scores. Sixty-three of 103 comparisons between psychodynamic psychotherapy and a nondynamic comparator were of "adequate" quality. Of 39 comparisons of a psychodynamic treatment and an "active" comparator, six showed dynamic treatment to be superior, five showed dynamic treatment to be inferior, and 28 showed no difference (few of which were powered for equivalence). Of 24 adequate comparisons of psychodynamic psychotherapy with an "inactive" comparator, 18 found dynamic treatment to be superior.

Conclusions.—Existing randomized controlled trials of psychodynamic psychotherapy are promising but mostly show superiority of psychodynamic psychotherapy to an inactive comparator. This would be sufficient to make psychodynamic psychotherapy an "empirically validated" treatment (per American Psychological Association Division 12 standards) only if further randomized controlled trials of adequate quality and sample size replicated findings of existing positive trials for specific disorders. We do not yet know what will emerge when other psychotherapies are subjected to this form of quality-based review.

▶ All fields of medicine and psychology are moving toward an evidence base for purposes of training, practice, and reimbursement. With the movement toward the use only of evidence-based practice, psychodynamic psychotherapy has fallen behind. Thus, examination of the evidence is important, not only for assessing the efficacy of this treatment approach but also for its very survival. Cognitive-behavioral approaches, in particular, have gained considerable support in recent years, in large part, because the proponents of this method have an extensive body of literature to support its effects. This article represents the efforts of a committee sponsored by the American Psychiatric Association to weigh the evidence of efficacy for psychodynamic psychotherapy. The group that took on this task started by developing a measure to assess the quality of the study under review. This was a good starting point because it reflects an attempt to systematize their task. Ultimately, they found that only about half of the studies they reviewed were adequate to the task. This, not surprisingly, was because many of the reports of studies they considered were conducted decades ago, when methodological approaches were less sophisticated than they are today. For example, 2 decades ago, researchers were not using intent-to-treat samples for analyses, whereas this is the standard in more recent studies. They point to a problem that is particular to a number of outcome studies that have led to the finding of several earlier comparative studies, that is, essentially the dodo bird verdict that "all have won and all must have prizes." This outcome means that psychotherapy is more helpful than no intervention but no one treatment is more effective than another for any particular disorder. The problem here has been that these studies were inadequately powered to detect differences, particularly when 2 active treatments were compared. Thus, the article winds up focusing a good deal more on the quality of existing studies rather than the ultimate efficacy of psychodynamic treatment versus other types of interventions. It is clear, however, that if practitioners of psycho-dynamic psychotherapy wish to remain viable, there needs to be a more extensive body of well-conducted outcome studies to demonstrate the benefits of this therapeutic approach. It seems likely that multisite studies will be needed to recruit enough research participants to assess differential effects among different types of approaches.

J. L. Krupnick, PhD

A New Parenting-Based Group Intervention for Young Anxious Children: Results of a Randomized Controlled Trial
Cartwright-Hatton S, McNally D, Field AP, et al (Univ of Manchester, UK; Central Manchester Foundation Trust, UK; et al)
J Am Acad Child Adolesc Psychiatry 50:242-251, 2011

Objective.—Despite recent advances, there are still no interventions that have been developed for the specific treatment of young children who have anxiety disorders. This study examined the impact of a new, cognitive–behaviorally based parenting intervention on anxiety symptoms.

Method.—Families of 74 anxious children (aged 9 years or less) took part in a randomized controlled trial, which compared the new 10-session, group-format intervention with a wait-list control condition. Outcome measures included blinded diagnostic interview and self-reports from parents and children.

Results.—Intention-to-treat analyses indicated that children whose parent(s) received the intervention were significantly less anxious at the end of the study than those in the control condition. Specifically, 57% of those receiving the new intervention were free of their primary disorder, compared with 15% in the control condition. Moreover, 32% of treated children were free of any anxiety diagnosis at the end of the treatment period, compared with 6% of those in the control group. Treatment gains were maintained at 12-month follow-up.

Conclusions.—This new parenting-based intervention may represent an advance in the treatment of this previously neglected group. Clinical trial registration information: Anxiety in Young Children: A Randomized Controlled Trial of a New Cognitive-Behaviourally Based Parenting Intervention; http://www.isrctn.org/; ISRCTN12166762.

▶ This randomized controlled trial represents an early, but important, assessment of a new treatment for young anxious children. As the authors point out, there are several evidence-based treatments for older children but no specific interventions for children age 9 or younger. Because anxiety disorders are highly prevalent among children and probably start quite early, this study provides evidence (Table 4) that an intervention aimed at this younger population works. What distinguishes this treatment from those that are aimed at older children is that the intervention is focused on parents. They were unable to provide at this stage definitive evidence that it was the specific techniques of the intervention

TABLE 4.—Means (SDs) and Effect Sizes of Outcome Measures Pre- and Postintervention and at Follow-up

	CBCL (DSM)			CBCL (Internalizing)			SCARED			MASC		
	Mean	SD	N	Mean	SD	N	Mean	SD	N	Mean	SD	N
Preintervention												
Intervention	73.56	8.44	34	66.59	7.61	34	31.88	13.30	34	57.57	9.85	23
Control	76.42	8.62	36	70.95	7.52	36	34.36	14.61	33	61.39	11.06	23
Postintervention												
Intervention	65.15	9.40	34	59.42	6.55	34	20.24	12.47	34	57.96	12.29	23
Control	71.78	9.91	36	67.03	9.35	36	30.85	15.04	33	58.13	12.92	23
Effect size, d (d_c)	0.41 (0.46)			0.48 (0.45)			1.01 (1.42)			−0.42 (−0.34)		
Follow-up												
Intervention	62.65	10.11	34	58.88	7.34	34	17.88	15.67	34	52.52	11.99	23
Control	67.56	9.58	36	64.12	9.47	36	24.94	15.45	33	54.48	11.18	23
Effect size, d (d_c)	0.19 (0.23)			0.10 (0.10)			0.35 (0.38)			−0.17 (0.19)		

Note: Effect size computed relative to preintervention means: d is based on pooled variance, whereas d_c is based on variance in control group. CBCL (Internalizing) = Child Behavior Checklist Internalizing Scale; CBCL (DSM) = Child Behavior Checklist DSM Anxiety Disorders score; MASC = Multidimensional Anxiety Scale for Children; SCARED = Screen for Child Anxiety Related Disorders (Parent version).

that provided the positive results as opposed to training in interacting with their children more or other nonspecific effects. Nevertheless, helping parents understand the nature of anxiety and what may give rise to anxiety disorders in their children would seem to be helpful. Interestingly, there was recently an article in *Science* that addressed the issue of how anxious children might learn better as well. It is heartening to see that attention is being paid to the specific needs of anxious children both in the home and in the school setting.

J. L. Krupnick, PhD

A Biobehavioral Home-Based Intervention and the Well-being of Patients With Dementia and Their Caregivers: The COPE Randomized Trial

Gitlin LN, Winter L, Dennis MP, et al (Thomas Jefferson Univ, Philadelphia, PA; et al)
JAMA 304:983-991, 2010

Context.—Optimal treatment to postpone functional decline in patients with dementia is not established.

Objective.—To test a nonpharmacologic intervention realigning environmental demands with patient capabilities.

Design, Setting, and Participants.—Prospective 2-group randomized trial (Care of Persons with Dementia in their Environments [COPE]) involving patients with dementia and family caregivers (community-living dyads) recruited from March 2006 through June 2008 in Pennsylvania.

Interventions.—Up to 12 home or telephone contacts over 4 months by health professionals who assessed patient capabilities and deficits; obtained blood and urine samples; and trained families in home safety, simplifying tasks, and stress reduction. Control group caregivers received 3 telephone calls and educational materials.

Main Outcome Measures.—Functional dependence, quality of life, frequency of agitated behaviors, and engagement for patients and well-being, confidence using activities, and perceived benefits for caregivers at 4 months.

Results.—Of 284 dyads screened, 270 (95%) were eligible and 237 (88%) randomized. Data were collected from 209 dyads (88%) at 4 months and 173 (73%) at 9 months. At 4 months, compared with controls, COPE patients had less functional dependence (adjusted mean difference, 0.24; 95% CI, 0.03-0.44; $P=.02$; Cohen $d=0.21$) and less dependence in instrumental activities of daily living (adjusted mean difference, 0.32; 95% CI, 0.09-0.55; $P=.007$; Cohen $d=0.43$), measured by a 15-item scale modeled after the Functional Independence Measure; COPE patients also had improved engagement (adjusted mean difference, 0.12; 95% CI, 0.07-0.22; $P=.03$; Cohen $d=0.26$), measured by a 5-item scale. COPE caregivers improved in their well-being (adjusted mean difference in Perceived Change Index, 0.22; 95% CI, 0.08-0.36; $P=.002$; Cohen $d=0.30$) and confidence using activities (adjusted mean difference, 0.81; 95% CI, 0.30-1.32; $P=.002$; Cohen $d=0.54$), measured by a 5-item scale. By 4 months, 64 COPE dyads (62.7%) vs 48 control group dyads (44.9%) eliminated 1 or more caregiver-identified problems ($\chi^2_1=6.72$, $P=.01$).

TABLE 2.—Comparison of Intervention (n = 102) and Control (n = 107) Group Patients and Caregivers at 4 Months[a]

| | Mean (SD) Score | | | | Adjusted Mean | | |
| | Baseline | | 4-Month Follow-up | | Difference Between | | |
	Control Group	Intervention Group	Control Group	Intervention Group	Groups (95% CI)	P Value	Cohen d
Patient outcomes							
Overall functional dependence[b]	2.8 (1.3)	3.0 (1.2)	3.3 (1.3)	3.7 (1.3)	0.24 (0.03 to 0.44)	.02	0.21
IADL dependence	1.8 (1.0)	1.8 (1.0)	2.5 (1.1)	2.8 (1.2)	0.32 (0.09 to 0.55)	.007	0.43
ADL dependence	4.1 (1.8)	4.3 (1.7)	4.3 (1.7)	4.6 (1.6)	0.16 (−0.09 to 0.42)	.21	
Activity engagement	2.0 (0.4)	1.9 (0.4)	1.9 (0.5)	2.0 (0.4)	0.12 (0.07 to 0.22)	.03	0.26
QOL-AD score	2.1 (0.5)	2.1 (0.4)	2.1 (0.5)	2.2 (0.5)	0.10 (0.00 to 0.20)	.06	0.14
ABID score	9.8 (10.7)	11.0 (14.6)	5.5 (8.0)	6.7 (10.6)	−0.65 (−3.05 to 1.74)	.59	
Caregiver outcomes							
Perceived change in well-being	2.8 (0.5)	2.7 (0.5)	2.9 (0.5)	3.1 (0.6)	0.22 (0.08 to 0.36)	.002	0.30
Confidence using activities[c]	7.0 (2.2)	6.6 (2.1)	6.9 (2.5)	7.5 (1.9)	0.81 (0.30 to 1.32)	.002	0.54

Abbreviations: ABID, Agitated Behaviors in Dementia scale; ADL, activities of daily living; CI, confidence interval; IADL, instrumental activities of daily living; QOL-AD, Quality of Life–Alzheimer Disease scale.

[a]Refer to the "Methods" section for descriptions of the scales used in all outcome measures. All analyses controlled for living arrangement (alone vs with caregiver) and baseline value of dependent variable. After adjustment for multiple comparisons by the method of Benjamini and Hochberg,[30] the P values for the 6 primary measures (not counting ADL and IADL subscales) were .006 for perceived change in well-being and confidence using activities, .04 for overall functional dependence and activity engagement, .07 for quality of life, and 0.59 for ABID score.

[b]This measure was assessed for 202 patients because 7 patients were placed in nursing homes and the caregivers were not asked functional dependence items at 4 months.

[c]This measure was assessed for 106 caregivers in the control group because 1 caregiver was unable to respond to items.

Conclusion.—Among community-living dyads, a nonpharmacologic bio-behavioral environmental intervention compared with control resulted in better outcomes for COPE dyads at 4 months. Although no group differences were observed at 9 months for patients, COPE caregivers perceived greater benefits.

Trial Registration.—clinicaltrials.gov Identifier: NCT00259454 (Table 2).

▶ The topic of this study is of considerable importance, given the aging of our society and the increasing number of individuals who care for family members with dementia in their homes. The psychological stress on such caregivers is immense and finding a way to help both patients with dementia and their caregivers is an important public health issue. This study is not one of psychotherapy per se, but it does describe a type of psychosocial intervention that shows promising results and at low cost.

One finding that I found particularly interesting was the significantly higher number of male caregivers who dropped out relative to the number of female caregivers. This supports other available data about the greater number of caregivers being women, a role that has been traditionally considered female. One must wonder about the continued reasons for this discrepancy with many more women in the workforce than was true decades ago. Maybe some thought could be given to ways to keep more male caregivers in programs such as this.

Another advantageous feature of this approach is that it is easy to administer. Table 2 indicates the ways in which this method was found effective.

J. L. Krupnick, PhD

A Randomized Clinical Trial of Acceptance and Commitment Therapy Versus Progressive Relaxation Training for Obsessive-Compulsive Disorder
Twohig MP, Hayes SC, Plumb JC, et al (Utah State Univ, Logan; Univ of Nevada, Reno)
J Consult Clin Psychol 78:705-716, 2010

Objective.—Effective treatments for obsessive-compulsive disorder (OCD) exist, but additional treatment options are needed. The effectiveness of 8 sessions of acceptance and commitment therapy (ACT) for adult OCD was compared with progressive relaxation training (PRT).

Method.—Seventy-nine adults (61% female) diagnosed with OCD (mean age = 37 years; 89% Caucasian) participated in a randomized clinical trial of 8 sessions of ACT or PRT with no in-session exposure. The following assessments were completed at pretreatment, posttreatment, and 3-month follow-up by an assessor who was unaware of treatment conditions: Yale-Brown Obsessive Compulsive Scale (Y-BOCS), Beck Depression Inventory—II, Quality of Life Scale, Acceptance and Action Questionnaire, Thought Action Fusion Scale, and Thought Control Questionnaire. Treatment Evaluation Inventory was completed at posttreatment.

TABLE 1.—Means and Standard Deviations for All Outcome Measures for the Two Conditions for Each Measurement Occasion

| | ACT | | | | | | PRT | | | | | |
| | Baseline (N = 41) | | Posttreatment (N = 36) | | Follow-up (N = 33) | | Baseline (N = 38) | | Posttreatment (N = 33) | | Follow-up (N = 31) | |
Measure	M	SD	M	SD	M	SD	M	SD	M	SD	M	SD
Outcome												
Y-BOCS	24.22	4.80	12.76	8.35	11.79	8.97	25.40	5.26	18.67	5.68	16.23	7.46
BDI-II	18.09	11.83	8.50	10.99	8.43	10.13	17.89	8.39	13.69[a]	9.83	10.89	8.06
QOLS	72.49	15.00	82.18	14.86	82.03	14.58	69.58	14.35	73.59[a]	12.42	73.19	17.01
Process												
AAQ-16	59.76	11.36	73.69	13.22	73.37	14.44	57.16	11.67	63.81[a]	7.69	67.13[b]	10.74
TCQ	65.54	12.23	56.11	10.76	56.74	9.66	65.04	8.04	61.80[a]	8.44	60.26	6.73
TAF–Morality	21.46	11.17	12.72	9.89	14.14	10.58	18.47	10.38	17.94[a]	9.49	18.13	9.53
TAF–Likelihood	9.76	8.21	5.47	6.47	6.90	7.56	7.76	7.66	6.22[a]	6.63	6.00	5.81

Note. ACT = acceptance and commitment therapy; PRT = progressive relaxation training; Y-BOCS = Yale–Brown Obsessive Compulsive Scale; BDI-II = Beck Depression Inventory–II; QOLS = Quality of Life Scale; AAQ-16 = Acceptance and Action Questionnaire (16-item version); TCQ = Thought Control Questionnaire; TAF = Thought Action Fusion.
[a]N = 32.
[b]N = 30.

Results.—ACT produced greater changes at posttreatment and follow-up over PRT on OCD severity (Y-BOCS: ACT pretreatment = 24.22, posttreatment = 12.76, follow-up = 11.79; PRT pretreatment = 25.4, posttreatment = 18.67, follow-up = 16.23) and produced greater change on depression among those reporting at least mild depression before treatment. Clinically significant change in OCD severity occurred more in the ACT condition than PRT (clinical response rates: ACT posttreatment = 46%—56%, follow-up = 46%—66%; PRT posttreatment = 13%—18%, follow-up = 16%—18%). Quality of life improved in both conditions but was marginally in favor of ACT at posttreatment. Treatment refusal (2.4% ACT, 7.8% PRT) and dropout (9.8% ACT, 13.2% PRT) were low in both conditions.

Conclusions.—ACT is worth exploring as a treatment for OCD (Table 1).

▶ I was particularly interested in reading this article because I had not to date heard about acceptance and commitment therapy (ACT) being used for any disorder outside of posttraumatic stress disorder. The ways in which the researchers might adapt the treatment for obsessive-compulsive disorder (OCD) was a topic worth investigating.

This randomized controlled trial included all the necessary ingredients of a well-designed trial. They used appropriate measures and statistical approaches to analyze their data. Their primary supervisors included the person who developed the method (Steven C. Hayes), so I would not expect the approach, if disseminated, to do as well, but clearly they had supervisors who were expert in teaching the method.

The authors make a good argument for developing an alternative method to exposure therapy with ritual prevention and cognitive procedures. As they point out, the former has a high dropout rate (25%), and it is underused in part because clinicians find it aversive.

I particularly like that the authors spelled out the overall philosophy of the method and provided session-by-session therapist behaviors. They were appropriately cautious about the approach, given that this method is in an early stage of development. Nevertheless, Table 1, reporting on outcomes, suggests that as the authors purport, ACT is worth exploring further as a treatment for OCD.

J. L. Krupnick, PhD

Cognitive Therapy vs Interpersonal Psychotherapy in Social Anxiety Disorder: A Randomized Controlled Trial
Stangier U, Schramm E, Heidenreich T, et al (Univ of Frankfurt, Germany; Univ of Freiburg, Germany; Univ of Applied Sciences, Esslingen, Germany; et al)
Arch Gen Psychiatry 68:692-700, 2011

Context.—Cognitive therapy (CT) focuses on the modification of biased information processing and dysfunctional beliefs of social anxiety disorder (SAD). Interpersonal psychotherapy (IPT) aims to change problematic interpersonal behavior patterns that may have an important role in the maintenance of SAD. No direct comparisons of the treatments for SAD in an outpatient setting exist.

Objective.—To compare the efficacy of CT, IPT, and a waiting-list control (WLC) condition.

Design.—Randomized controlled trial.

Setting.—Two academic outpatient treatment sites.

Patients.—Of 254 potential participants screened, 117 had a primary diagnosis of SAD and were eligible for randomization; 106 participants completed the treatment or waiting phase.

Interventions.—Treatment comprised 16 individual sessions of either CT or IPT and 1 booster session. Twenty weeks after randomization, post-treatment assessment was conducted and participants in the WLC received 1 of the treatments.

Main Outcome Measures.—The primary outcome was treatment response on the Clinical Global Impression Improvement Scale as assessed by independent masked evaluators. The secondary outcome measures were independent assessor ratings using the Liebowitz Social Anxiety Scale, the Hamilton Rating Scale for Depression, and patient self-ratings of SAD symptoms.

Results.—At the posttreatment assessment, response rates were 65.8% for CT, 42.1% for IPT, and 7.3% for WLC. Regarding response rates and Liebowitz Social Anxiety Scale scores, CT performed significantly better than did IPT, and both treatments were superior to WLC. At 1-year follow-up, the differences between CT and IPT were largely maintained, with significantly higher response rates in the CT vs the IPT group (68.4% vs 31.6%) and better outcomes on the Liebowitz Social Anxiety Scale. No significant treatment × site interactions were noted.

Conclusions.—Cognitive therapy and IPT led to considerable improvements that were maintained 1 year after treatment; CT was more efficacious than was IPT in reducing social phobia symptoms.

▶ This is a nicely conducted randomized, controlled trial comparing 2 manual-based treatments for social anxiety disorder. Of particular importance is that this is the first direct comparison of treatments for this disorder in an outpatient setting. Of note also is the fact that it was conducted in Germany, where so many psychotherapy studies are carried out in recent years. Indeed, 2 of the authors come from a department of psychiatry and psychotherapy. This study has much to recommend. There is a good number of subjects and randomization was stratified according to site, being careful to control for any site allegiance effects as well as presence or absence of comorbid depression. I found it interesting to observe, particularly in the case of interpersonal psychotherapy, how the general concepts of the intervention were adapted to fit the diagnostic category under review. One surprising feature was the rating of the therapeutic alliance after the first therapy session because most outcome studies look at early alliance after the third session. It was also interesting to read that, although both treatments were significantly more effective than a waiting-list control, cognitive therapy was more effective than interpersonal psychotherapy in reducing social phobia symptoms (Fig 2 in original article).

J. L. Krupnick, PhD

Treating fibromyalgia with mindfulness-based stress reduction: Results from a 3-armed randomized controlled trial
Schmidt S, Grossman P, Schwarzer B, et al (Univ Med Ctr, Freiburg, Germany; Univ of Basel Hosp, Switzerland; et al)
Pain 152:361-369, 2011

Mindfulness-based stress reduction (MBSR) is a structured 8-week group program teaching mindfulness meditation and mindful yoga exercises. MBSR aims to help participants develop nonjudgmental awareness of moment-to-moment experience. Fibromyalgia is a clinical syndrome with chronic pain, fatigue, and insomnia as major symptoms. Efficacy of MBSR for enhanced well-being of fibromyalgia patients was investigated in a 3-armed trial, which was a follow-up to an earlier quasi-randomized investigation. A total of 177 female patients were randomized to one of the following: (1) MBSR, (2) an active control procedure controlling for nonspecific effects of MBSR, or (3) a wait list. The major outcome was health-related quality of life (HRQoL) 2 months post-treatment. Secondary outcomes were disorder-specific quality of life, depression, pain, anxiety, somatic complaints, and a proposed index of mindfulness. Of the patients, 82% completed the study. There were no significant differences between groups on primary outcome, but patients overall improved in HRQoL at short-term follow-up ($P = 0.004$). Post hoc analyses showed that only MBSR manifested a significant pre-to-post-intervention improvement in HRQoL ($P = 0.02$). Furthermore, multivariate analysis of secondary measures indicated modest benefits for MBSR patients. MBSR yielded significant pre-to-post- intervention improvements in 6 of 8 secondary outcome variables, the active control in 3, and the wait list in 2. In conclusion, primary outcome analyses did not support the efficacy of MBSR in fibromyalgia, although patients in the MBSR arm appeared to benefit most. Effect sizes were small compared to the earlier, quasi-randomized investigation. Several methodological aspects are discussed, e.g., patient burden, treatment preference and motivation, that may provide explanations for differences. In a 3-armed randomized controlled trial in female patients suffering from fibromyalgia, patients benefited modestly from a mindfulness-based stress reduction intervention.

▶ In contrast with most studies that are reported in the mental health literature, this article actually reports negative results. The authors conducted a randomized, controlled trial on mindfulness-based stress reduction (MBSR) compared with a relaxation arm (an active control group) and a wait list, expecting to find significantly better results for the MBSR condition. They had conducted an earlier quasi-experimental study and found solid results for the MBSR. So why the lack of significant results in this larger study with more rigorous methodology? One would typically assign more weight to the study that is randomized, with better controls and stronger methodology. The authors speculate on why their disappointing results may have occurred, suggesting that the earlier study better conformed to more naturalistic conditions. They also add that wait-list patients who could choose either of the active treatments more frequently chose MSBR. This raised interesting questions about which study to put more stock in. Overall, it seems that despite different methodology that might have made it difficult to achieve their earlier, more promising results, the reader should be more inclined to have faith in the study with stronger methodology.

J. L. Krupnick, PhD

Prolonged Exposure Versus Dynamic Therapy for Adolescent PTSD: A Pilot Randomized Controlled Trial

Gilboa-Schechtman E, Foa EB, Shafran N, et al (Bar-Ilan Univ, Ramat-Gan, Israel; Univ of Pennsylvania, Philadelphia; et al)
J Am Acad Child Adolesc Psychiatry 49:1034-1042, 2010

Objective.—To examine the efficacy and maintenance of developmentally adapted prolonged exposure therapy for adolescents (PE-A) compared with active control time-limited dynamic therapy (TLDP-A) for decreasing posttraumatic and depressive symptoms in adolescent victims of single-event traumas.

Method.—Thirty-eight adolescents (12 to 18 years old) were randomly assigned to receive PE-A or TLDP-A.

Results.—Both treatments resulted in decreased posttraumatic stress disorder and depression and increased functioning. PE-A exhibited a greater decrease of posttraumatic stress disorder and depression symptom severity and a greater increase in global functioning than did TDLP-A. After treatment, 68.4% of adolescents beginning treatment with PE-A and 36.8% of those beginning treatment with TLDP-A no longer met diagnostic criteria for posttraumatic stress disorder. Treatment gains were maintained at 6- and 17-month follow-ups.

Conclusions.—Brief individual therapy is effective in decreasing posttraumatic distress and behavioral trauma-focused components enhance efficacy.

Clinical Trial Registry Information.—Prolonged Exposure Therapy Versus Active Psychotherapy in Treating Post-Traumatic Stress Disorder in Adolescents, URL: http://clinicaltrials.gov, unique identifier: NCT00183690.

▶ This is a well-conducted study, with a couple of aspects that are particularly useful. First, the prolonged exposure (PE) method, long found effective with adults, has been adapted for adolescents, and this study reflects an early attempt to assess its efficacy. It is also useful that the comparison treatment in this instance was another active treatment, rather than the wait-list control condition that has frequently been used. That being said, there were other aspects that aroused concern in terms of the balance between the 2 treatments being investigated. For example, the PE approach was taught by a developer of the method, with a longer period of training for PE than for time-limited dynamic therapy (TLDP). I also wondered whether a better TLDP might have been the one developed by Horowitz and colleagues rather than the brief dynamic approach that was used since the former approach was designed with a focus on stressful life events rather than the more generalized perspective used in the latter. It may be that the investigators were interested in comparing and contrasting a trauma-focused approach with a nontrauma—focused treatment, but it seems to me that the deck would not have been stacked to the same degree if both approaches used a trauma focus.

J. L. Krupnick, PhD

Six-Year Follow-up of a Preventive Intervention for Parentally Bereaved Youths: A Randomized Controlled Trial
Sandler I, Ayers TS, Tein J-Y, et al (Arizona State Univ, Tempe; et al)
Arch Pediatr Adolesc Med 164:907-914, 2010

Objective.—To evaluate the efficacy of the Family Bereavement Program (FBP) to prevent mental health problems in parentally bereaved youths and their parents 6 years later.

Design.—Randomized controlled trial.

Setting.—Arizona State University Prevention Research Center from November 2002 to July 2005.

Participants.—Two hundred eighteen bereaved youths (89.34% of 244 enrolled in the trial 6 years earlier) and 113 spousally bereaved parents.

Interventions.—The FBP includes 12 group sessions for caregivers and youths; the literature control (LC) condition includes bereavement books for youths and caregivers.

Main Outcome Measures.—Comparisons of youths in the FBP and LC on a measure of mental disorder diagnosis, 5 measures of mental health problems, and 4 measures of competent functioning; and comparisons of spousally bereaved parents on 2 measures of mental health problems.

Results.—Youths in the FBP as compared with those in the LC had significantly lower externalizing problems as reported by caregivers and youths (adjusted mean, -0.06 vs 0.13, respectively; $P = .02$) and on teacher reports of externalizing problems (adjusted mean, 52.69 vs 56.27, respectively; $P = .001$) and internalizing problems (adjusted mean, 47.29 vs 56.27, respectively; $P = .002$), and they had higher self-esteem (adjusted mean, 33.93 vs 31.91, respectively; $P = .005$). Parents in the FBP had lower depression scores than those in the LC (adjusted mean, 5.48 vs 7.83, respectively; $P = .04$). A significant moderated program effect indicated that for youths with lower baseline problems, the rate of diagnosed mental disorder was lower for those in the FBP than in the LC.

Conclusion.—This study demonstrates efficacy of the FBP to reduce mental health problems of bereaved youths and their parents 6 years later.

TABLE 2.—Family Bereavement Program Intervention Main Effects at 6-Year Follow-Up

Measure	Actual Proportion or Actual Mean (95% CI)[a]		P Value	
	FBP	LC	Cohen d[b]	False Discovery Rate
Diagnosis of mental disorder or substance abuse disorder, %	33.64 (24.81 to 42.47)	41.05 (31.16 to 50.94)	.28	.28
Mental health problems				
Externalizing disorder, %[c]	15.45 (8.70 to 22.20)	27.37 (18.40 to 36.34)	.04 (OR=1.57)	.09
Externalizing problems, mean				
Caregiver and adolescent/young adult report	−0.07 (−0.20 to 0.05)	0.13 (0.01 to 0.25)	.02 (d=0.31)	.05
Teacher report[d]	52.39 (50.57 to 54.21)	56.28 (54.65 to 57.91)	.001 (d=0.59)	.01
Internalizing disorder, %[c]	15.45 (8.70 to 22.20)	13.68 (6.77 to 20.59)	.76	.77
Internalizing problems, mean				
Caregiver and adolescent/young adult report	−0.03 (−0.14 to 0.09)	0.03 (−0.09 to 0.14)	.57	.69
Teacher report[d]	48.12 (46.12 to 50.11)	52.35 (50.42 to 54.28)	.002 (d=0.57)	.01
Competence, mean				
Self-esteem	33.91 (32.96 to 34.87)	31.90 (30.95 to 32.84)	.005 (d=0.40)	.02
Academic	3.02 (2.88 to 3.16)	2.98 (2.82 to 3.15)	.62	.69
Peer	3.28 (3.19 to 3.37)	3.16 (3.07 to 3.25)	.11	.18
Grade point average	2.52 (2.29 to 2.75)	2.43 (2.18 to 2.67)	.63	.69
Risky behaviors				
Substance abuse disorders, %	10.00 (4.39 to 15.61)	13.68 (6.77 to 20.59)	.68	.88
Marijuana or alcohol use, mean	2.56 (2.22 to 2.91)	2.50 (2.13 to 2.87)	.89	.89
Polydrug use, mean	1.57 (1.21 to 1.94)	1.74 (1.25 to 2.22)	.62	.88
Sexual partners, mean, No.	2.89 (1.79 to 3.98)	2.06 (1.36 to 2.77)	.21	.63
Mental health problems of spousally bereaved caregiver, score, mean[e]				
BDI	6.05 (4.37 to 7.73)	7.40 (5.36 to 9.45)	.04 (d=0.40)	.04
PERI	1.88 (1.73 to 2.02)	2.04 (1.86 to 2.21)	.03 (d=0.42)	.04

Abbreviations: BDI, Beck Depression Inventory; CI, confidence interval; FBP, Family Bereavement Program; LC, literature control; OR, odds ratio; PERI, Psychiatric Epidemiology Research Interview.
[a]The CIs for the actual proportions and means did not control for the baseline covariate and did not reflect the full-information maximum likelihood estimate of intervention effect.
[b]Cohen d is reported only for the findings with $P \leq .05$.
[c]The modules for internalizing and externalizing problems were categorized by I.S., T.S.A., and S.W., who are trained as clinical psychologists. Internalizing disorders include agoraphobia, eating disorder, generalized anxiety disorder, bipolar depression, major depressive disorder, obsessive-compulsive disorder, panic disorder, posttraumatic stress disorder, social phobia, and specific phobia. Externalizing disorders include attention-deficit/hyperactivity disorder, conduct disorder with antisocial personality disorder considered, and oppositional defiant disorder.
[d]For 122 students who were still enrolled in junior or senior high school at least 1 month prior to the data collection, we were successful in collecting teacher reports for 117 youths. We obtained teacher reports for 112 youths from teachers in English/language, social studies/history or government, math/science, or any other major subject and used the mean of the scores for the 2 teachers. We obtained only 1 teacher report for 5 youths.
[e]The sample size was 113.

Trial Registration.—clinicaltrials.gov Identifier: NCT01008189 (Table 2).

▶ This randomized controlled trial provides long-term (6 years) follow-up on the efficacy of a prevention program for bereaved youth and their parents. The most significant contribution of this article is its report on the degree to which gains are maintained. Since most studies have follow-up assessments that are no longer than 18 months to 2 years, the fact that these researchers followed up their sample for 6 years is impressive.

The article describes a well-conceptualized approach to preventing mental health problems in children and families that have experienced parental bereavement. This trauma is one with considerable potential for instigating anxiety, mood, and behavioral problems, and prevention is always preferable to treatment of a disorder. The ways in which the intervention focuses on strengthening caregiver-youth relationships and maintaining discipline in the face of loss seem particularly effective. Given that surviving parents are also grieving, there is a great risk that they won't pay as much attention to their children's problems as they are developing. This intervention helps adult survivors deal with their own problems while being more attuned to their grieving children. Table 2 identifies the many ways the program helped bereaved families.

J. L. Krupnick, PhD

Bereavement, Complicated Grief, and *DSM*, Part 1: Depression
Zisook S, Reynolds CF III, Pies R, et al (Univ of California San Diego; Univ of Pittsburgh Graduate School of Public Health, PA; Tufts Univ School of Medicine, Boston, MA; et al)
J Clin Psychiatry 71:955-956, 2010

Background.—Before 1980 when the *Diagnostic and Statistical Manual of Mental Disorders*, Third Edition (*DSM-III*), was published, bereavement was not considered part of psychiatry's official terminology. Recent bereavement was mentioned only as an exclusion when diagnosing major depressive episode (MDE) and as a V-code, indicating a condition prompting clinical attention but not a mental disorder. This distinction continued in the *Diagnostic and Statistical Manual of Mental Disorders*, Fourth Edition, Text Revision (*DSM-IV-TR*). The *International Statistical Classification of Diseases and Related Health Problems, Tenth Revision* (*ICD-10*) would classify bereavement as a major depressive disorder (MDD). In the *DSM-IV-TR*, a recently bereaved person with MDD symptoms is not diagnosed with MDD or MDE unless he or she exhibits guilt, suicidal thoughts, worthlessness, psychomotor retardation, marked functional impairment, and psychotic features. Evidence was reviewed to determine if such a distinction is valid.

Bereavement/Depression Connection.—Bereavement is considered one of the universal stressors likely to lead to major depression. MDE symptoms are found in about a third of widows or widowers after 1 month and about a fourth after 7 months; they last a year or more in 10% to 15% of persons. Clinicians can be confused about the grief/MDE relationship because in each condition persons exhibit low mood, sadness, and social withdrawal. To avoid overdiagnosing MDE, the *DSM-IV-TR* has continued the distinction between bereaved and depressed individuals when no other symptoms are noted. Many grief experts question the need to wait for 2 full months before diagnosing as normal a major depressive syndrome in the context of grief.

Analysis.—Current reviews note similarities in clinical and behavioral characteristics, comorbidities, course, and treatment response between bereavement-related depressive syndromes and non-n-bereavement-related MDD. Similarities are also seen between bereavement-related major depressive syndromes and other life-event-n-related depressions in terms of demographics, clinical characteristics, intensity, familiality, course, associated features, and treatment response. The overall symptom profile of persons who are depressed and their risk for recurrence of depressive symptoms are similar whether bereavement is involved or not. Bereaved persons actually have had a longer duration of illness than non-bereaved individuals. One study also found that persons excluded from a diagnosis of MDE because of the *DSM-IV-TR* stance are more severely depressed than non-bereaved MDD controls. No support was found for recommending the special treatment outlined in the *DSM-IV-TR.*

Conclusions.—The evidence indicates that either all depressive episodes soon after a stressful life event not associated with morbid feelings of worthlessness, psychomotor slowness, suicidal ideation, psychotic features, or marked and prolonged functional impairment should not be considered MDE or no bereavement exclusion should be in the *DSM-V.* The *ICD-10* method of diagnosing MDD when all symptomatic, duration, and severity criteria are met appears more clinically accurate. The V-code bereavement should be eliminated or not used when symptoms are better characterized as MDD, adjustment disorder, post-traumatic stress disorder (PTSD), or complicated grief.

▶ This article is very brief, but it is well worth reading. It takes on recent discussions about how to handle bereavement, currently listed as a V-code, nondiagnosis according to *Diagnostic and Statistic Manual of Mental Disorders*, Fourth Edition, Text Revision (DSM-IV-TR) criteria, at least for 2 months subsequent to loss of a loved one. There have been caveats to this categorization, for example, even if the individual being assessed suffers from such symptoms as guilt, suicidal thoughts, marked functional impairment, and psychotic features, meeting the usual criteria for major depressive disorder does not apply unless symptoms persist for longer than 2 months. Among the arguments against this convention for DSM-V is the wish to keep DSM and *International Statistical Classification of Diseases and Health Related Problems* (ICD) diagnoses comparable, with the problem being that ICD-10 and ICD-11 do not exclude the diagnosis of major depression in the face of a recent bereavement. Another argument is that 2 recent reviews note the similarities between bereavement-related depression and other non-bereavement-related depression.

My argument against the bereavement exclusion used to be that 2 months seemed like a totally arbitrary length of time to allow for bereavement-related distress. Typically, most people who lose a loved one grieve for quite a bit longer than this. The arguments against treatment during this time, however, are more compelling reasons to remove bereavement as a V-code. Because the most recent research, including 3 secondary data analyses of large population-based databases, demonstrate no significant differences between bereavement-related depression and depression triggered by other circumstances across a range of demographic and clinical characteristics, it is difficult to disagree that all major depression should be regarded as a diagnosable disorder, worthy of clinical attention and insurance reimbursement.

J. L. Krupnick, PhD

Clinical and Psychosocial Predictors of Suicide Attempts and Nonsuicidal Self-Injury in the Adolescent Depression Antidepressants and Psychotherapy Trial (ADAPT)
Wilkinson P, Kelvin R, Roberts C, et al (Cambridge Univ, England, UK; Manchester Univ, England, UK; Royal Manchester Children's Hosp, Pendlebury, England, UK)
Am J Psychiatry 168:495-501, 2011

Objective.—The authors assessed whether clinical and psychosocial factors in depressed adolescents at baseline predict suicide attempts and nonsuicidal self-injury over 28 weeks of follow-up.

Method.—Participants were 164 adolescents with major depressive disorder taking part in the Adolescent Depression Antidepressants and Psychotherapy Trial (ADAPT). Clinical symptoms, family function, quality of current personal friendships, and suicidal and nonsuicidal self-harm were assessed at baseline. Suicidal and nonsuicidal self-harm thoughts and behaviors were assessed during 28 weeks of follow-up.

Results.—High suicidality, nonsuicidal self-injury, and poor family function at entry were significant independent predictors of suicide attempts over the 28 weeks of follow-up. Nonsuicidal self-injury over the follow-up period was independently predicted by nonsuicidal self-injury, hopelessness, anxiety disorder, and being younger and female at entry.

Conclusions.—Both suicidal and nonsuicidal self-harm persisted in depressed adolescents receiving treatment in the ADAPT study. A history of nonsuicidal self-injury prior to treatment is a clinical marker for subsequent suicide attempts and should be as carefully assessed in depressed youths as current suicidal intent and behavior.

▶ It is indeed startling to read that suicide is the third leading cause of death in adolescents in the United States and the second leading cause in the rest of the developed world. These statistics underscore the importance of good assessment of adolescents most at risk for suicide. It was very discouraging to read that so many trials of interventions for suicidal adolescents have proven to be ineffective as well. For example, dialectical behavior therapy, which has empirical evidence of being efficacious with self-harming adults, showed no better results than treatment as usual in reducing suicidal or nonsuicidal self-harm in adolescents. Thus, even with good assessment, much work still needs to be done in developing interventions that can make more of an impact with this population. The biggest surprise of this study was the finding that both suicidal and nonsuicidal self-harm are significant risks for suicide attempts later. There is a good deal in the literature about self-injury in adolescents, particularly among those with borderline personality, but this is usually discussed in terms of its use to reduce anxiety or to modify problematic affective states. This study suggests that this type of self-harm should be paid heed in addition as an important predictor of later suicide attempts. The role of impaired family functioning and the somewhat promising results of a couple of family-based interventions suggest that perhaps family treatment might be a more promising route for treatment than individual or group therapies.

J. L. Krupnick, PhD

Girls who Cut: Treatment in an Outpatient Psychodynamic Psychotherapy Practice with Adolescent Girls and Young Adult Women
Ruberman L (Bronx Children's Psychiatric Ctr & Montefiore Med Ctr, NY)
Am J Psychother 65:117-132, 2011

The observation of deficits in the capacity for mature emotional self-regulation in girls who cut is noted in the literature (Daldin, 1990; Novick & Novick, 1991; Nock et al., 2008). The acquisition of the ability to respond in a healthy manner to stress and challenge, either from outside or inside the self, is one of the most important tasks of early development; girls who cut have not accomplished this developmental task or are seriously compromised in their efforts to do so. The connection between this observation, the psychosexual developmental antecedents of this deficit, and psychodynamic approaches to treatment are explored in the literature and in case reviews.

▶ I found this article to be fascinating and clinically very useful. The review of the literature was of particular interest, especially in its citing of studies that link self-injurious behavior with impulsivity and such behavior as tattooing. The link to eating disorders and other problems associated with the body makes sense in the way it is put together in the author's analysis. This article cited other recent data that link nonsuicidal self-injury with increased frequency of suicide attempts, a finding that places great importance on addressing this issue.

The case examples that were explicated were useful in understanding the meaning of this behavior in clinical practice. However, it was a bit puzzling to contrast one example of a girl who cut, whose problems centered around feeling rejected by her mother, with another case in which the girl's relationship with her mother was the only one in her family in which she felt safe, although that may have led to difficulties with individuation from this parent. Nevertheless, the psychodynamic exploration and interpretation of this challenging behavior provided insightful and applicable ways of understanding and treating girls who engage in cutting themselves.

J. L. Krupnick, PhD

Impact of the 2004 Food and Drug Administration Pediatric Suicidality Warning on Antidepressant and Psychotherapy Treatment for New-Onset Depression
Valluri S, Zito JM, Safer DJ, et al (Univ of Maryland, Baltimore; Johns Hopkins Med Institutions, Baltimore, MD)
Med Care 48:947-954, 2010

Objective.—To assess the national impact of the March 2004 Food and Drug Administration (FDA) antidepressant suicidality warning on the outpatient treatment of new-onset depression in youth.

Method.—A repeated measures, longitudinal design in a cohort of youth diagnosed with new-onset depression was used to assess pre- and post-FDA warning effects. US commercial insurance enrollees in the i3 INNOVUS database from January 2003 through December 2006 were examined. The study population included youth 2- to 17-years old with a new-onset depression diagnosis from July 2003 through June 2006 (N = 40,309). The main independent variables were the warning period (post- vs. pre-FDA warning) and age group (children vs. adolescents). The main outcome measures were youth with antidepressant dispensings and psychotherapy visits measured in 30-day intervals across 36 months following a new-onset diagnosis of any depressive disorder (N = 40,309) and specifically major depressive disorder (MDD) (N = 11,532).

Results.—Compared to youth with a new-onset diagnosis of depression in the pre-FDA warning period, youth with new-onset diagnosis of depression during the postwarning period had (1) A significantly lower likelihood of antidepressant use: (odds ratio [OR] = 0.85 [0.81−0.89]); When youth with the diagnosis of depression were separated into those with MDD and those with less severe depression diagnoses, only the latter had a significant postwarning antidepressant decline. (2) A significant increase in the odds of a psychotherapy visit (children, OR = 1.31 [1.23−1.40]; adolescents OR = 1.19 [1.15−1.24]).

Conclusions.—The FDA suicidality warning was associated with an overall decrease in antidepressant treatment for youth with a clinician-reported diagnosis of depression, but not for those with MDD. Also, following the warning, psychotherapy without medication increased (Table 1).

▶ This is an article with considerable clinical relevance. It explores whether psychiatrists stopped or decreased the use of antidepressant medication after the Food and Drug Administration required the warning about increased suicidality in children and adolescents. This was a matter of some concern among clinicians working with adolescents in particular since the rates of suicide among adolescents had significantly declined with the use of such medication.

Table 1 shows that a significant number of youths receive a depression diagnosis in the United States as well as the changes in treatments preceding and following the warning. Fortunately, the results show that the decline in use of medication is only for those with less severe diagnoses. This is reassuring because it means that those with the greatest need for pharmaceutical intervention still

TABLE 1.—Demographic and Clinical Characteristics of Youth With New-Onset Depression (N = 40,309)

Characteristic	Prewarning (July 2003–February 2004) N = 9428	%	Postwarning (March 2004–June 2006) N = 30881	%	P
Gender					0.088
Male	4358	46	13,962	45	
Age group					0.026
Children (2–12 yr)	2368	25	7409	24	
Adolescents (13–17 yr)	7060	75	23,472	76	
Region					<0.0001
Northeast	886	9	3419	11	
Midwest	3615	38	10,841	35	
South	3567	38	11,940	39	
West	1360	14	4681	15	
Median mo of enrollment (range)	38 (12–48)		38 (12–48)		
Other psychiatric diagnoses in 180 d prior to new-onset depression diagnosis					
ADHD	1080	11	3207	10	0.003
Anxiety	841	9	2807	9	0.616
Bipolar	67	1	267	1	0.149
CD/ODD	370	4	1160	4	0.455
Other psychiatric diagnosis	612	6	2267	7	0.005
Treatments for depression in 180 d after a new-onset depression diagnosis					
Either antidepressants or psychotherapy	7496	80	24,168	78	0.001
Antidepressant use, any*	4004	42	10,658	35	<0.0001
SSRI/SNRI use, any	3585	38	9123	30	<0.0001
Antidepressant use, only†	1496	16	3597	12	<0.0001
Psychotherapy visits, any	6000	64	20,571	67	<0.0001
Psychotherapy visits, only	3492	37	13,660	44	<0.0001

ADHD indicates attention-deficit/hyperactivity disorder; CD/ODD, conduct disorder/oppositional defiant disorder; SSRI, selective serotonin reuptake inhibitor; SNRI, serotonin-norepinephrine reuptake inhibitor.
*"Antidepressant use, any" refers to antidepressant use regardless of psychotherapy visits.
†"Antidepressant use, only" refers to antidepressant use without any psychotherapy visit.

received it. Perhaps those with less severe depression could benefit from psychotherapy only. Given the absence of knowledge about long-term effects of prolonged medication use in children, trying psychotherapy first with such children might serve their longer-term health interests.

J. L. Krupnick, PhD

Conjoint IPT for Postpartum Depression: Literature Review and Overview of a Treatment Manual

Carter W, Grigoriadis S, Ravitz P, et al (Women's College Hosp, Toronto, Ontario, Canada; Univ of Toronto, Ontario, Canada; et al)
Am J Psychother 64:373-392, 2010

Distress about the quality of a woman's relationship with her partner has consistently emerged as a risk factor for Postpartum Depression (PPD). In addition to having an increased likelihood of developing PPD, women who are distressed about their relationships, experience more severe depressive symptoms of greater duration, and are more vulnerable to the development of mental health problems. The emotional well-being of partners of depressed mothers is also affected, signalling the need for interventions that incorporate the woman as well as her partner. Few interventions have been designed for women simultaneously experiencing PPD and relationship distress in a conjoint format. This article describes a newly developed Interpersonal Psychotherapy (IPT) conjoint approach to treating PPD in the context of relationship distress. The existing literature on PPD is reviewed, as well as relationship distress and psychotherapy interventions for PPD with couples. This is followed by a description of an IPT conjoint approach to treating PPD with relationship distress.

▶ This article describes a new variation of interpersonal psychotherapy (IPT), that is, conjoint IPT for postpartum depression (PPD). It really is a nice amalgam of various existing IPT approaches, including the original IPT for depression, IPT for PPD (as an individual treatment), and IPT for couples with relationship distress. While it seems likely that women with PPD could be seen in any of the other forms of IPT, this approach is useful in its specific focus on couples in which the wife has PPD. Individual IPT for depression allows up to 4 conjoint sessions, but in that approach and in the IPT for women with PPD, the focus is only on the depressed mother. Also, in the study by Stewart and O'Hara on IPT for PPD, only first-time mothers were treated, whereas conjoint IPT for PPD includes families with other children. What is particularly useful about this article is the way it takes the reader through each of the stages of this treatment, nicely explicating what the primary issues and techniques are likely to be. With this article in hand, it would not be difficult to conduct this type of intervention if a clinician is already familiar with the IPT approach. Given the very important role played by the couple relationship in PPD, it also makes sense to have a full treatment focused on this relationship, with both participants present. While other IPT researchers have added in more focus on attachment theory and its centrality in this approach relative to the original IPT for depression manual, I was glad to see that these researchers also emphasized the importance of assessing the couples' attachment capacities and pointed out the ways in which attachment issues might be activated in the face of becoming parents, either for the first time or not. The treatment, as described, adds a useful addition to the psychosocial approaches that can be used to treat PPD.

J. L. Krupnick, PhD

Clinical Consensus Strategies for Interpersonal Problems Between Young Adults and Their Parents
Eubanks-Carter C, Burckell LA, Goldfried MR (Stony Brook Univ, NY)
J Consult Clin Psychol 78:212-224, 2010

Objective.—Research that identifies areas of agreement among expert therapists can complement findings from clinical trials by highlighting common practices as well as innovations. The present study accessed

TABLE 2.—Clinical Situations Involving Young Adults Experiencing Interpersonal Problems With Their Parents

SASB-Based Pattern	Background	Situation
1. Affiliative child, hostile and withdrawn parent	The client is a 31-year-old, married, multiracial woman. She is seeking treatment for anxiety related to current work and family stressors, in particular, her estrangement from her father. The client reports that her father has been distant and rejecting of her ever since he and her mother divorced, over 20 years ago. He has two other children by a second marriage and has close relationships with both of them.	In session, the client reports that she and her husband are now planning to have their first child. She would like to reestablish a relationship with her father so that her child can have a grandfather. The client says that she has called her father several times over the past few weeks. She has invited him to join her for dinner and other activities. However, he has declined all of her offers and said that he prefers to have limited contact with her. The client feels confused, sad, and hurt by her father's behavior.
2. Neglectful parent, resentful child	The client is a 30-year-old, Latina woman, seeking therapy for depression following a break-up with a boyfriend. The client grew up with a drug-addicted father and an irresponsible, childlike mother.	In session, the client says that her mother keeps asking her to listen to her problems and give her advice and support. But when the client tries to talk to her mother about how she feels and how hard things have been since she broke up with her boyfriend, her mother does not pay attention and changes the subject back to herself. The client feels frustrated and angry with her mother. But then she feels guilty and feels that her mother really needs her emotional support.
3. Suffocating parent, hostile child	The client is a 30-year-old, white woman. The client divorced recently, and she and her 8-year-old son are now living with her parents while she tries to get back on her feet financially. The client's mother is very helpful with the client's son, babysitting while the client looks for work, helping the son with his homework, and cooking dinner for the entire family. The client has greatly appreciated her mother's help.	In session, the client says that she wants to have more time to herself, to pursue her own interests and develop more of a social life. She is planning to move out of her parents' house as soon as she secures a job. However, her mother keeps suggesting that they spend more time together, such as meeting in the city for lunch and going shopping together on the weekend. So far, the client has avoided spending more time with her mother by telling her that she is too busy with job interviews. The client feels guilty about not being there for her mother after all that her mother has done for her.
4. Critical parent, hostile child	The client is a 25-year-old, white female. She works full-time and supports herself financially. The client's mother told the client that she should enter therapy because she was making so many "bad decisions" with her life.	In session, the client says that her mother insists that she work in an office setting. To please her mother, the client has tried to hold down office jobs. However, she has not been successful—she has had five different jobs since she graduated from college three years ago. The client feels guilty about her lack of success. But she also feels frustrated with her mother, who she says is "driving me crazy" by "trying to run my life." The client wants to learn how to say "no" to her mother, but she is afraid that her mother will become angry with her.

5. Self-neglectful child, enmeshed parent	The client is an 18-year-old, white woman who lives with her mother and stepfather. The client is depressed, irritable, and has a history of cutting herself but is not suicidal. She was enrolled in a community college, but recently withdrew because she was failing. She was also recently fired from a job.	The client reports that her mother became angry when she learned that the client had been fired. She accused the client of being irresponsible and gave her an ultimatum to get a job or leave the house. The client says that she feels incompetent and doubts that she will be able to find and keep another job. The client also says that she is furious with her mother for threatening to kick her out of the house. She is planning to move out and live with her father, whom her mother cannot stand.
6. Independent child, hostile and enmeshed parent	The client is a 22-year-old, white man seeking treatment for anxiety and depression. The client recently graduated from college, and is living with his parents while he looks for a job.	In session, the client reports that he recently came out to his parents. He said that they were very upset, and told him that homosexuality violated their religious beliefs. They also expressed concern about how their friends would react to the news. Since then, neither the client nor his parents have talked about what happened. The client says that the atmosphere at home is very stressful, and everyone is on edge.

Note. SASB = Structural Analysis of Social Behavior.

consensus among expert therapists on the effectiveness of clinical strategies for treating young adults experiencing interpersonal problems with their parents.

Method.—This study drew on the behavioral–analytic model (Goldfried & D'Zurilla, 1969) and the methodology of the *Expert Consensus Guideline Series* (Frances, Kahn, Carpenter, Ross, & Docherty, 1996). In Phase I, 54 therapists (mean age = 60.32 years; 55.6% women, 44.4% men; 96.3% White/European American) provided clinical situations involving young adult clients and their parents. In Phase II, 171 therapists (mean age = 59.45 years; 47.4% women, 52.0% men; 91.8% White/European American) proposed responses to the situations, and more general clinical strategies underlying the responses were identified. In Phase III, 134 peer-nominated expert therapists (a mean of 22.33 therapists per situation; mean age = 55.46 years; 61.2% women, 34.3% men; 91.0% White/European American) rated the effectiveness of these clinical strategies.

Results.—Results indicated that the experts reached consensus on strategies rated as highly effective; in particular, they agreed on the value of exploring clients' emotional experience and providing validation. Participants reached greater agreement on strategies for use in future sessions than strategies for immediate use. Exploratory analyses revealed correlations between experts' theoretical orientations and their ratings.

Conclusions.—The findings provide converging evidence of the value of exploring emotions and validating clients and, further, demonstrate the feasibility of this method for accessing clinicians' experience (Table 2).

▶ An ongoing source of frustration to psychotherapy researchers over many decades has been the lack of attention paid to their findings by practicing clinicians. There has been a problematic disconnect between researchers providing scientific evidence about psychosocial interventions and the integration of such findings into clinical practice. The study described in this article attempts to bridge that chasm by using clinical consensus strategies to identify findings that might be perceived as more clinically relevant than those reported in randomized controlled trials. It responds to the suggestions of the American Psychological Association Presidential Task Force on Evidence-Based Practice (2006) that advocated for a broader view of how practice can be linked to research.

The study describes a 3-phase process in which questionnaires were sent to randomly selected social workers and psychologists. In phase 1, these clinicians were asked to describe situations between a client and his or her parents that were discussed in actual therapy sessions. It is unfortunate that the return rate of this mailing was only 16.36%, indicating that only a small proportion of potential respondents answered. Phase 2 involved sending out more questionnaires, asking respondents to think about how they might advise a colleague who was seeking consultation. Phase 3 involved sending peer-nominated expert clinicians the responses generated in Phase 2 to rate the effectiveness of the strategies that were recommended. These methods are creative and provide an interesting way to try to ascertain what can be recommended for certain types of clinical situations.

I did have some questions about various aspects of the study. For example, the clients about whom the researchers sought more information were those identified as young adults, defined as individuals between the ages of 18 and 35 years. While the ages of 18 to 30 years might be understandable as falling within this category, it seems to me that extending young adulthood all the way up to 35 is a bit of a stretch! While I liked the examples that were given in Table 2 that provided some examples of the interpersonal patterns that were rated, I did not always agree that the vignette fits the designated pattern, eg, the self-neglectful child and enmeshed parent. As the authors point out, since objective data were not required to identify the effective clinicians, it was not clear how the people who referred them knew that they tended to obtain good psychotherapy outcomes. Finally, it would have been desirable to have had respondents who were not so overwhelmingly European Americans. One can only wonder if somewhat different perspectives might have been provided by a more diverse group of clinicians. Overall, however, this is a well-conducted study that advances the field in terms of attempts to learn how to make psychotherapy more effective.

J. L. Krupnick, PhD

Advances in Psychotherapy for Children and Adolescents with Eating Disorders
Lock J, Fitzpatrick KK (Stanford Univ School of Medicine, CA)
Am J Psychother 63:287-303, 2009

There is a significant lag in the development of evidence based approaches for eating disorders in children and adolescents despite the fact that these disorders typically onset during these developmental periods. Available studies suggest that psychotherapy is the best available approach to these disorders. Specific studies support the use of family based interventions, adolescent focused individual therapy, and developmentally adapted cognitive behavioral therapy in this age group. The current report summarizes the available evidence supportive of each of these treatment modalities, as well as, provides a description of the rationale and principle therapeutic targets and intervention types. Future directions in psychotherapy research in child and adolescent eating disorders are discussed.

▶ What is most striking about this review article, which summarizes the state of the evidence about psychotherapy for children and adolescents with eating disorders, is the limited amount of scientific evidence available for these serious disorders. As the authors point out, mortality rates for anorexia nervosa are among the highest for any psychiatric disorder (8%-12% of patients) and problems with bulimia nervosa are distressingly high among high school and college girls. As is typical with regard to the treatment of many disorders, however, controlled trials of treatments for adults are much more common than such trials for children and adolescents. This continues to be the case despite the fact that many disorders, including eating disorders, begin prior to adulthood.

There are 2 aspects of this article that bear particular attention. One is the attention that is paid to the differences between child/adolescent treatment versus adult treatment. Given the developmental issues that must be attended to when treating children and adolescents, this is an important distinction. The role played by parents/families seems to be an important and differentiating characteristic. The other feature of the article that is particularly useful is the explication of the features that comprise each of the interventions that have thus far been found effective. The fuller description of each approach is something that is not usually available in reports of comparative treatments.

It is encouraging to see that some approaches to these tenacious problems are achieving good results. It is also promising that a number of trials of interventions with this age group are about to conclude or are just getting started. The more scientific evidence there is, the more likely it is that clinicians addressing these disorders in youth will be likely to choose an approach with a strong evidence base.

J. L. Krupnick, PhD

Common Skills that Underlie the Common Factors of Successful Psychotherapy

Karson M, Fox J (Univ of Denver, CO)
Am J Psychother 64:269-281, 2010

Key common factors across psychotherapy approaches are important to therapeutic effectiveness. We identify some common skills of the therapist that are specific to the psychotherapy role. Describing these common skills and contrasting them to the professional clinical and social roles helps to clarify our vision of the therapy role and to articulate its associated skills. Such descriptions assist faculty members who are training students who seek to learn the therapeutic role and skills.

▶ This is a good article to use for training psychotherapists. Since common factors are present across a range of psychotherapies, the skills it teaches and demonstrates are useful regardless of one's theoretical orientation. Since the authors seem to have a psychodynamic perspective, however, it would be useful for them to describe in some instances how a particular discussion could be approached from another theoretical viewpoint. They do this at some points. For example, in the section on the psychotherapist's role, they note that an observation the therapist makes about the therapy relationship could be articulated in terms of the patient's belief about people in general.

What is particularly interesting about this article is that the authors discuss therapeutic skills that are not typically described in other articles on this topic. In particular, I found the distinction they make between the professional and therapeutic frame a useful one. Of greatest interest, and one that makes this article especially pleasurable to read for the practicing clinician, are the vignettes that are provided that suggest ways the therapist might respond. When the patient makes a comment that comes from his/her social role, it identifies the response the therapist can give that indicates the therapeutic role. Other authors have differentiated the therapeutic stance from the appropriate response of a friend or family member, but this article is more specific in describing these differences.

J. L. Krupnick, PhD

Does negative religious coping accompany, precede, or follow depression among Orthodox Jews?
Pirutinsky S, Rosmarin DH, Pargament KI, et al (Columbia Univ, NY; McLean Hosp, Belmont, MA; Bowling Green State Univ, OH)
J Affect Disord 132:401-405, 2011

Background.—Cross sectional research suggests that negative religious coping (e.g., anger at God and religious disengagement) strongly correlates with depression and anxiety. However, causality is difficult to establish as negative coping can accompany, cause, or result from distress. Among Orthodox Jews, some studies have found correlations between negative religious coping and anxiety and depression, while others found that high levels of negative coping related with decreased distress. We therefore examined longitudinal relationships between negative coping and depressive symptoms among Orthodox Jews.

Methods.—Participants (80 Orthodox Jews) completed the Jewish Religious Coping Scale and the Center for Epidemiologic Studies' Depression Scale at two times. Using Structural Equation Modeling, we compared four models describing possible causal patterns.

Results.—Negative religious coping and depressive symptoms were linearly related. Furthermore, a model including negative coping as a predictor of future depression fit the data best and did not significantly differ from a saturated model.

Limitations.—This research was limited by reliance on self-report measures, an internet sample, and examination of only negative religious coping.

Conclusions.—Consistent with a "primary spiritual struggles" conceptualization, negative religious coping appears to precede and perhaps cause future depression among Orthodox Jews. Clinical interventions should target spiritual struggles, and more research integrating this construct into theory and practice is warranted.

▶ The question that is posed in this study is whether religious coping accompanies, precedes, or follows depression among Orthodox Jews, with the results showing that negative religious coping precedes and possibly causes the depression that follows (Table 1). Finding the longitudinal pattern of what occurs first and what follows is quite interesting in terms of understanding what might be causal in the case of depression in this demographic. It is not surprising that negative religious coping provides the impetus for depression in this group given, as the authors observe, Orthodox Judaism's profound integration of religion into everyday cognition, emotion, and behavior. In other words, religion is at the heart of their lives. When such individuals fail to see

TABLE 1.—Zero-order Pearson Correlations Between All Study Variables

| | Time 1 | | Time 2 | |
	Depression	Negative Coping	Depression	Negative Coping
Time 1				
Depression	—			
Negative coping	.38*	—		
Time 2				
Depression	62*	.44*	—	
Negative coping	.41*	.90*	.49*	—
M	24.89	8.67	23.46	8.06
SD	7.99	3.76	9.12	3.58
Range	10—48	4—19	9—60	4—19

*$p<0.001$.

God as a protector or a source of comfort, it would be fair to think that their world order would be highly disrupted, leading to a loss of everything that they hold most dear. I did question, however, the authors' comment about clinical interventions targeting spiritual struggles within this population—not because I don't believe that such a focus might be useful, but because I would suspect that these issues might be more likely to be taken up with religious leaders rather than mental health clinicians.

J. L. Krupnick, PhD

Quasi-experimental study on the effectiveness of psychoanalysis, long-term and short-term psychotherapy on psychiatric symptoms, work ability and functional capacity during a 5-year follow-up
Knekt P, the Helsinki Psychotherapy Study Group (Social Insurance Institution, Helsinki, Finland; et al)
J Affect Disord 132:37-47, 2011

Background.—Psychotherapy is apparently an insufficient treatment for some patients with mood or anxiety disorder. In this study the effectiveness of short-term and long-term psychotherapies was compared with that of psychoanalysis.

Methods.—A total of 326 psychiatric outpatients with mood or anxiety disorder were randomly assigned to solution-focused therapy, short-term psychodynamic and long-term psychodynamic psychotherapies. Additionally, 41 patients suitable for psychoanalysis were included in the study. The patients were followed from the start of the treatment and assessed 9 times during a 5-year follow-up. The primary outcome measures on symptoms were the Beck Depression Inventory, the Hamilton Depression and Anxiety Rating Scales, and the Symptom Check List, anxiety scale. Primary work ability and functional capacity measures were the Work Ability Index, the Work-subscale of the Social Adjustment Scale, and the Perceived Psychological Functioning Scale.

Results.—A reduction in psychiatric symptoms and improvement in work ability and functional capacity was noted in all treatment groups during the 5-year follow-up. The short-term therapies were more effective than psychoanalysis during the first year, whereas the long-term therapy was more effective after 3 years of follow-up. Psychoanalysis was most effective at the 5-year follow-up, which also marked the end of the psychoanalysis.

Conclusions.—Psychotherapy gives faster benefits than psychoanalysis, but in the long run psychoanalysis seems to be more effective. Results from trials, among patients suitable for psychoanalysis and with longer follow-up, are needed before firm conclusions about the relative effectiveness of psychoanalysis and psychotherapy in the treatment of mood and anxiety disorders can be drawn.

▶ This article caught my attention because it included long-term psychodynamic psychotherapy as well as psychoanalysis among the 4 treatments it was comparing. This is such a rarity in psychotherapy studies these days that I thought it warranted further attention. Of course, the study was conducted in Finland, where the reimbursement system is completely different from that in the United States. It is curious how studies of long-term psychotherapy and psychoanalysis are most likely to come from Germany or Scandinavia in the current era. This study also reminded me of the many complexities involved in comparing long-term and short-term treatments. For example, patients who received psychoanalysis were the only ones who chose their treatment condition, whereas the others were randomized. The use of psychotropic medication was much more common among the short-term therapy recipients. Those who selected psychoanalysis were more motivated and more highly educated. In other words, there were significant differences among the patients at the outset of treatment. The findings make sense if one thinks that longer term, more intensive treatment should have more significant, sustained effects. The problem with the comparison, however, is that all the groups seemed to do best when their particular treatment ended. So those in briefer treatments did well in the first year of treatment when their therapies were conducted and concluded. Those in long-term psychotherapy did best at the 3-year mark when their therapies concluded, and those in psychoanalysis did best at the 5-year mark when their treatment ended. Those in psychoanalysis may have achieved better results at that point, but by that time, those in the shorter-term treatments had been away from treatment for more than 4 years, allowing plenty of time for relapse of depression or anxiety. Maybe a fairer test of each method would be to assess how patients are functioning 6 months or a year after finishing treatment, with these time points varying depending on when their therapy was completed. Also, the goals of each of the treatments are likely quite different, with the goal of a treatment such as solution-based therapy being focused primarily on symptoms, and the goal of psychoanalysis being nothing less than personality restructuring, modification of defenses, and analysis of deeper psychic structures. So it's a bit like comparing apples and oranges, but the authors should be applauded for making the attempt.

J. L. Krupnick, PhD

Mediators of Psychotherapy Outcome

A Tripartite Learning Conceptualization of Psychotherapy: The Therapeutic Alliance, Technical Interventions, and Relearning

Scaturo DJ (Syracuse Vet Ctr, NY)
Am J Psychother 64:1-27, 2010

One problem in conceptualizing the various explanatory factors in psychotherapy has been the lack of a common theoretical language by which to construe these various aspects of treatment. This article integrates a broad range of theoretical contributions within the wider context of a learning theory perspective of essential psychotherapeutic processes. A ripartite model of psychotherapy is outlined that incorporates the contributions of the emotional learning that takes place in the therapeutic alliance, the cognitive aspects of the therapist's technical interventions that are intended to accelerate change, and the behavioral elements of relearning that take place in the patient's world beyond the consulting room.

▶ This would be an excellent article to assign to students of psychotherapy for training purposes. It nicely lays out the primary areas of consideration in psychosocial intervention: the working relationship with the patients, the

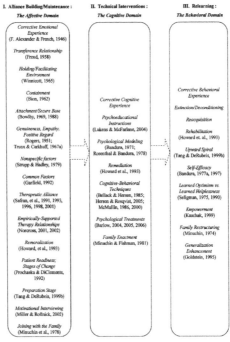

FIGURE 1.—Tripartite learning conceptualization of psychotherapy. (Reprinted from Scaturo DJ. A tripartite learning conceptualization of psychotherapy: the therapeutic alliance, technical interventions, and relearning. *Am J Psychother.* 2010;64:1-27. © Association for the Advancement of Psychotherapy.)

types of technical interventions that compose the core of different approaches, and the types of relearning that take place in therapeutic encounters. It is particularly useful in describing how this conceptualization has pan-theoretical applicability. Thus, these are not components that are particular to one or another school of thought but rather encompass the broad dimensions of the activities that compose any and all types of psychotherapy. Fig 1 identifies the particular concepts, behaviors, and attitudes that compose the proposed tripartite learning. These include the affective domain that is the territory of alliance building and maintenance, the cognitive domain that is associated with technical interventions, and the behavioral domain that falls under relearning. Both Fig 1 and the article as a whole also provide a useful overview of the field of psychotherapy, with references that include some of the classics of psychotherapy and psychotherapy research.

J. L. Krupnick, PhD

Attachment Style in the Prediction of Recovery Following Group Treatment of Combat Veterans With Post-Traumatic Stress Disorder
Forbes D, Parslow R, Fletcher S, et al (Univ of Melbourne, Victoria, Australia; et al)
J Nerv Ment Dis 198:881-884, 2010

Post-traumatic stress disorder (PTSD) can be difficult to treat, with gains often particularly modest in combat veterans. Although group-based treatments are commonly delivered for veterans, little is known about factors influencing their outcomes. Attachment style is known to be associated with psychopathology after trauma and is critical to group-based interventions, but has not yet been investigated in relation to treatment outcome. A better understanding of factors that influence outcome is critical in optimizing the effectiveness of such interventions. This study investigated attachment style as a predictor of outcome for 103 veterans attending group-based treatment for combat-related PTSD. Measures included the Clinician Administered PTSD Scale, PTSD Checklist, and Relationship Styles Questionnaire. Path analyses indicated preoccupied attachment style strongly negatively predicted outcome following treatment. The preoccupied attachment style impedes recovery in group-based treatment for veterans with PTSD. Potential mechanisms underlying this finding are discussed. The results suggest that greater attention should be paid at initial assessment to attachment style of veterans before entering PTSD treatment, particularly group-based interventions.

▶ It is interesting that attachment style is now being considered as a potential predictor variable in studies of cognitive and behavioral treatment. This has been considered a variable of importance for quite some time in the interpersonal psychotherapy literature as well as psychodynamic psychotherapy, that is, treatments that place more emphasis on relatedness and problems with relationships. Finding that individuals with posttraumatic stress disorder who have a preoccupied attachment style do not do well in cognitive and behavioral therapies extends the importance of awareness of such issues, even in treatments that do not specifically target relationship problems. It also raises the issue of whether other treatment approaches, that is, those that do more specifically target the attachment difficulties that patients with this style present might be a better choice for these patients. This gets to the heart of one of the main questions in psychotherapy research, that is, which treatment is best for which patient? Clearly even treatments that focus on maladaptive cognitions might not be the best choice for patients whose problems are in the relational domain. Although this was only a preliminary study in this area, needing replication with another larger study, it points to the importance of initial assessment of patients, even in areas which might not seem to be relevant to the task at hand. The authors do a nice job of explaining why the particular presentation of patients with preoccupied attachment styles might preclude their getting maximum benefit from a treatment that focuses on exposure to feared thoughts and memories. Just as practitioners of treatments that focus on relationships need to assess their patients' cognitive styles, so do practitioners of cognitive and behavioral treatments need to assess their patients' relational/attachment styles. Both are part of a comprehensive assessment that might help determine which treatment approach would be the more effective with a given individual, regardless of the patient's specific diagnostic category.

J. L. Krupnick, PhD

Predictors of Patient and Caregiver Distress in an Adult Sample With Bipolar Disorder Seeking Family Treatment
Lee AMR, Simeon D, Cohen LJ, et al (Beth Israel Med Ctr, NY)
J Nerv Ment Dis 199:18-24, 2011

Little is known about the potentially unique sources of distress in populations seeking family-oriented treatment for bipolar disorder. The present study aimed to characterize this new treatment population by measuring depression, anxiety, quality of life, knowledge of bipolar disorder, therapeutic alliance, and mental illness stigma in 43 bipolar patients and 41 caregivers at family treatment intake. In all, 50% of patients and 27.6% of caregivers had significant depressive symptoms, whereas 51.2% of patients and 45.5% of caregivers had significant anxiety symptoms. Caregiver anxiety was inversely related to patient anxiety, stigma, and poor alliance. Treatment nonadherence was associated with more anxiety and stigma in patients and less anxiety in caregivers. In summary, family-oriented bipolar treatment seekers are significantly distressed at intake, and may benefit from lowering anxiety and stigma in patients and raising awareness and concern in caregivers. Future research should further clarify the complex relationships between caregiver and patient symptoms and attitudes (Table 4).

▶ Because family-oriented treatment identifies the family as the identified patient, it makes sense to explore what the sources of distress are for both the

TABLE 4.—Correlations Between Caregiver Distress Variables and Patient and Caregiver Treatment Targets

Caregiver Distress Variables	Patient Treatment Targets	df	r	p	Caregiver Treatment Targets	df	r	p
cCES-D	pBK	28	0.13	0.487	cBK	28	0.02	0.909
	pISMI	27	0.09	0.655	cISMI	26	0.26	0.192
	pPA	24	−0.30	0.150	—	—	—	—
cSTAI	pBK	32	0.19	0.292	cBK	23	0.02	0.937
	pISMI	31	−0.40	0.024*	cISMI	22	0.10	0.657
	pPA	27	−0.41	0.030*	—	—	—	—
cQ-LES-Q	pBK	29	0.14	0.456	cBK	29	0.11	0.547
	pISMI	29	−0.12	0.520	cISMI	28	−0.13	0.500
	pPA	26	−0.01	0.968	—	—	—	—

*$p < 0.05$.

family member with the psychiatric disorder, in this case bipolar spectrum disorders, and the family members who are participating in treatment because of this individual. Several studies, particularly about patients with schizophrenia, have found that family behavior has played an important role in helping or creating conditions that lead to relapse. I have a couple of methodological quibbles with the study design: (1) The researchers chose to make up their own alliance scale when there are existing measures with a good deal of data and (2) they used only a screening measure for depression rather than a diagnostic instrument to determine diagnosis. The study was exploratory, however, and the sample size was relatively small. In light of this, maybe gold standards in measure selection are not necessary. The most interesting part of the study is the finding that caregivers reporting more anxiety were linked to patients who were less depressed and reported better quality of life. As shown in Table 4, the researchers also found that more caregiver anxiety was associated with patients experiencing better alliance and less stigma. The authors of the article are quite creative in speculating about what might account for these surprising results.

J. L. Krupnick, PhD

Working with Parents: Implications for Individual Psychotherapeutic Work with Children and Adolescents
Ruberman L (Bronx Children's Psychiatric Ctr & Montefiore Med Ctr, NY)
Am J Psychother 63:345-362, 2009

Child psychotherapists recognize that working with parents is an indispensable part of working individually with child and adolescent patients. Children and adolescents are typically referred by their parents or other concerned adults. What tends to differ among clinicians is their approach to parents rather than the conviction of the importance of the parents' involvement. Historically, it was the "child guidance" movement early in the 20th century that initially impacted how clinicians work with parents and how this parent work can be integrated with individual child work. A different, but equally significant, impact came from the field of child psychoanalysis, despite the fact that "parent work" had not been the primary interest of its authors. This paper reviews 100 years of clinical writings in child psychoanalysis, highlighting its legacy for modern psychotherapists. In addition, I present several cases that stress the parent-child relationship in individual child and adolescent treatment to illustrate a clinically flexible approach to involving parents.

▶ Reading this article was a pleasure. It provides a review, primarily psychoanalytic/psychodynamic in perspective, of the history of psychotherapeutic work with children and their parents. Beginning with the child guidance movement of the early 20th century, it highlights the growth and evolution of psychotherapy with children and writing about their treatment. It nicely summarizes the main findings and conclusions of most of the major theoreticians and clinicians working in this area, from the early observations of analysts in Freud's circle to the more recent thinking of attachment theorists. Much of their writing influences not only current treatment with children and adolescents but has also been influential in thinking about and treating adult patients.

The author provides a number of clinical examples of work with parents of children with different types of problems and of different ages, including work with parents who are resistant to involvement in the therapeutic process. The different ways of conceptualizing the nature of the difficulties and intervening with parents is very useful. These examples provide a vivid description of various ways the child clinician can help his/her patient through direct work with a parent.

J. L. Krupnick, PhD

Cultural and Social Factors

National Trends in Outpatient Psychotherapy
Olfson M, Marcus SC (Columbia Univ, NY; New York State Psychiatric Inst; Univ of Pennsylvania, Philadelphia; et al)
Am J Psychiatry 167:1456-1463, 2010

Objective.—The authors investigated recent trends in the use of outpatient psychotherapy in the United States.

Method.—Service use data from two representative surveys of the U.S. general population, the 1998 (N=22,953) and 2007 (N=29,370) Medical Expenditure Panel Surveys, were analyzed, focusing on individuals who made more than one outpatient psychotherapy visit during that calendar year. The authors computed rates of any psychotherapy use; percentages of persons treated for mental health conditions with only psychotherapy, only psychotropic medication, or their combination; the mean number of psychotherapy visits of persons receiving psychotherapy; and psychotherapy expenditures.

TABLE 2.—U.S. National Trends in the Estimated Number and Percentage of Patients Treated With Psychotherapy, Psychotropic Medication, and Their Combination, by Treated Mental Health Condition Group, 1998 and 2007[a]

Treated Mental Health Condition (Ns for 1998 and 2007 MEPS)	1998 (Estimated N or %)	2007 (Estimated N or %)	Analysis z or Adjusted Odds Ratio[b]	p or 95% CI
Any mental health condition (N=1,407, N=2,203)	16,110,790	23,268,345	z=6.86	p<0.0001
Psychotherapy only (%)	15.9	10.5	0.66	0.48−0.90
Psychotherapy and medication (%)	40.0	32.1	0.73	0.59−0.90
Medication only (%)	44.1	57.4	1.63	1.32−2.00
Depressive disorders (N=560, N=860)	6,616,640	8,839,124	z=4.03	p<0.0001
Psychotherapy only (%)	8.5	6.3	0.59	0.48−1.27
Psychotherapy and medication (%)	50.5	42.5	0.78	0.59−1.03
Medication only (%)	41.0	51.2	1.39	1.04−1.86
Bipolar disorders (N=64, N=143)	706,423	1,504,390	z=4.10	p<0.0001
Psychotherapy only (%)	0	1.4	—	
Psychotherapy and medication (%)	88.6	67.5	0.26	0.09−0.77
Medication only (%)	11.4	31.1	3.54	1.21−10.40
Anxiety disorders (N=220, N=557)	2,608,363	6,027,100	z=8.24	p<0.0001
Psychotherapy only (%)	19.5	9.1	0.41	0.22−0.79
Psychotherapy and medication (%)	42.2	35.4	0.78	0.50−1.21
Medication only (%)	38.3	55.5	1.96	1.23−3.11
Adjustment disorders (N=120, N=157)	1,512,068	1,670,049	z=0.65	p=0.52
Psychotherapy only (%)	26.5	30.7	1.45	0.66−3.19
Psychotherapy and medication (%)	27.9	18.7	0.70	0.34−1.44
Medication only (%)	45.6	50.6	0.99	0.50−1.95
Schizophrenia disorders (N=47, N=77)	515,957	714,597	z=1.48	p=0.13
Psychotherapy only (%)	8.4	5.7	0.46	0.09−2.28
Psychotherapy and medication (%)	75.4	68.7	0.76	0.26−2.22
Medication only (%)	16.2	25.6	1.81	0.54−6.11
Childhood-onset disorders (N=243, N=362)	2,575,672	3,628,568	z=3.08	p=0.002
Psychotherapy only (%)	13.1	8.5	0.52	0.24−1.11
Psychotherapy and medication (%)	40.7	33.4	0.72	0.45−1.14
Medication only (%)	46.2	58.1	1.76	1.11−2.78
Other mental disorders (N=95, N=118)	1,097,806	1,258,266	z=0.82	p=0.21
Psychotherapy only (%)	20.2	10.6	0.39	0.13−1.23
Psychotherapy and medication (%)	39.9	38.7	1.01	0.45−2.28
Medication only (%)	39.9	50.7	1.60	0.68−3.76
Mental health-related conditions (N=330, N=514)	3,441,420	5,374,918	z=4.74	p<0.0001
Psychotherapy only (%)	24.2	8.8	0.36	0.17−0.77
Psychotherapy and medication (%)	25.3	20.3	0.78	0.47−1.27
Medication only (%)	50.5	70.9	2.14	1.37−3.34

[a]Data based on the 1998 and 2007 Medical Expenditure Panel Surveys (MEPS).
[b]Adjusted for age, sex, race/ethnicity, and insurance.

Results.—The percentage of persons using outpatient psychotherapy was 3.37% in 1998 and 3.18% in 2007 (adjusted odds ratio=0.95, 95% CI=0.82−1.09). Among individuals receiving outpatient mental health care, use of only psychotherapy (15.9% and 10.5% in 1998 and 2007, respectively; adjusted odds ratio=0.66, 95% CI=0.48−0.90) as well as psychotherapy and psychotropic medication together (40.0% and 32.1%; adjusted odds ratio=0.73, 95% CI=0.59−0.90) declined while use of only psychotropic medication increased (44.1% and 57.4%; adjusted odds ratio=1.63, 95% CI=1.32–2.00). Declines occurred in annual psychotherapy visits per psychotherapy patient (mean values, 9.7 and 7.9; adjusted $\beta=-1.53$, p<0.0001), mean expenditure per psychotherapy visit ($122.80 and $94.59; $\beta=28.21$, p<0.0001), and total national psychotherapy expenditures ($10.94 and $7.17 billion; z=2.61, p=0.009).

Conclusions.—During the decade from 1998 to 2007, the percentage of the general population who used psychotherapy remained stable. Over the same period, however, psychotherapy assumed a less prominent role in outpatient mental health care as a large and increasing proportion of mental health outpatients received psychotropic medication without psychotherapy (Table 2).

▶ It is interesting to read about the trends in mental health treatment, although the findings (Table 2) do not yield any big surprises. By looking at large-scale representative surveys, the authors found that the rate of psychotherapy use in the United States has remained quite stable from 1998 to 2007. There is a small minority of individuals who seek out psychosocial treatment, and the majority of those seek individual psychotherapy over family or group treatment.

The authors provide many good reasons for the trends, for example, an increase in people receiving psychotropic medication alone. They discuss issues such as stigma that, for all of the well-known people who have acknowledged that they suffer from mental illness and have received treatment, continue to play an important role in people's reluctance to seek help in the specialty mental health sector. Not only do pharmaceutical companies now advertise medications on television and in magazines, reaching a very wide audience, but also most people obtain psychotropic medications from their primary care physicians. Thus, people are influenced by advertising, and to obtain medication, they don't actually have to see a mental health professional. As the authors point out, there is also less of a burden to taking medications only. It is less expensive than taking medication and attending psychotherapy sessions, and it does not involve all of the logistics that weekly (or more) face-to-face encounters require. Thus, it was not surprising to see that more people are taking medication for mental disorders, but this increase is not evident in use of psychotherapy. Surely insurance coverage being limited for psychotherapy, especially among managed care companies, must play an important role in this as well.

J. L. Krupnick, PhD

3 Alcohol and Substance Abuse

Introduction

A major problem in the field is that fundamental advances such as new medications developed from translational bench research that have good effectiveness, such as naltrexone and suboxone, are not being used nearly enough by clinicians. What good will all of our new research be if it does not get to benefit the patient, who is suffering from an addiction and a dual diagnosis? A greater emphasis on evidence-based treatment in the addiction psychiatry field is long overdue.

It is also worth mentioning the increasing recognition of craving as an important factor in relapse and how it is triggered by both pleasurable and painful memories.

Richard J. Frances, MD

Neuroscience Advances

"A Disease Like Any Other"? A Decade of Change in Public Reactions to Schizophrenia, Depression, and Alcohol Dependence
Pescosolido BA, Martin JK, Long JS, et al (Indiana Univ, Bloomington; Columbia Univ, NY)
Am J Psychiatry 167:1321-1330, 2010

Objective.—Clinicians, advocates, and policy makers have presented mental illnesses as medical diseases in efforts to overcome low service use, poor adherence rates, and stigma. The authors examined the impact of this approach with a 10-year comparison of public endorsement of treatment and prejudice.

Method.—The authors analyzed responses to vignettes in the mental health modules of the 1996 and 2006 General Social Survey describing individuals meeting DSM-IV criteria for schizophrenia, major depression, and alcohol dependence to explore whether more of the public 1) embraces neurobiological understandings of mental illness; 2) endorses treatment from providers, including psychiatrists; and 3) reports community acceptance or rejection of people with these disorders. Multivariate analyses examined whether acceptance of neurobiological causes increased treatment support and lessened stigma.

Results.—In 2006, 67% of the public attributed major depression to neurobiological causes, compared with 54% in 1996. High proportions of respondents endorsed treatment, with general increases in the proportion endorsing treatment from doctors and specific increases in the proportions endorsing psychiatrists for treatment of alcohol dependence (from 61% in 1996 to 79% in 2006) and major depression (from 75% in 1996 to 85% in 2006). Social distance and perceived danger associated with people with these disorders did not decrease significantly. Holding a neurobiological conception of these disorders increased the likelihood of support for treatment but was generally unrelated to stigma. Where associated, the effect was to increase, not decrease, community rejection.

Conclusions.—More of the public embraces a neurobiological understanding of mental illness. This view translates into support for services but not into a decrease in stigma. Reconfiguring stigma reduction strategies may require providers and advocates to shift to an emphasis on competence and inclusion.

▶ The authors conclude that the general public increasingly perceives mental illness as a neurobiological entity. Perhaps the most relevant question is what caused these positive and dramatic changes, including acceptance of a disease model and positive views toward treatment, especially evidence-based treatment. Are these changes related to new science advances and the public seeing effective results from treatments and from positive changes in attitude? Are scientific spokespeople and media efforts, such as Charley Rose's series on the brain, having positive effects? Are institutes such as the National Institute on Drug Abuse, National Institute on Alcohol Abuse and Alcoholism, and National Institute of Mental Health becoming more effective at illuminating science and better informing the public about "brain diseases"? Did organizations such as the American Academy of Addiction Psychiatry, American Psychiatric Association, and the American College of Psychiatrists play a role in public and medical education that effected these improvements? My guess is all of these plus the fact that people "vote with their feet" and gravitate toward those treatments that really do help and make a difference in their lives.

R. J. Frances, MD

Association of Frontal and Posterior Cortical Gray Matter Volume With Time to Alcohol Relapse: A Prospective Study
Rando K, Hong K-I, Bhagwagar Z, et al (Yale Univ School of Medicine, New Haven, CT; Yale Child Study Ctr, New Haven, CT)
Am J Psychiatry 168:183-192, 2011

Objective.—Alcoholism is associated with gray matter volume deficits in frontal and other brain regions. Whether persistent brain volume deficits in abstinence are predictive of subsequent time to alcohol relapse has not been established. The authors measured gray matter volumes in healthy volunteers and in a sample of treatment-engaged, alcohol-dependent patients after 1 month of abstinence and assessed whether smaller frontal gray matter volume was predictive of subsequent alcohol relapse outcomes.

Method.—Forty-five abstinent alcohol-dependent patients in treatment and 50 healthy comparison subjects were scanned once using high-resolution (T_1-weighted) structural MRI, and voxel-based morphometry was used to assess regional brain volume differences between the groups. A prospective study design was used to assess alcohol relapse in the alcohol-dependent group for 90 days after discharge from 6 weeks of inpatient treatment.

Results.—Significantly smaller gray matter volume in alcohol-dependent patients relative to comparison subjects was seen in three regions: the medial frontal cortex, the right lateral prefrontal cortex, and a posterior region surrounding the parietal-occipital sulcus. Smaller medial frontal and parietal-occipital gray matter volumes were each predictive of shorter time to any alcohol use and to heavy drinking relapse.

Conclusions.—These findings are the first to demonstrate that gray matter volume deficits in specific medial frontal and posterior parietal-occipital brain regions are predictive of an earlier return to alcohol use and relapse risk, suggesting a significant role for gray matter atrophy in poor clinical outcomes in alcoholism. Extent of gray matter volume deficits in these regions could serve as useful neural markers of relapse risk and alcoholism treatment outcome.

▶ An old pathology professor of mine said, "Them that has, gets." This article finds with magnetic resonance evidence that alcohol-dependent patients have significantly smaller gray matter volume than control subjects and that those with greater deficits have poor clinical outcomes with increased risk of relapse (Fig 2 in the original article). However, try to explain this to a brilliant young alcoholic, and you will often hear many excuses and reasons not to worry. "I'm too smart already," and "who cares what happens tomorrow I want to live today." On the other hand, showing some the pictures can be like showing a smoker a black lung and increase their motivation to quit. The issue of treating these patients with vitamins and searching for neuroprotective pharmacologic approaches should also be considered and researched. These brain changes have many levels of effects on emotions, memory, judgment, social skills, and other factors that have an impact on these patients' lives.

R. J. Frances, MD

Childhood Risk Factors for Young Adult Substance Dependence Outcome in Offspring from Multiplex Alcohol Dependence Families: A Prospective Study

Hill SY, Steinhauer SR, Locke-Wellman J, et al (Univ of Pittsburgh School of Medicine, PA)
Biol Psychiatry 66:750-757, 2009

Background.—Age of onset to begin drinking is a known risk factor for alcohol dependence. Factors have been identified that contribute to age of onset to begin regular drinking. These include reduced P300, increased postural sway, and personality variation. A longitudinal study spanning childhood to young adulthood provided the opportunity to determine if these same factors would predict the presence and onset of substance use disorders (SUD).

Methods.—Multiplex families were identified through two or more alcohol-dependent brothers. Offspring from these multiplex or control families ($n = 133$) were followed annually during childhood. Using childhood predictors previously identified as risk factors for age of onset to begin drinking, SUD outcome by young adulthood was modeled.

Results.—Familial risk status was a significant predictor of young adult SUD outcome as a main effect and as an interaction with P300 amplitude recorded before the age of 13. In adolescence (age 15), increased postural sway and familial risk predicted the SUD outcome by age 22. Analysis comparing the presence of one or both risk factors showed that those above the median for sway and below the median for P300 amplitude had substantially increased odds of developing SUD (odds ratio = 8.08 [confidence interval = 1.52–42.83]).

Conclusions.—Our findings indicate that among the factors predicting age of onset to begin regular drinking, P300 predicts SUD outcome across an 11-year span. The present findings provide the longest follow-up to date demonstrating that neurobiological factors in childhood are among the most salient predictors of young adult SUD outcome.

▶ The search for biological and behavioral markers predictive from childhood of the risk for later addictive problems is of great relevance for targeting prevention programs and informing high-risk families what to watch for. Later onset of the use of substances such as alcohol and nicotine is protective against later development of addiction, even in families high at risk for problems. This 11-year longitudinal study of risk factors finds that both the P300 electroencephalogram marker and increased body sway are predictors of outcome after 11 years. With an 8-fold increase in problems when the marker is present, this is rapidly becoming a clinically significant finding. As public policy hopefully shifts in favor of prevention and early case finding, any and all measures should be taken that can find valid biological, genetic, and behavioral markers and develop effective prevention programs that will slow or prevent disease onset. Families at high risk should take measures to encourage the delay of onset of use by any means they can devise.

R. J. Frances, MD

Decision-Making Deficits Linked to Real-life Social Dysfunction in Crack Cocaine-Dependent Individuals

Cunha PJ, Bechara A, de Andrade AG, et al (Univ of São Paulo College of Medicine, Brazil; Univ of Southern California, Los Angeles, CA)
Am J Addict 20:78-86, 2011

Crack cocaine-dependent individuals (CCDI) present abnormalities in both social adjustment and decision making, but few studies have examined this association. This study investigated cognitive and social performance of 30 subjects (CCDI × controls); CCDI were abstinent for 2 weeks. We used the Social Adjustment Scale (SAS), Wisconsin Card Sorting Test (WCST), and Iowa Gambling Task (IGT). Disadvantageous choices on the IGT were associated with higher levels of social dysfunction in CCDI, suggesting the ecological validity of the IGT. Social dysfunction and decision making may be linked to the same underlying prefrontal dysfunction, but the nature of this association should be further investigated.

▶ This study finds a relationship between cocaine-induced abnormalities in cognitive function that affect both social adjustment and decision making and are mediated by the effects of cocaine on the prefrontal cortex (Fig 2). These effects last long after the last use of the drug. Clinically, this leads to risk-taking behavior, poor choices related to money, and poor social choices that frequently destabilizes marital relationships and families and puts society at risk in a host of ways, including increased criminal behavior. In my own private practice, I have seen a number of high-level Wall Street executives with cocaine problems rapidly make and lose fortunes and wreck their family lives as a result of their cocaine use. But because of their successes, it is hard to convince them of the damage to their judgment caused by their drug use. It is also difficult and frightening to imagine the indirect negative effects this kind of behavior is having on a large scale on our national economy.

R. J. Frances, MD

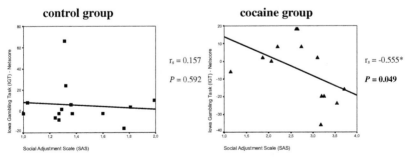

FIGURE 2.—Correlation between decision making and social adjustment among the control group and the cocaine group. *Notes: r_s:* Spearman correlation coefficient; **P* value < .05. (Reprinted from Cunha PJ, Bechara A, de Andrade AG, et al. Decision-making deficits linked to real-life social dysfunction in crack cocaine-dependent individuals. *Am J Addict.* 2011;20:78-86. John Wiley and Sons (www.interscience.wiley.com).)

Neural Correlates of Affect Processing and Aggression in Methamphetamine Dependence

Payer DE, Lieberman MD, London ED (Univ of California, Los Angeles (UCLA))
Arch Gen Psychiatry 68:271-282, 2011

Context.—Methamphetamine abuse is associated with high rates of aggression but few studies have addressed the contributing neurobiological factors.

Objective.—To quantify aggression, investigate function in the amygdala and prefrontal cortex, and assess relationships between brain function and behavior in methamphetamine-dependent individuals.

Design.—In a case-control study, aggression and brain activation were compared between methamphetamine-dependent and control participants.

Setting.—Participants were recruited from the general community to an academic research center.

Participants.—Thirty-nine methamphetamine-dependent volunteers (16 women) who were abstinent for 7 to 10 days and 37 drug-free control volunteers (18 women) participated in the study; subsets completed self-report and behavioral measures. Functional magnetic resonance imaging (fMRI) was performed on 25 methamphetamine-dependent and 23 control participants.

Main Outcome Measures.—We measured self-reported and perpetrated aggression and self-reported alexithymia. Brain activation was assessed using fMRI during visual processing of facial affect (affect matching) and symbolic processing (affect labeling), the latter representing an incidental form of emotion regulation.

Results.—Methamphetamine-dependent participants self-reported more aggression and alexithymia than control participants and escalated perpetrated aggression more following provocation. Alexithymia scores correlated with measures of aggression. During affect matching, fMRI showed no differences between groups in amygdala activation but found lower activation in methamphetamine-dependent than control participants in the bilateral ventral inferior frontal gyrus. During affect labeling, participants recruited the dorsal inferior frontal gyrus and exhibited decreased amygdala activity, consistent with successful emotion regulation; there was no group difference in this effect. The magnitude of decrease in amygdala activity during affect labeling correlated inversely with self-reported aggression in control participants and perpetrated aggression in all participants. Ventral inferior frontal gyrus activation correlated inversely with alexithymia in control participants.

Conclusions.—Contrary to the hypotheses, methamphetamine-dependent individuals may successfully regulate emotions through incidental means (affect labeling). Instead, low ventral inferior frontal gyrus activity may contribute to heightened aggression by limiting emotional insight.

▶ This article, using functional magnetic resonance imaging, finds that lack of emotional insight as a result of methamphetamine effects on the ventral inferior frontal gyrus area of the brain contributes to heightened aggression in methamphetamine-dependent individuals (Fig 3 in original article). It was surprising that methamphetamine-dependent individuals were able to regulate emotions and that this emotional insight deficit accounted for the increased aggression. The recent increased use of stimulants of many chemical varieties is becoming more prevalent, and combined with readily available dangerous weapons, including automatic guns, this poses a real societal danger. Also, we are seeing an increased tendency in many localities to liberalize drug laws and law enforcement, and the rapidly changing fads of new drugs coming out of laboratories may also increase the hazard to the public and especially to vulnerable younger people. They often may not be fully aware of the risks they are taking and inflicting on others when they use these dangerous drugs. Whether this kind of research can lead to pharmacologic or other treatment methods to counter the brain effects of the amphetamines is another fruitful area for further research.

R. J. Frances, MD

In Vivo Imaging of Cerebral Serotonin Transporter and Serotonin$_{2A}$ Receptor Binding in 3,4-Methylenedioxymethamphetamine (MDMA or "Ecstasy") and Hallucinogen Users

Erritzoe D, Frokjaer VG, Holst KK, et al (Copenhagen University Hospital Rigshospitalet, Denmark; Univ of Copenhagen, Denmark; et al)
Arch Gen Psychiatry 68:562-576, 2011

Context.—Both hallucinogens and 3,4-methylenedioxy-methamphetamine (MDMA or "ecstasy") have direct agonistic effects on postsynaptic serotonin$_{2A}$ receptors, the key site for hallucinogenic actions. In addition, MDMA is a potent releaser and reuptake inhibitor of presynaptic serotonin.

Objective.—To assess the differential effects of MDMA and hallucinogen use on cerebral serotonin transporter (SERT) and serotonin$_{2A}$ receptor binding.

Design.—A positron emission tomography study of 24 young adult drug users and 21 nonusing control participants performed with carbon 11 (^{11}C)—labeled 3-amino-4-[2-[(di(methyl)amino)methyl]phenyl] sulfanyl-benzonitrile (DASB) and fluorine 18 (^{18}F)—labeled altanserin, respectively. Scans were performed in the user group after a minimum drug abstinence period of 11 days, and the group was subdivided into hallucinogen-preferring users (n = 10) and MDMA-preferring users (n = 14).

Participants.—Twenty-four young adult users of MDMA and/or hallucinogenic drugs and 21 nonusing controls.

Main Outcome Measures.—In vivo cerebral SERT and serotonin$_{2A}$ receptor binding.

Results.—Compared with nonusers, MDMA-preferring users showed significant decreases in SERT nondisplaceable binding potential (neocortex, −56%; pallidostriatum, −19%; and amygdala, −32%); no significant changes were seen in hallucinogen-preferring users. Both cortical and pallidostriatal SERT nondisplaceable binding potential was negatively correlated with the number of lifetime MDMA exposures, and the time of abstinence from MDMA was positively correlated with subcortical, but not cortical, SERT binding. A small decrease in neocortical serotonin$_{2A}$ receptor binding in the serotonin$_{2A}$ receptor agonist users (both user groups) was also detected.

Conclusions.—We found evidence that MDMA but not hallucinogen use is associated with changes in the cerebral presynaptic serotonergic transmitter system. Because hallucinogenic drugs primarily have serotonin$_{2A}$ receptor agonistic actions, we conclude that the negative association between MDMA use and cerebral SERT binding is mediated through a direct presynaptic MDMA effect rather than by the serotonin$_{2A}$ agonistic effects of MDMA. Our cross-sectional data suggest that subcortical, but not cortical, recovery of SERT binding might take place after several months of MDMA abstinence.

▶ This is a really cool and certainly important study. It has major public health implications, as it carries a powerful message: drugs (actually in this case, only ecstasy) rot the brain. The study, which is elegantly and meticulously conducted, provides in vivo neuroimaging evidence that methylenedioxymethamphetamine (ecstasy) burns out the brain's serotonergic system (Figs 1 and 2 in the original article). This is consistent with the clinical evidence of the neurotoxicity of ecstasy as well as its evident clinical manifestations of serotonergic perturbations. I guess what I found particularly surprising was the relative absence of effect with other hallucinogenic drugs. These appeared relatively benign in terms of reducing cortical binding to the serotonergic marker. This study also shows direct effect between the duration and amount of ecstasy use. The neurotoxic damage to the cortical serotonergic is also compelling. It's kind of surprising to me that the media did not pick up on this one.

P. F. Buckley, MD

Risk Factors

Accounting for the association between childhood maltreatment and alcohol-use disorders in males: a twin study
Young-Wolff KC, Kendler KS, Ericson ML, et al (Univ of Southern California, Los Angeles, CA; Virginia Commonwealth Univ, Richmond)
Psychol Med 41:59-70, 2011

Background.—An association between childhood maltreatment and subsequent alcohol abuse and/or dependence (AAD) has been found in multiple studies of females. Less is known about the association between childhood maltreatment and AAD among males, and the mechanisms that underlie this association in either gender. One explanation is that childhood maltreatment increases risk for AAD. An alternative explanation is that the same genetic or environmental factors that increase a child's risk for being maltreated also contribute to risk for AAD in adulthood.

Method.—Lifetime diagnosis of AAD was assessed using structured clinical interviews in a sample of 3527 male participants aged 19-56 years from the Virginia Adult Twin Study of Psychiatric and Substance Use Disorders. The sources of childhood maltreatment-AAD association were estimated using both a matched case-control analysis of twin pairs discordant for childhood maltreatment and bivariate twin modeling.

Results.—Approximately 9% of participants reported childhood maltreatment, defined as serious neglect, molestation, or physical abuse occurring before the age of 15 years. Those who experienced childhood maltreatment were 1.74 times as likely to meet AAD criteria compared with males who did not experience childhood maltreatment. The childhood maltreatment-AAD association largely reflected environmental factors in common to members of twin pairs. Additional exploratory analyses provided evidence that AAD risk associated with childhood maltreatment was significantly attenuated after adjusting for measured family-level risk factors.

Conclusions.—Males who experienced childhood maltreatment had an increased risk for AAD. Our results suggest that the childhood maltreatment-AAD association is attributable to broader environmental adversity shared between twins.

▶ This is the first study that looks at environmental, genetic, and the 2 factors jointly as contributors to the causation of how childhood maltreatment leads to increased risk of subsequent alcohol abuse/dependence (AAD) in males. Although the contribution of child abuse to AAD in women has been widely reported, there has been less attention paid to this problem in males and this large N twin study provides ways to parcel out the genetic versus environmental impacts that might lead to the 1.7 increased odds ratio in males of developing AAD when childhood maltreatment has preceded onset of AAD problems. The finding of the principal role of environmental factors in the risk of AAD with childhood mistreatment, which can be attenuated after adjusting for family-level risk factors, provides hope that intervention at various levels making environmental adjustments could lead to reduced childhood mistreatment and reduced AAD. One point I found myself questioning was the report here that only 9% of participants reported childhood maltreatment. I wondered whether the real percentage might be much higher given the tendency to deny and underreport serious childhood problems especially in families with AAD. The methodology of using twin registries to parcel out genetic, environmental, and combined vulnerabilities and risk factors has been fruitful, and this group of researchers deserves great credit for having been leaders and pioneers in applying this kind of research in addiction and other areas of psychiatry.

R. J. Frances, MD

Addiction as a Systems Failure: Focus on Adolescence and Smoking
Baler RD, Volkow ND (Natl Insts of Health, Bethesda, MD)
J Am Acad Child Adolesc Psychiatry 50:329-339, 2011

Objective.—Scientific advances in the field of addiction have forever debunked the notion that addiction reflects a character flaw under voluntary control, demonstrating instead that it is a bona fide disease of the brain. The aim of this review is to go beyond this consensus understanding and explore the most current evidence regarding the vast number of genetic, developmental, and environmental factors whose complex interactions modulate addiction risk and trajectory.

Method.—Focusing on childhood and adolescent smoking as a paradigm, we review the important risk factors for the development of addictions, starting at the level of genetics and closing with a focus on sociocultural and policy factors.

Results.—A critical review of the pertinent literature provides a detailed view of the cumulative power of risk and protection factors across different phenomenological levels to modulate the risk of undesirable outcomes, particularly for young people. The result represents a compelling argument for the need to engage in comprehensive, multilevel approaches to promoting health.

Conclusions.—Today, the field of medicine understands more about disease than about health; however it need not be that way. The view of drug addiction as a systems failure should help refocus our general approach to developing dynamic models and early comprehensive interventions that optimize the ways in which we prevent and treat a complex, developmental disorder such as drug addiction.

▶ This article is a sophisticated review of how addiction as a model disease can be looked at with a systems approach, including factors such as genetic, developmental, environmental, social, and cultural, all of which all are necessary components of a full understanding of the disease and for developing a means of intervening (Fig 1 in the original article). For example, a greater understanding of the genetics of smoking and its influence on adolescence is revealing a polygenic contribution, which may eventually lead to personalized pharmacologic interventions tailored to the individual's genetic makeup. Interventions focused on child development and family and peer groups, as well as those aimed at a societal level, are other system levels that are important to bring to bear when attacking the complexities of drug addiction. The complexity and multiplicity of systems involved is one of the things that make a career choice of working in the addiction field so interesting. To fully understand addiction, one must learn about so much on so many levels! Few have done so with the skill and persistence of Nora Volkow.

R. J. Frances, MD

Patterns and Predictors of Alcohol Use in Male and Female Urban Police Officers
Ballenger JF, Best SR, Metzler TJ, et al (Dept of Veterans Affairs Med Ctr, San Francisco, CA; et al)
Am J Addict 20:21-29, 2010

In a large sample of urban police officers, 18.1% of males and 15.9% of females reported experiencing adverse consequences from alcohol use and 7.8% of the sample met criteria for lifetime alcohol abuse or dependence. Female officers had patterns of alcohol use similar to male officers and substantially more than females in the general population. Critical incident exposure and posttraumatic stress disorder (PTSD) symptoms were not associated with level of alcohol use. Greater psychiatric symptoms were related to adverse consequences from alcohol use. There was a noteworthy gender by work stress interaction: greater routine work stress related to lower current alcohol use in female officers.

▶ There are many reasons why studying alcohol and addiction problems in critical professions is important, and this well-done large study of urban police in America sheds light on the drinking issues faced by police. It is not surprising that police have more problems with alcohol than the general population. The sensation-seeking, risk-taking aspects of the profession make the choice of becoming a police officer a natural one for those genetically prone to addiction. In addition, the stresses of the job, whether leading to posttraumatic stress disorder or not, along with a culture of drinking among law enforcement professionals, could contribute to these high rates. Police and firefighters tend not to drink during the day; however, when later realizing the dangers they faced, strong whiskey may seem like a good idea to them. The most striking finding in this study was the very high rates of alcohol use and risk for problem drinking in women compared with the general population. Is this a particular hazard for women police officers alone or for women acculturated to the drinking culture in fields that in the past had been predominantly occupied by men? Given the fact that police carry guns, are trusted to behave responsibly, and need to have good self-control, the prevention, early detection, and treatment of alcohol problems in police should be a high priority. Police employee assistance programs and health benefits have been weakened in recent years and more attention needs to be paid to funding these efforts.

R. J. Frances, MD

Association Between Opioid Prescribing Patterns and Opioid Overdose-Related Deaths

Bohnert ASB, Valenstein M, Bair MJ, et al (Serious Mental Illness Treatment Resource and Evaluation Ctr, Ann Arbor, MI; Dept of Veterans Affairs, HSR&D Ctr of Excellence, Indianapolis, IN; et al)
JAMA 305:1315-1321, 2011

Context.—The rate of prescription opioid-related overdose death increased substantially in the United States over the past decade. Patterns of opioid prescribing may be related to risk of overdose mortality.

Objective.—To examine the association of maximum prescribed daily opioid dose and dosing schedule ("as needed," regularly scheduled, or both) with risk of opioid overdose death among patients with cancer, chronic pain, acute pain, and substance use disorders.

Design.—Case-cohort study.

Setting.—Veterans Health Administration (VHA), 2004 through 2008.

Participants.—All unintentional prescription opioid overdose decedents (n = 750) and a random sample of patients (n = 154 684) among those individuals who used medical services in 2004 or 2005 and received opioid therapy for pain.

TABLE 1.—Characteristics of the Sample of Veterans Health Administration Patients Receiving Opioid Therapy

	No. (%)		
Characteristic	Opioid Overdose Decedents (n = 750)	All Others (n = 154 684)	P Value
Male sex	700 (93.3)	144 304 (93.3)	.96
Age, y			
18-29	31 (4.1)	3995 (2.6)	<.001
30-39	60 (8.0)	8407 (5.4)	
40-49	313 (41.7)	23 888 (15.4)	
50-59	297 (39.6)	50 216 (32.5)	
60-69	38 (5.1)	29 985 (19.4)	
≥70	11 (1.5)	38 183 (24.7)	
Race			
Black	52 (6.9)	25 409 (16.4)	<.001
White	625 (83.3)	110 965 (71.7)	
Other/missing	73 (9.7)	18 310 (11.8)	
Hispanic ethnicity	23 (3.1)	6342 (4.1)	.15
Pain-related diagnoses[a]			
Cancer	91 (12.1)	36 712 (23.7)	<.001
Chronic bodily pains	588 (78.4)	107 158 (69.3)	<.001
Headache	90 (12.0)	10 208 (6.6)	<.001
Neuropathy	32 (4.3)	8339 (5.4)	.17
Injuries and acute pain	222 (29.6)	29 522 (19.1)	<.001
Other diagnoses[a]			
Substance use disorders	296 (39.5)	15 195 (9.8)	<.001
Other psychiatric disorders	498 (66.4)	51 929 (33.6)	<.001
COPD, CVD, and sleep apnea	467 (62.3)	123 025 (79.5)	<.001

Abbreviations: COPD, chronic obstructive pulmonary disease; CVD, cardiovascular disease.

[a]All conditions were measured in the year up to and including the first opioid fill during the observation period and are not mutually exclusive.

TABLE 2.—Unadjusted Rate of Prescription Opioid Overdose Death by Opioid Dose and Fill Type

	Overdose Deaths, No.	Person-Months	Overdose Death Rate per 1000 Person-Months (95% CI)
Patients With Chronic Noncancer Pain Diagnoses			
Maximum prescribed daily opioid dose, mg/d			
0	243	2 729 022.7	0.09 (0.08-0.10)
1-<20	44	395 205.0	0.11 (0.08-0.15)
20-<50	108	458 296.2	0.24 (0.19-0.28)
50-<100	86	129 491.6	0.66 (0.53-0.82)
≥100	125	100 479.3	1.24 (1.04-1.48)
Fill types			
Regularly scheduled only	115	323 304.7	0.36 (0.29-0.43)
As needed only	152	672 276.0	0.23 (0.19-0.27)
Simultaneous as needed and regularly scheduled	96	87 891.5	1.09 (0.88-1.33)
Patients With Cancer Diagnoses			
Maximum prescribed daily opioid dose, mg/d			
0	32	859 278.3	0.04 (0.03-0.05)
1-<20	7	91 108.9	0.08 (0.03-0.16)
20-<50	14	96 778.6	0.14 (0.08-0.24)
50-<100	14	28 809.7	0.49 (0.27-0.82)
≥100	24	24 380.1	0.98 (0.63-1.46)
Fill types			
Regularly scheduled only	11	68 153.9	0.16 (0.08-0.29)
As needed only	31	151 865.6	0.20 (0.14-0.29)
Simultaneous as needed and regularly scheduled	17	21 057.9	0.81 (0.47-1.29)
Patients With Acute Pain Diagnoses			
Maximum prescribed daily opioid dose, mg/d			
0	97	786 769.5	0.12 (0.10-0.15)
1-<20	17	81 006.8	0.21 (0.12-0.34)
20-<50	33	95 109.1	0.36 (0.25-0.50)
50-<100	41	29 080.7	1.13 (0.78-1.59)
≥100		22 537.9	1.82 (1.31-2.47)
Fill types			
Regularly scheduled only	42	65 163.2	0.64 (0.46-0.87)
As needed only	52	142 311.5	0.37 (0.27-0.48)
Simultaneous as needed and regularly scheduled	31	20 259.8	1.53 (1.04-2.17)
Patients With Substance Use Disorder Diagnoses			
Maximum prescribed daily opioid dose, mg/d			
0	159	378 244.9	0.42 (0.36-0.49)
1-<20	24	44 630.0	0.54 (0.34-0.80)
20-<50	42	53 584.0	0.78 (0.56-1.06)
50-<100	27	17 019.2	1.59 (1.05-2.31)
≥100	44	14 809.2	2.97 (2.16-3.99)
Fill types			
Regularly scheduled only	44	38 722.0	1.14 (0.83-1.53)
As needed only	59	78 314.2	0.75 (0.57-0.97)
Simultaneous as needed and regularly scheduled	34	13 006.3	2.61 (1.81-3.65)

Abbreviation: CI, confidence interval.

Main Outcome Measure.—Associations of opioid regimens (dose and schedule) with death by unintentional prescription opioid overdose in subgroups defined by clinical diagnoses, adjusting for age group, sex, race, ethnicity, and comorbid conditions.

Results.—The frequency of fatal overdose over the study periodamongindividuals treated with opioids was estimated to be 0.04%. The risk of overdose death was directly related to the maximum prescribed daily dose of opioid medication. The adjusted hazard ratios (HRs) associated with a maximum prescribed dose of 100 mg/d or more, compared with the dose category 1 mg/d to less than 20 mg/d, were as follows: among those with substance use disorders, adjusted HR = 4.54 (95% confidence interval [CI], 2.46-8.37; absolute risk difference approximation [ARDA] = 0.14%); among those with chronic pain, adjusted HR = 7.18 (95% CI, 4.85-10.65; ARDA = 0.25%); among those with acute pain, adjusted HR = 6.64 (95% CI, 3.31-13.31; ARDA = 0.23%); and among those with cancer, adjusted HR = 11.99 (95% CI, 4.42-32.56; ARDA = 0.45%). Receiving both as-needed and regularly scheduled doses was not associated with overdose risk after adjustment.

Conclusion.—Among patients receiving opioid prescriptions for pain, higher opioid doses were associated with increased risk of opioid overdose death (Tables 1 and 2).

▶ This is a great example of the value of the Veterans Affairs (VA) database and electronic medical records for conducting health services research that can directly inform clinical care. Obviously, the choice of topic is highly significant and of great relevance, especially to patients in the VA, a great number of whom have pain problems. The data are intuitive (Tables 1 and 2) in the sense that those patients who are prescribed more opioids are more likely to have overdose-related deaths. On the other hand, the data do not discriminate as to whether these deaths are caused by unintentional overdose or intentional suicide; this is important in describing which patients are most at risk, so that, for instance, clinicians could be more judicious in prescribing the amount and/or formulation of opioids for some given subgroups of patients. This work is most welcome in such a stellar journal as *JAMA*, especially as quality and safety take a more center stage role in research activities at academic medical centers.

P. F. Buckley, MD

Dual Diagnosis

Long-term Antipsychotic Treatment and Brain Volumes: A Longitudinal Study of First-Episode Schizophrenia
Ho B-C, Andreasen NC, Ziebell S, et al (Univ of Iowa Carver College of Medicine)
Arch Gen Psychiatry 68:128-137, 2011

Context.—Progressive brain volume changes in schizophrenia are thought to be due principally to the disease. However, recent animal studies indicate that antipsychotics, the mainstay of treatment for schizophrenia patients, may also contribute to brain tissue volume decrement. Because antipsychotics are prescribed for long periods for schizophrenia patients

TABLE 2.—Random Regression Coefficient Mixed Models: Fixed Effects of Follow-up Duration, APS Treatment, Illness Severity, and Substance Misuse on MRI Brain Volumes in 211 Schizophrenia Patients[a]

Regions of Interest	Follow-up Duration[b] b[g] (SE)	F (P)	APS Treatment[c] b (SE)	F (P)	Illness Severity[d] b (SE)	F (P)	Substance Misuse[e] b (SE)	F (P)	APS × Time[f] b (SE)	F (P)
Total cerebral tissue	−1.62 (0.37)	18.80 (<.001)	−0.11 (0.07)	2.39 (.12)	0.49 (0.26)	3.65 (.06)	4.81 (4.67)	1.06 (.30)	−0.03 (0.01)	4.29 (.04)
Total cerebral GM	−1.80 (0.26)	46.61 (<.001)	−0.15 (0.05)	8.11 (.005)	0.39 (0.18)	4.38 (.04)	1.56 (3.32)	0.22 (.64)	0.008 (0.01)	0.74 (.39)
Frontal GM	−1.04 (0.13)	62.44 (<.001)	−0.07 (0.03)	6.67 (.01)	0.27 (0.10)	6.94 (.01)	0.99 (1.83)	0.29 (.59)	0.0005 (0.005)	0.01 (.93)
Temporal GM	−0.15 (0.06)	6.43 (.01)	−0.03 (0.01)	4.33 (.04)	0.07 (0.05)	1.86 (.17)	−1.00 (0.88)	1.29 (.26)	0.001 (0.002)	0.18 (.67)
Parietal GM	−0.47 (0.07)	45.48 (<.001)	−0.03 (0.01)	4.75 (.03)	0.09 (0.06)	2.20 (.14)	0.56 (1.07)	0.27 (.60)	0.003 (0.003)	1.17 (.28)
Total cerebral WM	0.16 (0.32)	0.27 (.61)	0.05 (0.06)	0.66 (.42)	0.19 (0.24)	0.68 (.41)	2.98 (4.27)	0.49 (.49)	−0.04 (0.01)	10.34 (.001)
Frontal WM	−0.18 (0.13)	2.03 (.16)	0.01 (0.03)	0.13 (.72)	0.07 (0.11)	0.37 (.54)	1.16 (1.97)	0.34 (.56)	−0.01 (0.005)	6.11 (.01)
Temporal WM	0.05 (0.05)	1.17 (.28)	0.01 (0.01)	1.50 (.22)	0.02 (0.04)	0.30 (.58)	−0.16 (0.76)	0.05 (.83)	−0.006 (0.002)	8.08 (.005)
Parietal WM	0.18 (0.08)	5.39 (.02)	0.03 (0.02)	3.19 (.08)	0.06 (0.07)	0.65 (.42)	1.70 (1.31)	1.67 (.20)	−0.01 (0.003)	13.40 (<.001)
Lateral ventricles	0.27 (0.06)	24.27 (<.001)	−0.01 (0.01)	0.68 (.41)	0.00 (0.06)	0.01 (.94)	2.44 (1.03)	5.60 (.02)	0.003 (0.002)	3.79 (.05)
Sulcal CSF	2.01 (0.23)	78.78 (<.001)	−0.02 (0.04)	0.27 (.61)	−0.16 (0.21)	0.56 (.45)	0.14 (3.77)	0.00 (.97)	0.02 (0.01)	6.95 (.01)
Caudate	−0.01 (0.00)	8.92 (.003)	0.00 (0.00)	0.47 (.49)	0.00 (0.00)	0.69 (.41)	0.03 (0.07)	0.17 (.68)	−0.0003 (0.0001)	4.27 (.04)
Putamen	−0.03 (0.01)	7.73 (.01)	0.01 (0.00)	21.32 (<.001)	−0.01 (0.01)	0.70 (.40)	0.06 (0.14)	0.20 (.66)	0.0008 (0.0004)	5.63 (.02)
Thalamus	−0.05 (0.01)	30.86 (<.001)	0.00 (0.00)	0.44 (.51)	0.00 (0.01)	0.14 (.71)	0.13 (0.12)	1.08 (.30)	−0.0006 (0.0003)	3.67 (.06)
Cerebellum	0.00 (0.04)	0.00 (.95)	0.01 (0.01)	0.31 (.58)	−0.10 (0.08)	1.54 (.22)	−3.25 (1.39)	5.48 (.02)	−0.0053 (0.0017)	9.28 (.002)

Abbreviations: APS, antipsychotic; CSF, cerebrospinal fluid; GM, gray matter; MRI, magnetic resonance imaging; WM, white matter.
[a] Covariates: intracranial volume at intake scan, sex, imaging protocol, and age at intake scan; random effects: follow-up duration and an intercept term to model within-patient correlations in brain volumes across time (unstructured covariance structure).
[b] Interscan interval since initial MRI brain scan (days).
[c] Lifetime APS treatment up to the time of MRI scan acquisition (mean daily APS treatment; chlorpromazine milligram equivalents per day).
[d] Mean Global Assessment Scale score during follow-up period.
[e] Mean severity of alcohol and illicit substance misuse during follow-up period (6-point rating scale: 0, none; 1, occasional use; 2, occasional heavy use; 3, mild impairment; 4, moderate impairment; and 5, severe impairment).
[f] Antipsychotic treatment × follow-up duration interaction term.
[g] Estimate of regression coefficient or slope.

and have increasingly widespread use in other psychiatric disorders, it is imperative to determine their long-term effects on the human brain.

Objective.—To evaluate relative contributions of 4 potential predictors (illness duration, antipsychotic treatment, illness severity, and substance abuse) of brain volume change.

Design.—Predictors of brain volume changes were assessed prospectively based on multiple informants.

Setting.—Data from the Iowa Longitudinal Study.

Patients.—Two hundred eleven patients with schizophrenia who underwent repeated neuroimaging beginning soon after illness onset, yielding a total of 674 high-resolution magnetic resonance scans. On average, each patient had 3 scans ($\geq$2 and as many as 5) over 7.2 years (up to 14 years).

Main Outcome Measure.—Brain volumes.

Results.—During longitudinal follow-up, antipsychotic treatment reflected national prescribing practices in 1991 through 2009. Longer follow-up correlated with smaller brain tissue volumes and larger cerebrospinal fluid volumes. Greater intensity of antipsychotic treatment was associated with indicators of generalized and specific brain tissue reduction after controlling for effects of the other 3 predictors. More antipsychotic treatment was associated with smaller gray matter volumes. Progressive decrement in white matter volume was most evident among patients who received more antipsychotic treatment. Illness severity had relatively modest correlations with tissue volume reduction, and alcohol/illicit drug misuse had no significant associations when effects of the other variables were adjusted.

Conclusions.—Viewed together with data from animal studies, our study suggests that antipsychotics have a subtle but measurable influence on brain tissue loss over time, suggesting the importance of careful risk-benefit review of dosage and duration of treatment as well as their off-label use (Table 2).

▶ This study has several counterintuitive but important findings. First, if our current medications were altering the course of the disease of schizophrenia, one might have hoped that they would reverse or slow down some of the decrement of white matter that occurs with progression of the disease. On the contrary, in this study, when controlled for several other factors, including substance abuse, which is very common in schizophrenia, medications in a dose-related way further decrease brain volumes. In addition, it is surprising that alcohol and substance use did not also have an association as one might have expected (Table 2). Other studies have found substances of abuse to also cause decreased brain volumes. We need to find drugs that will promote neurogenisis and that might alter the process of severe mental illnesses, and we are farther away from that goal than I'd hoped.

R. J. Frances, MD

The Emerging Link Between Alcoholism Risk and Obesity in the United States

Grucza RA, Krueger RF, Racette SB, et al (Washington Univ School of Medicine, St Louis, MO)

Arch Gen Psychiatry 67:1301-1308, 2010

Context.—The prevalence of obesity has risen sharply in the United States in the past few decades. Etiologic links between obesity and substance use disorders have been hypothesized.

Objective.—To determine whether familial risk of alcohol dependence predicts obesity and whether any such association became stronger between the early 1990s and early 2000s.

Design.—We conducted analyses of the repeated cross-sectional National Longitudinal Alcohol Epidemiologic Survey (1991-1992) and National Epidemiologic Survey on Alcohol and Related Conditions (2001-2002).

Setting.—The noninstitutionalized US adult population in 1991-1992 and 2001-2002.

Participants.—Individuals drawn from population-based, multistage, random samples (N = 39 312 and 39 625).

Main Outcome Measure.—Obesity, defined as a body mass index (calculated from self-reported data as weight in kilograms divided by height in meters squared) of 30 or higher and predicted from family history of alcoholism and/or problem drinking.

Results.—In 2001-2002, women with a family history of alcoholism (defined as having a biological parent or sibling with a history of alcoholism or alcohol problems) had 49% higher odds of obesity than those without a family history (odds ratio, 1.48; 95% confidence interval, 1.36-1.61; $P < .001$), a highly significant increase ($P < .001$) from the odds ratio of 1.06 (95% confidence interval, 0.97-1.16) estimated for 1991-1992. For men in 2001-2002, the association was significant (odds ratio, 1.26; 95% confidence interval, 1.14-1.38; $P < .001$) but not as strong as for women. The association and the secular trend for women were robust after adjustment for covariates, including sociodemographic variables, smoking status, alcohol use, alcohol or drug dependence, and major depression. Similar trends were observed for men but did not meet statistical significance criteria after adjustment for covariates.

Conclusions.—These results provide epidemiologic support for a link between familial alcoholism risk and obesity in women and possibly in men. This link has emerged in recent years and may result from an interaction between a changing food environment and predisposition to alcoholism and related disorders (Table 2).

▶ There is growing evidence of a link between obesity and alcoholism risk, especially in women (Table 2). This study found a 49% higher odds ratio of obesity when a family history of alcoholism is also present in women, and a 1.26 odds ratio in men, which was less strong. The idea that looking for a dopamine high as a common denominator in addiction is among the factors

TABLE 2.—Prevalence of Obesity by FHA: 1991-1992 and 2001-2002

| | NLAES (1991-1992) | | | | NESARC (2001-2002) | | | |
| | | Prevalence, % (SE) | | OR (95% CI) | | Prevalence, % (SE) | | OR (95% CI) |
	No. of Participants	No FHA	FHA	(FHA vs No FHA)	No. of Participants	No FHA	FHA	(FHA vs No FHA)
Women	22 182	15.4 (0.4)	16.1 (0.5)	1.06 (0.97-1.16)	21 975	20.8 (0.5)	28.0 (0.7)	1.48 (1.36-1.61)[a,b]
Men	17 130	13.9 (0.4)	14.9 (0.6)	1.08 (0.97-1.22)	17 650	21.4 (0.6)	25.5 (0.7)	1.26 (1.14-1.38)[a,c]
Total	39 312	14.6 (0.3)	15.6 (0.4)	1.08 (1.00-1.15)[d]	39 625	21.1 (0.5)	26.9 (0.5)	1.37 (1.28-1.47)[a,b]

Abbreviations: CI, confidence interval; FHA, family history of alcoholism; NESARC, National Epidemiologic Survey on Alcohol and Related Conditions; NLAES, National Longitudinal Alcohol Epidemiologic Survey; OR, odds ratio.
[a]P<.001.
[b]NESARC OR differs from NLAES with P<.001.
[c]NESARC OR differs from NLAES with P=.05.
[d]P=.05.

that has led many to want to include binge eating as an addictive disorder. There may be other intervening variables and stressors in these families that account for the increase. For example, daughters and sisters of alcoholics frequently have suffered physical or emotional abuse or neglect, which may also make them more prone to depression and to overeat in addition to a higher vulnerability to substance abuse.

R. J. Frances, MD

Assessing the Prevalence of Nonmedical Prescription Opioid Use in the General Canadian Population: Methodological Issues and Questions
Fischer B, Nakamura N, Ialomiteanu A, et al (Simon Fraser Univ, Vancouver, British Columbia; Centre for Addiction and Mental Health, Toronto, Ontario; et al)
Can J Psychiatry 55:606-609, 2010

Objective.—To assess the prevalence of nonmedical prescription opioid use (NMPOU) in the Canadian general adult population in the context of rising overall prescription opioid (PO) consumption and related problems in North America.

Method.—The prevalence of NMPOU was assessed as a multiitem construct in the Canadian Alcohol and Drug Use Monitoring Survey (CADUMS; $n = 16\,672$), an ongoing cross-sectional monthly random digit dialing telephone survey representative of the general Canadian population, aged 15 years and older. CADUMS data were collected between April and December of 2008 with a response rate of 43.5%.

Results.—About 22% of CADUMS respondents reported PO use in the last year, while 0.5% reported NMPOU during the same time frame. PO use was significantly higher among women than among men, and highest in the group aged 25 to 54 years. NMPOU was similar among men and women, and highest in the group aged 15 to 24 years.

Conclusions.—CADUMS data indicate an extremely low rate of NMPOU, especially given the levels of overall PO use, other PO-use related problems, and NMPOU levels estimated in the general US population where NMPOU has been assessed to be 10 times higher than in Canada. NMPOU survey item construction and response rates appear to strongly influence and potentially compromise NMPOU survey data. Existing NMPOU data and survey methods need to be validated for this important indicator in Canada, where increasing PO use and problem levels have been recognized as a significant and rising public health problem.

▶ Well, Canada may be a clean country but even so, the results of this study are remarkable! The study reports an abuse rate of opioids at 0.5% among a broad-based sample (16 672) of the Canadian population. I have highlighted this study not so much for its findings but rather as a good illustration of the difficulties in conducting epidemiological field trials! In essence, this study sought to replicate for Canada, the previously published North American Study of Household

Drug use that was conducted several years ago by the Substance Abuse and Mental Health Services Administration. However, this Canadian study had a disappointing response rate of approximately 43%. Additionally, it sampled young teenagers who were likely, for obvious reasons, to underreport any opioid abuse. Indeed, one might ask whether a telephone survey to obtain this kind of information could be valid anyway. If I was called up out of the blue, I certainly wouldn't give this information over the phone. This is a tricky line of research.

P. F. Buckley, MD

Identifying prescription opioid use disorder in primary care: Diagnostic characteristics of the Current Opioid Misuse Measure (COMM)
Meltzer EC, Rybin D, Saitz R, et al (Boston Univ School of Medicine, MA; Boston Univ School of Public Health, MA)
Pain 152:397-402, 2011

The Current Opioid Misuse Measure (COMM), a self-report assessment of past-month aberrant medication-related behaviors, has been validated in specialty pain management patients. The performance characteristics of the COMM were evaluated in primary care (PC) patients with chronic pain. It was hypothesized that the COMM could identify patients with prescription drug use disorder (PDD). English-speaking adults awaiting PC visits at an urban, safety-net hospital, who had chronic pain and had received any opioid analgesic prescription in the past year, were administered the COMM. The Composite International Diagnostic Interview served as the "gold standard," using DSM-IV criteria for PDD and other substance use disorders (SUDs). A receiver operating characteristic (ROC) curve demonstrated the COMM's diagnostic test characteristics. Of the 238 participants, 27 (11%) met DSM-IV PDD criteria, whereas 17 (7%) had other SUDs, and 194 (82%) had no disorder. The mean COMM score was higher in those with PDD than among all others (ie, those with other SUDs or no disorder, mean 20.4 [SD 10.8] vs 8.4 [SD 7.5], $P < .0001$). A COMM score of ≥ 13 had a sensitivity of 77% and a specificity of 77% for identifying patients with PDD. The area under the ROC curve was 0.84. For chronic pain patients prescribed opioids, the development of PDD is an undesirable complication. Among PC patients with chronic pain-prescribed prescription opioids, the COMM is a promising tool for identifying those with PDD (Table 2).

▶ I found this a particularly interesting study, addressing an important clinical question: is there a reliable questionnaire to detect prescription drug abuse among patients receiving health care (in this instance primary care)? The results are generally encouraging. This scale, the Current Opioid Misuse Measure (COMM), fared well with a COMMscore above 13, achieving a sensitivity of 77% and a specificity of 77% for detecting prescription drug users. Of course, the study has many drawbacks: the one short evaluation, the overreliance on medical records, and the relatively small group of patients who met the criteria

TABLE 2.—COMM Prediction Score vs DSM-IV Diagnosis

COMM Score	Sensitivity	Specificity	PPV	NPV	Positive Likelihood Ratio	Negative Likelihood Ratio
7	0.961	0.484	0.196	0.989	1.866	0.079
8	0.884	0.540	0.201	0.972	1.924	0.213
9	0.846	0.595	0.215	0.967	2.094	0.258
10	0.807	0.646	0.230	0.962	2.284	0.297
11	0.802	0.681	0.25	0.964	2.538	0.282
12	0.807	0.712	0.269	0.965	2.805	0.270
13	0.769	0.767	0.303	0.962	3.311	0.300
14	0.692	0.813	0.327	0.952	3.704	0.3784
15	0.692	0.843	0.367	0.954	4.421	0.364
16	0.615	0.858	0.363	0.944	4.351	0.447
17	0.576	0.873	0.375	0.940	4.569	0.484

for drug use anyway. Nevertheless, these results are encouraging. One could anticipate the COMM being used as a screening tool in high-risk hospital patients, especially those frequenting pain clinics.

P. F. Buckley, MD

Methamphetamine Self-Administration Produces Attentional Set-Shifting Deficits and Alters Prefrontal Cortical Neurophysiology in Rats

Parsegian A, Glen WB Jr, Lavin A, et al (Med Univ of South Carolina, Charleston)
Biol Psychiatry 69:253-259, 2011

Background.—Chronic methamphetamine abusers exhibit deficits in tasks requiring intact prefrontal cortex function, and prefrontal cortex dysfunction has been implicated in the loss of control over drug use. This study used a combination of behavioral and electrophysiologic assessments in rats with a history of long access methamphetamine self-administration to determine methamphetamine-induced changes in prefrontal cortex-dependent attentional set-shifting performance, drug-seeking, and prefrontal cortex neuronal activity.

Methods.—Male Long-Evans rats self-administered methamphetamine (.02 mg/infusion, intravenous) or received yoked saline infusions for 6 hours a day for 14 days. Cognitive flexibility was assessed using an attentional set-shifting task before 2 weeks of self-administration and 1 day after self-administration. Animals then underwent 11 days of abstinence, followed by three subsequent tests for context-induced drug seeking. Finally, animals were anesthetized, and single-unit in vivo extracellular recordings were performed in the dorsomedial prefrontal cortex.

Results.—Methamphetamine-experienced rats showed escalated drug intake and context-induced drug-seeking following abstinence. During the extradimensional set-shift component, meth-experienced rats showed selective impairments that were identical to deficits produced by excitotoxic lesions of the prefrontal cortex. Rats with a history of chronic methamphetamine intake also exhibited higher basal firing frequency and a significantly greater proportion of burst-firing cells in the prefrontal cortex compared with yoked-saline controls.

Conclusions.—Prefrontal cortex-specific alterations in neuronal function may play a key role in methamphetamine-induced attentional deficits and drug-seeking. These data support the possibility that targeting prefrontal cortex pathology may improve treatment outcome in methamphetamine addiction (Figs 3 and 4).

▶ This is a really elegant series of experiments combining both pharmacologic perturbation with electrophysiological study in rats. Although it is not a knockout mouse susceptible to methamphetamine, the investigators have succeeded in producing the mouse-equivalent of the chronic methamphetamine addict. They then show difficulties in prefrontal cortical performance that are only

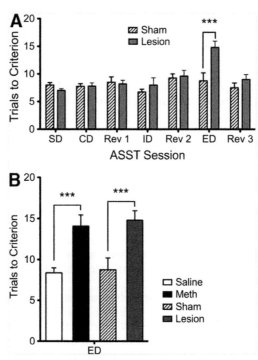

FIGURE 3.—Excitotoxic lesions of the medial prefrontal cortex (PFC) produce a selective deficit in extradimensional set-shifting. (A) Rats with bilateral excitotoxic lesions of the medial PFC showed poorer ED performance relative to sham-lesioned animals (***$p < .001$). (B) Direct comparison of PFC-lesioned rats with chronic meth-experienced rats shows a striking parallel in the ED deficit (significantly different from respective control group; ***$p < .001$). CD, complex discrimination; ED, extradimensional shift; ID, intradimensional shift; rev one, reversal 1; rev two, reversal 2; rev three, reversal 3; SD, simple discrimination. (Reprinted from Biological Psychiatry, Parsegian A, Glen WB Jr, Lavin A, et al. Methamphetamine self-administration produces attentional set-shifting deficits and alters prefrontal cortical neurophysiology in rats. *Biol Psychiatry.* 2011;69:253-259. Copyright 2011, with permission from Society of Biological Psychiatry.)

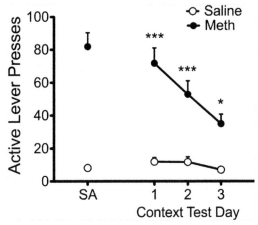

FIGURE 4.—Context-induced methamphetamine (Meth) seeking after abstinence from self-administration (SA). Lever pressing during the context tests resulted in no drug reinforcement or cue presentation. Active lever responding remained elevated for the three daily test trials (post-SA Days 12, 13, and 14) in meth-experienced animals compared with yoked-saline subjects (*$p < .05$; ***$p < .001$) but showed an extinction pattern between Days 1 and 3 ($p < .05$). (Reprinted from Biological Psychiatry, Parsegian A, Glen WB Jr, Lavin A, et al. Methamphetamine self-administration produces attentional set-shifting deficits and alters prefrontal cortical neurophysiology in rats. *Biol Psychiatry.* 2011;69:253-259. Copyright 2011, with permission from Society of Biological Psychiatry.)

partially attenuated by the cessation of methamphetamine. The studies are logical in thought and sequence. The methodology is excellent. These studies parallel other clinical investigations from this outstanding addictions research program at the Medical University of South Carolina.

P. F. Buckley, MD

Opioid Formulations Designed to Resist/Deter Abuse
Raffa RB, Pergolizzi JV Jr (Temple Univ School of Pharmacy, Philadelphia, PA; Johns Hopkins Univ School of Medicine, Baltimore, MD)
Drugs 70:1657-1675, 2010

Physicians who prescribe opioid analgesics for patients with moderate to severe chronic pain face a balancing act in the wake of the current publicity regarding abuse (nonmedical use) of prescription pain killers. There is a spectrum of opioid abuse ranging from those who misuse the drug by not following doctors orders to those who take the drugs to achieve a high or divert the drugs to the street market for profit. Formulations of opioid analgesics designed to resist or deter abuse have been proposed, and are now either on the market or in the pipeline. These are innovative formulations that make the drug less convenient or less desirable to abusers. This article examines three such new products along with clinical studies that report on their safety and effectiveness. These drugs include extended-release morphine with sequestered naloxone

(Embeda®), controlled-release oxycodone in a high-viscosity hard gelatin capsule (Remoxy®) and an immediate-release oxycodone tablet with subtherapeutic niacin as an aversive agent (Acurox® with niacin tablets).

Extended-release morphine with sequestered naltrexone offers a pharmacological barrier in that pellets of morphine surround an internal core of naltrexone (ratio 100:4 of morphine: naltrexone), which is released if the tablet is compromised by chewing or crushing. The hard gelatin capsule of controlled-release oxycodone was designed to resist tampering and the drug cannot be extracted with a needle. The immediate-release oxycodone formulation with subtherapeutic niacin uses a gel-forming ingredient designed to inhibit inhalation and prevent extraction of the drug for injection. The subtherapeutic niacin is intended to induce flushing and other unpleasant effects if the drug is taken in an excessive quantity. While these drugs hold individual promise, it remains undetermined if they can truly prevent abuse. Drug-seeking individuals are extremely resourceful and show little loyalty to a particular drug when other drugs are available. It is possible that abuse-deterring formulations may divert such individuals to find other drugs that are easier to compromise. Nevertheless, these formulations are important innovations and warrant further study to assess their appropriate role as analgesics.

▶ Everybody knows that opioid abuse is a hot topic at this moment. The deaths of celebrities from overdoses, whether intended or unintended, have been greeted with public rage and real concern as to why such lethal drugs are readily accessible. This review article gives a glimpse of what might be in store for future drug seekers. The article describes both antitamper profiles and the pharmacological properties (including efficacy) of 3 novel delivery systems for opioids. The rationale and approaches seem very reasonable. As the article describes, the Food and Drug Administration does not support distinct claims for deterency in the product label unless these are proven unequivocally in well-conducted targeted studies. As you might imagine, studying this area is a researcher's nightmare. Accordingly, if any of these drugs do make it and come to market, they will be without a formal claim that they can deter abuse. Also, of course, drug abusers have no respect for such innovations, and they are notoriously adept at finding new ways of abuse. Nevertheless, this is a very interesting article at the interface between drug development and public policy.

P. F. Buckley, MD

Provision of Pain- and Symptom-Relieving Drugs for HIV/AIDS in Sub-Saharan Africa
Harding R, Powell RA, Kiyange F, et al (King's College London, UK; African Palliative Care Association Kampala, Uganda)
J Pain Symptom Manage 40:405-415, 2010

Context.—Although pain and burdensome symptoms among HIV-infected persons can be effectively managed, the availability of opioids and other symptom-controlling drugs is a particular challenge in sub-Saharan Africa.

Objectives.—This study aimed to identify current drug availability and prescribing practices in 12 sub-Saharan African countries and to examine the barriers and potential facilitators for use of opioids and other key HIV/AIDS symptom-controlling drugs.

Methods.—This was a cross-sectional survey, integrating data from palliative care facilities and competent authorities within ministries of health in 12 African countries.

Results.—Of 62 responding facilities, problems were reported in accessing named nonopioids, with a small number of facilities unable to dispense

Factors hampering roll out & challenges	Suggested responses & solutions
Political o Store supplies are unreliable o Lack of political will o Lack of national policy and motivation o Bureaucracy	*Political* o Advocacy to MoH to raise awareness o Public education o Change prescribing rules o PWA lobbying o Government take responsibility for central purchase & distribution o License nurses to prescribe o Legislative change
Clinical o Professionals lack knowledge on HIV pain, assessment, and management o Professionals fear opioids o Lack of professional training o Lack of clinician interest in the dying o Public opioid fear	*Clinical* o Focus on training palliative not supportive care o Focus on training in opioid use in HIV not just cancer o Graft onto existing providers o Provide a shorter prescribing course for non-specialists o Better HBC training?
Site-specific o Lack of storage facilities o Rural distance from suppliers o Specialist palliative care excludes other organizations	*Site-specific* o Closer collaboration with doctors? o Better clinical supervision o Access to state pharmacies o Roll-out to rural areas? o Improve primary / secondary integration? o Improve networking with existing prescribers o More storage cupboards
Resources o Lack of prescribers and pharmacists o Costs o Lack of facilities to follow patients up at home	*Resources* o Identify sources of opioid funding o More pharmacists o Evaluation of opioid expansion

FIGURE 2.—Challenges and responses: data integration. (Reprinted from the Journal of Pain and Symptom Management, Harding R, Powell RA, Kiyange F, et al. Provision of pain- and symptom-relieving drugs for HIV/AIDS in sub-Saharan Africa. *J Pain Symptom Manage.* 2010;40:405-415. Copyright 2010, with permission from the U.S. Cancer Pain Relief Committee.)

TABLE 2.—Comparison of Competent Authorities and Site Data: Opioid Availability

	Morphine	Pethidine	Codeine	Tramadol	Nitrazepam	Methadone	Fentanyl	Tilidine	Etorphine
Kenya (n = 6)	• ✓	• X	• ✓	• X			• ✓		
Ethiopia (n = 1)	• X	• X	• X						
Tanzania (n = 4)	• ✓	✓	• ✓	✓					• X
Uganda (n = 8)	• ✓		• ✓	✓	• X				
Namibia (n = 1)	• X	• X	• X			• X	• X	• X	

• = noted by Competent Authority as present in country; ✓ = mentioned by at least one facility in country; X = not mentioned by any facility.

them. Less than half the facilities were currently prescribing opioids of any strength. Further problems were identified in terms of the availability and supply continuity of named antiemetics and anxiolytics. The data identified a number of systemic problems, suggesting that opioid supply issues are similar to less controlled drugs, such as antiemetics. Among competent authorities, there was no agreement on whether further opioid expansion was possible. Integration of data from care facilities and competent authorities highlighted a disparity in the understanding of the availability of specific drugs, with competent authorities naming drugs that were not listed by any responding facility in their respective country.

Conclusion.—This study shows that opioid expansion needs to balance supply and skills: Currently there are insufficient trained clinical personnel to prescribe, and supply is unreliable. Efforts to expand supply should ensure that they do not weaken current systems (Fig 2 and Table 2).

▶ This is a sad tale of chaos in the care of people with human immunodeficiency virus/acquired immunodeficiency syndrome (HIV/AIDS) in Africa. It details a pattern of great inconsistency in access availability and in competency to deliver analgesic medications that may be a necessary part of the care of people in Africa. The availability of drugs in different countries is clearly documented (Table 2). The problems that contribute to this dismal situation are well categorized (Fig 2). They are myriad and complex. These also juxtapose the care for HIV/AIDS and likely also drug availability patterns thereupon, although this was not the actual subject of this report.

P. F. Buckley, MD

Risks for possible and probable opioid misuse among recipients of chronic opioid therapy in commercial and medicaid insurance plans: The TROUP Study

Sullivan MD, Edlund MJ, Fan M-Y, et al (Univ of Washington, Seattle; Univ of Arkansas for Med Sciences, Little Rock; et al)
Pain 150:332-339, 2010

The use of chronic opioid therapy (COT) for chronic non-cancer pain (CNCP) has increased dramatically in the past two decades. There has also been a marked increase in the abuse of prescribed opioids and in accidental opioid overdose. Misuse of prescribed opioids may link these trends, but has thus far only been studied in small clinical samples. We therefore sought to validate an administrative indicator of opioid misuse among large samples of recipients of COT and determine the demographic, clinical, and pharmacological risks associated with possible and probable opioid misuse. A total of 21,685 enrollees in commercial insurance plans and 10,159 in Arkansas Medicaid who had at least 90 days of continuous opioid use 2000—2005 were studied for one year. Criteria were developed for possible and probable opioid misuse using administrative claims data concerning excess days supplied of short-acting and long-acting opioids,

TABLE 2.—Factors Associated with Possible and Probable Opioid Misuse; HealthCore

Variables	Possible Misuse				Probable Misuse			
	Odds Ratio	95% CI	Wald's Chisq	P-Value	Odds Ratio	95% CI	Wald's Chisq	P-Value
Age: 18–30	3.56	3.11, 4.09	326.819	<0.001	15.95	11.73, 21.67	313.043	<0.001
Age: 31–40	2.89	2.60, 3.21	382.312	<0.001	9.86	7.43, 13.07	252.119	<0.001
Age: 41–50	2.15	1.95, 2.37	234.928	<0.001	5.31	4.02, 7.00	139.624	<0.001
Age: 51–64	1.45	1.32, 1.60	56.561	<0.001	2.21	1.66, 2.93	29.824	<0.001
Reference: age ≥65								
Female	1.06	1.01, 1.12	5.027	0.025	1.09	0.98, 1.21	2.740	<0.001
Reference: male								
CNCP: joint	0.91	0.85, 0.98	6.479	0.011	0.94	0.82, 1.07	0.899	<0.001
CNCP: back	1.13	1.07, 1.19	17.902	<0.001	1.11	1.00, 1.23	3.782	<0.001
CNCP: head	1.22	1.14, 1.31	32.069	<0.001	1.58	1.41, 1.78	58.891	<0.001
CNCP: neck	1.00	0.93, 1.07	0.004	0.952	0.93	0.81, 1.06	1.295	<0.001
Reference: no CNCP diagnosis								
# Non-tracer pain	1.08	1.06, 1.11	41.601	<0.001	1.19	1.14, 1.24	63.131	<0.001
Reference: no non-tracer pain								
Charlson score	0.98	0.95, 1.00	2.888	0.089	0.96	0.91, 1.02	1.814	<0.001
MH: 1	1.07	0.99, 1.15	3.144	0.076	1.04	0.91, 1.18	0.279	<0.001
MH: ≥2	1.12	0.99, 1.26	3.390	0.066	1.15	0.95, 1.40	2.046	<0.001
Reference: no mental health diagnosis								
SA/alcohol	1.38	1.10, 1.72	8.080	0.004	1.77	1.27, 2.47	11.303	<0.001
SA/opioid	1.39	1.00, 1.93	3.929	0.047	3.53	2.39, 5.21	40.113	<0.001

SA/non-opioid	1.75	1.38, 2.22	21.199	<0.001	1.78	1.27, 2.48	11.291	<0.001
Reference: no SA diagnosis								
Sedative/hypnotics days supply/30 d	1.02	1.02, 1.03	64.585	<0.001	1.04	1.03, 1.05	65.140	<0.001
Reference: <30 d supply								
Opioid daily dose: median-120	1.65	1.56, 1.74	315.925	<0.001	2.68	2.39, 3.00	284.748	<0.001
Opioid daily dose: >120	2.37	2.13, 2.65	241.722	<0.001	6.70	5.60, 8.03	426.878	<0.001
Reference: opioid daily dose < median								
Opioid type: Schedule II short only	1.35	1.14, 1.59	12.437	<0.001	1.08	0.77, 1.50	0.197	<0.001
Opioid type: Schedule II long only	0.99	0.88, 1.11	0.040	0.842	0.42	0.33, 0.54	47.152	<0.001
Opioid type: non-Schedule II + Schedule II short	3.06	2.66, 3.52	248.668	<0.001	5.19	4.26, 6.32	267.503	<0.001
Opioid type: non-Schedule II + Schedule II long	1.66	1.51, 1.82	113.453	<0.001	1.88	1.61, 2.19	65.532	<0.001
Opioid type: Schedule II short + long	1.65	1.41, 1.92	40.230	<0.001	1.39	1.08, 1.78	6.725	<0.001
Opioid type: all 3 types	3.47	2.83, 4.26	142.631	<0.001	7.44	5.81, 9.52	254.018	<0.001
Reference: Non-Schedule II only								

opioid prescribers and opioid pharmacies. We estimated possible misuse at 24% of COT recipients in the commercially insured sample and 20% in the Medicaid sample and probable misuse at 6% in commercially insured and at 3% in Medicaid. Among non-modifiable factors, younger age, back pain, multiple pain complaints and substance abuse disorders identify patients at high risk for misuse. Among modifiable factors, treatment with high daily dose opioids (especially >120 mg MED per day) and short-acting Schedule II opioids appears to increase the risk of misuse. The consistency of the findings across diverse patient populations and the varying levels of misuse suggest that these results will generalize broadly, but await confirmation in other studies (Table 2).

▶ This is a wonderful and in many ways classical pharmacoepidemiological study of opioid misuse derived from 2 large administrative claims data sets. The results are self-evident and point to a substantial pattern of prescription opioid abuse (Table 2). While the proportions of abuse and possible abuse may differ between the Arkansas Medicaid claims database and the larger health care database, the pattern is essentially the same. It is surprising perhaps that mental health and current addiction diagnoses were not highlighted more prominently, although these diagnoses' preopioid prescriptions are identified as risk factors. The pattern of back pain and headaches as pain types most associated with misuse also rings true. On the other hand, this is an analysis of claims data, and no patients were interviewed nor were the actual clinical records reviewed. However, these types of studies are invaluable for providing the big picture but are generally less robust when it comes to more granular perspectives.

P. F. Buckley, MD

Substance misuse treatment for high-risk chronic pain patients on opioid therapy: A randomized trial
Jamison RN, Ross EL, Michna E, et al (Brigham & Women's Hosp, Boston, MA)
Pain 150:390-400, 2010

Chronic pain patients who show aberrant drug-related behavior often are discontinued from treatment when they are noncompliant with their use of opioids for pain. The purpose of this study was to conduct a randomized trial in patients who were prescribed opioids for noncancer back pain and who showed risk potential for or demonstration of opioid misuse to see if close monitoring and cognitive behavioral substance misuse counseling could increase overall compliance with opioids. Forty-two patients meeting criteria for high-risk for opioid misuse were randomized to either standard control (High-Risk Control; $N = 21$) or experimental compliance treatment consisting of monthly urine screens, compliance checklists, and individual and group motivational counseling (High-Risk Experimental; $N = 21$). Twenty patients who met criteria indicating low potential for misuse were recruited to a low-risk control group (Low-Risk Control). Patients were followed for 6 months and completed pre- and post-study questionnaires and monthly electronic diaries. Outcomes consisted of the percent with a positive Drug Misuse Index (DMI), which was a composite score of self-reported drug misuse (Prescription Drug Use Questionnaire), physician-reported abuse behavior (Addiction Behavior Checklist), and abnormal urine toxicology results. Significant differences were found between groups with 73.7% of the High-Risk Control patients demonstrating positive scores on the DMI compared with 26.3% from the High-Risk Experimental group and 25.0% from the Low-Risk Controls ($p < 0.05$). The results of this study demonstrate support for the benefits of a brief behavioral intervention in the management of opioid compliance among chronic back pain patient at high-risk for prescription opioid misuse.

▶ Remarkable! The results of this small study show a dramatic reduction in abuse of opioids in the active treatment groups who received cognitive, behavioral, and motivational intervention. Although the methodology seems apt, the assessments for abuse were not equal across the 3 groups (see Fig 2 in the original article). Also, the control group received no intervention and was simply followed up over time. These attributes may have contributed to the whopping effect seen for outcomes between the 2 groups that received therapy and the control group that did not receive any intervention. It's an interesting study. It suggests that psychotherapeutic intervention can have powerful effects in opioid-using patients with chronic pain. Many, however, would dispute this assertion.

P. F. Buckley, MD

Comorbidity

A Pilot Study of Neurocognitive Function in Older and Younger Cocaine Abusers and Controls

Kalapatapu RK, Vadhan NP, Rubin E, et al (Columbia Univ, NY)
Am J Addict 20:228-239, 2011

This pilot study compared basic neurocognitive functioning among older and younger cocaine abusers and control participants, as a preliminary assessment of whether specific cognitive deficits exist in an aged cocaine-abusing population. We hypothesized an interaction between aging and cocaine abuse, such that older cocaine abusers would exhibit decreased neuropsychological test performance relative to both younger cocaine abusers and older control participants. Four groups (n = 20 each) were examined: older cocaine abusers (ages 51–70), younger cocaine abusers (ages 21–39), and two nonillicit substance-using control groups. Basic neuropsychological and psychiatric measures were administered to all participants. Older participants performed more poorly than younger participants on the Mini-Mental State Examination (MMSE, $p < .01$), Digit Span Backward ($p < .01$), and Trail Making Test (TMT) Parts A and B ($p < .01$). Cocaine abusers performed more poorly than controls on TMT A ($p < .01$). Older and younger cocaine abusers used similar amounts of cocaine ($p > .05$). Older cocaine abusers performed more poorly than older control participants and younger cocaine abusers on the Digit Span Forward ($p < .0125$). Older cocaine abusers also performed more poorly than younger cocaine abusers on TMT A ($p < .0125$). This study provides preliminary evidence that older cocaine abusers use a significant amount of cocaine and that there is an interaction between aging and cocaine abuse on psychomotor speed, attention, and short-term memory. Future examination of neurocognitive function in older cocaine abusers is clearly warranted.

▶ The issue of cocaine abuse effects on the elderly brain is only beginning to be studied, and important questions as to whether cocaine abuse hastens dementia, leads to a more rapid aging of the brain, and the kinds of impairments caused and possible treatments are areas needing more study. Not surprisingly, this study finds more neurocognitive impairment in older cocaine abusers compared both with peers and with younger cocaine abusers. Psychomotor speed, attention, and short-term memory problems are important indicators of the damage of cocaine to an aging brain. The degree of heavy use in the elderly was found to be similar to that of younger cocaine abusers. Increasingly, the public is interested in factors that can lead to healthy aging, preventing and postponing dementia, and lifestyles that promote the protection of the brain. High among healthy brain strategies are abstaining from harmful levels of alcohol use, refraining from substance abuse, preserving healthy supportive and active relationships with family and friends, and having an active mental life.

R. J. Frances, MD

Pharmacologic Treatment

Prescription Pain Medication Dependence
Dodrill CL, Helmer DA, Kosten TR (Baylor College of Medicine, Houston, TX)
Am J Psychiatry 168:466-471, 2011

Treating patients like Mr. J and his wife for opioid addiction requires a consistent, empathic clinician who can detect prescription opioid use and engage the patient, treat the pain, and facilitate abstinence. Chronic pain complicates management of opioid abuse, and treatment benefits from collaboration among a psychiatrist, pain management specialist, physical therapist, and psychotherapist to achieve an optimal balance of pain control and improved functioning. Use of the buprenorphine/naloxone combination will likely play an increasingly important role in the treatment of individuals with chronic pain and opioid abuse.

▶ This article reviews the benefits of treating patients who have a combination of prescription opioid dependence with pain management using Suboxone, a combination of buprenorphine and naloxone. The rapid rise of prescription drug abuse has been alarming, and those who are addicted to opioids are often reluctant to seek out treatment in methadone programs. Suboxone has turned out to be a safer and less stigmatized way to maintain or detoxify patients with this problem and is usually done as an outpatient procedure.

Patients report high satisfaction with the treatment, and addiction psychiatrists have found it quite useful. This article gives good advice on how to induce and start buprenorphine when needed. The Drug Enforcement Agency is visiting every doctor who prescribes the medication, which feels onerous, but the visits are usually benign. Although diversion of OxyContin has been significant, I have not seen significant diversion of buprenorphine.

R. J. Frances, MD

Prescription Pain Medication Dependence
Dodrill CL, Helmer DA, Kosten TR (Baylor College of Medicine, Houston, TX)
Am J Psychiatry 168:466-471, 2011

Treating patients like Mr. J and his wife for opioid addiction requires a consistent, empathic clinician who can detect prescription opioid use and engage the patient, treat the pain, and facilitate abstinence. Chronic pain complicates management of opioid abuse, and treatment benefits from collaboration among a psychiatrist, pain management specialist, physical therapist, and psychotherapist to achieve an optimal balance of pain control and improved functioning. Use of the buprenorphine/naloxone combination will likely play an increasingly important role in the treatment of individuals with chronic pain and opioid abuse (Fig 1).

▶ This is a provocative and highly illustrative clinical vignette that depicts the difficulties, clinically "in the trenches," with providing care for patients with prescription pain medication dependence. The article also hits hard on the responsibility of clinicians to detect and have aberrant behaviors related to prescription pain addiction on the radar screen (Fig 1). The case report also focused on a Veterans Affairs patient, which is of significance given the high rates of both addiction disorders and mental illness comorbidities in soldiers

1. Requests for higher medication doses
2. Early refills
3. Requests for specific pain medications
4. Extra medication because of travel or inability to attend more frequent visits
5. Lost medication
6. Multiple unsanctioned dose escalations
7. Unexpected urine toxicology results showing no opioids, indicating diversion
8. Deterioration in work or social functioning
9. Resistance to change or to discontinuation of opioids despite adverse effects
10. Refusal to comply with random drug screens
11. Concurrent abuse of alcohol or illicit drugs
12. Use of multiple physicians and pharmacies

FIGURE 1.—Aberrant medication-related behaviors[a]. [a] From reference 20. (Reprinted with permission from the American Journal of Psychiatry, Dodrill CL, Helmer DA, Kosten TR. Prescription pain medication dependence. *Am J Psychiatry*. 2011;168:466-471. © 2011. American Psychiatric Association)

returning home from war. It is important for us to understand what we can and cannot do by Food and Drug Administration regulation. The authors have done a very nice job laying out the scenarios.

P. F. Buckley, MD

A Double-Blind, Randomized Trial of Sertraline for Alcohol Dependence: Moderation by Age and 5-Hydroxytryptamine Transporter-Linked Promoter Region Genotype
Kranzler HR, Armeli S, Tennen H, et al (Univ of Connecticut School of Medicine, Farmington; Fairleigh Dickinson Univ, Teaneck, NJ; et al)
J Clin Psychopharmacol 31:22-30, 2011

Late-onset/low-vulnerability alcoholics (LOAs) appear to drink less when treated with a selective serotonin reuptake inhibitor than placebo, whereas early-onset/high-vulnerability alcoholics (EOAs) show the opposite effect. We conducted a 12-week, parallel-group, placebo-controlled trial of the efficacy of sertraline in alcohol dependence (AD). We compared the effects in LOAs versus EOAs and examined the moderating effects of a functional polymorphism in the serotonin transporter gene. Patients (N = 134, 80.6% male, 34.3% EOAs) with *Diagnostic and Statistical Manual of Mental Disorders-IV* AD received up to 200 mg of sertraline (n = 63) or placebo (n = 71) daily. We used urn randomization, and patients were genotyped for the tri-allelic 5-hydroxytryptamine transporter protein linked promoter region polymorphism. Planned analyses included main and interaction effects of medication group, age of onset ($\leq$25 years vs >25 years), and genotype (L'/L' vs S' carriers) on drinking outcomes. Results showed that the moderating effect of age of onset on the response to sertraline was conditional on genotype. There were no main or interaction effects among S' allele carriers. However, in L' homozygotes, the effects of medication group varied by age of onset ($P = 0.002$). At the end of treatment, LOAs reported fewer drinking and heavy drinking days when treated with sertraline ($P = 0.011$), whereas EOAs had fewer drinking and heavy drinking days when treated with placebo ($P < 0.001$). The small cell sizes and high rate of attrition, particularly for L' homozygotes, render these findings preliminary and their replication in larger samples necessary. Because AD is common, particularly in medical settings, and selective serotonin reuptake inhibitors are widely prescribed by practitioners, these findings have potential public health significance and warrant further evaluation.

▶ Many years ago, Donald Goodwin, MD, had the hypothesis that alcoholics were born 2 martinis short of normal and that their serotonin levels were set a bit low, with alcohol first increasing and then with high doses causing depletion of central serotonin and mood dysregulation (Fig 2). The idea that selective serotonin reuptake inhibitors (SSRIs) would be effective in treating primary alcoholism followed but did not pan out, although they help with unipolar depression associated with alcoholism. This study finds in a small sample the

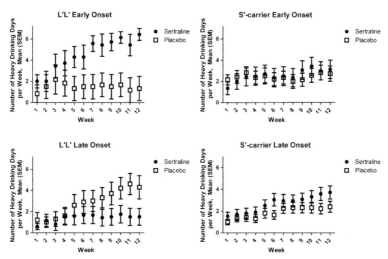

FIGURE 2.—Number of HDDs by Study week, age of onset of alcohol dependence, medication group, and 5-HTTLPR genotype. Values are mean ($\pm$ SEM) and reflect drinking behavior during the week identified on the x axis. As in the analyses, the figures include the intent-to-treat sample and imputed values for missing data. The decrease in DDs from baseline to week 1 is not shown in the figure, but can be ascertained using data from Table 1. (Reprinted from Kranzler HR, Armeli S, Tennen H, et al. A double-blind, randomized trial of sertraline for alcohol dependence: moderation by age and 5-hydroxytryptamine transporter-linked promoter region genotype. *J Clin Psychopharmacol.* 2011;31:22-30.)

promising finding that both late-onset and specific genetics related to an SSRI may be markers for the treatment effectiveness of SSRIs in alcoholism (Fig 2). This area of research is important for both addictions and depression and may lead to the long-promised dawn of an era of genetically informed targeted psychopharmacology with the addition of genome analysis as it becomes more clinically useful, affordable, and available. Also, newer pharmacological agents may be able to better target specific ways alcohol and serotonin regulation interact for individuals with specific genetic alleles. The more we understand about the pathophysiology and gene expression of psychiatric illnesses in relation to addiction, the better we will be able to design more effective future treatments.

R. J. Frances, MD

A Double-Blind, Randomized Trial of Sertraline for Alcohol Dependence: Moderation by Age and 5-Hydroxytryptamine Transporter-Linked Promoter Region Genotype
Kranzler HR, Armeli S, Tennen H, et al (Univ of Connecticut School of Medicine, Farmington; Fairleigh Dickinson Univ, Teaneck, NJ; et al)
J Clin Psychopharmacol 31:22-30, 2011

Late-onset/low-vulnerability alcoholics (LOAs) appear to drink less when treated with a selective serotonin reuptake inhibitor than placebo, whereas early-onset/high-vulnerability alcoholics (EOAs) show the opposite effect. We conducted a 12-week, parallel-group, placebo-controlled trial of the efficacy of sertraline in alcohol dependence (AD). We compared the effects in LOAs versus EOAs and examined the moderating effects of a functional polymorphism in the serotonin transporter gene. Patients (N = 134, 80.6% male, 34.3% EOAs) with *Diagnostic and Statistical Manual of Mental Disorders-IV* AD received up to 200 mg of sertraline (n = 63) or placebo (n = 71) daily. We used urn randomization, and patients were genotyped for the tri-allelic 5-hydroxytryptamine transporter protein linked promoter region polymorphism. Planned analyses included main and interaction effects of medication group, age of onset (≤25 years vs > 25 years), and genotype (L′/L′ vs S′ carriers) on drinking outcomes. Results showed that the moderating effect of age of onset on the response to sertraline was conditional on genotype. There were no main or interaction effects among S′ allele carriers. However, in L′ homozygotes, the effects of medication group varied by age of onset (P = 0.002). At the end of treatment, LOAs reported fewer drinking and heavy drinking days when treated with sertraline (P = 0.011), whereas EOAs had fewer drinking and heavy drinking days when treated with placebo (P < 0.001). The small cell sizes and high rate of attrition, particularly for L′ homozygotes, render these findings preliminary and their replication in larger samples necessary. Because AD is common, particularly in medical settings, and selective serotonin reuptake inhibitors are widely prescribed by practitioners, these findings have potential public health significance and warrant further evaluation (Fig 1).

▶ Finding a medication that has both a robust and a reliable treatment effect for alcoholism is a major challenge. There are now several studies that have shown

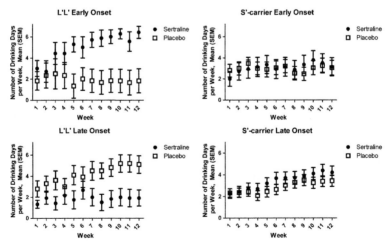

FIGURE 1.—Number of DDs by study week, age of onset of alcohol dependence, medication group, and 5-HTTLPR genotype. Values are mean (TSEM) and reflect drinking behavior during the week identified on the x axis. As in the analyses, the figures include the intent-to-treat sample and imputed values for missing data. The decrease in DDs from baseline to week 1 is not shown in the figure, but can be ascertained using data from Table 1. (Reprinted from Kranzler HR, Armeli S, Tennen H, et al. A double-blind, randomized trial of sertraline for alcohol dependence: moderation by age and 5-hydroxytryptamine transporter-linked promoter region genotype. *J Clin Psychopharmacol.* 2011;31:22-30.)

some benefit for sertraline (and now less for other selective serotonin-norepinephrine reuptake inhibitors) in patients with alcohol dependence. However, as in much of psychopharmacology, the effect is modest and it is hard to predict which group of patients is more likely to benefit over others. This complicated analysis of serotonin transporter gene polymorphism in relation to both alcohol dependence and severity of disorder (using earlier age of onset as a well-established proxy for severity) shows an interesting effect of interaction between drug, earlier age of onset, and genetic liability. Although, of course, still a good way off from clinical practice, the implications of this study are clear. This group also does great work in alcoholism. The study methodology here is exemplary.

P. F. Buckley, MD

Pharmacogenetic Approach at the Serotonin Transporter Gene as a Method of Reducing the Severity of Alcohol Drinking

Johnson BA, Ait-Daoud N, Seneviratne C, et al (Univ of Virginia, Charlottesville; Univ of Texas Health Science Ctr at San Antonio; Univ of Maryland, Baltimore)
Am J Psychiatry 168:265-275, 2011

Objective.—Severe drinking can cause serious morbidity and death. Because the serotonin transporter (5-HTT) is an important regulator of neuronal 5-HT function, allelic differences at that gene may modulate

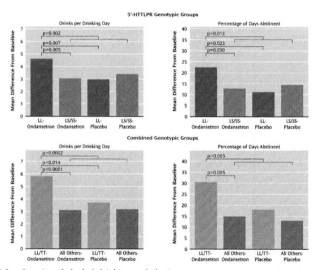

FIGURE 2.—Severity of alcohol drinking and abstinence rates among genotypic variants in the serotonin transporter gene before and during treatment with ondansetron or placebo[a]. [a] Numbers of participants in the genotypic groups are listed in Table 2. 5'-HTTLPR=5'-regulatory region of the serotonin transporter gene. (Reprinted with permission from the American Journal of Psychiatry, Johnson BA, Ait-Daoud N, Seneviratne C, et al. Pharmacogenetic approach at the serotonin transporter gene as a method of reducing the severity of alcohol drinking. *Am J Psychiatry.* 2011;168:265-275. © 2011. American Psychiatric Association.)

TABLE 1.—Biological Information on SLC6A4 Polymorphisms Examined in the Study[a]

Physical Position	Chromosome Position (NCBI Genome Build)	Alleles	Minor Allele Frequency				p Values for Deviation From Hardy-Weinberg Equilibrium[c]			Primers and Probe Sequences/Context Sequence ID of ABI Primers and Probes	Number of Missing Data Points
			CEU[b]	Pooled[c]	White[c]	Hispanic[c]	Pooled	White	Hispanic		
Promoter	25,588,443: 25,588,485 (36.1)	L/S	0.450	0.438	0.424	0.447	0.461	0.850	0.461	Forward: TCCT CCGCTTTGGCG CCTCTTCC Reverse: TGGGGGTTGCAGGGGA GATCCTG	0
Exon 15 (3′-UTR)	25,549,137 (36.3)	G/T	0.433	0.430	0.440	0.424	0.457	0.544	0.827	C_7473190_10	7

[a]The pooled sample consists of samples from individuals of Caucasian and Hispanic origin. L=long allele; S=short allele; ABI=Applied Biosystems; NCBI=National Center for Biotechnology Information; 3′-UTR=3′-untranslated region.
[b]CEU=European ancestry sample from the HapMap project.
[c]Data from this study.

the severity of alcohol consumption and predict therapeutic response to the 5-HT$_3$ receptor antagonist, ondansetron.

Method.—The authors randomized 283 alcoholics by genotype in the 5′-regulatory region of the 5-HTT gene (LL/LS/SS), with additional genotyping for another functional single-nucleotide polymorphism (T/G), rs1042173, in the 3′-untranslated region, in a double-blind controlled trial. Participants received either ondansetron (4 µg/kg twice daily) or placebo for 11 weeks, plus standardized cognitive-behavioral therapy.

Results.—Individuals with the LL genotype who received ondansetron had a lower mean number of drinks per drinking day (−1.62) and a higher percentage of days abstinent (11.27%) than those who received placebo. Among ondansetron recipients, the number of drinks per drinking day was lower (−1.53) and the percentage of days abstinent higher (9.73%) in LL compared with LS/SS individuals. LL individuals in the ondansetron group also had a lower number of drinks per drinking day (−1.45) and a higher percentage of days abstinent (9.65%) than all other genotype and treatment groups combined. For both number of drinks per drinking day and percentage of days abstinent, 5′-HTTLPR and rs1042173 variants interacted significantly. LL/TT individuals in the ondansetron group had a lower number of drinks per drinking day (−2.63) and a higher percentage of days abstinent (16.99%) than all other genotype and treatment groups combined.

Conclusions.—The authors propose a new pharmacogenetic approach using ondansetron to treat severe drinking and improve abstinence in alcoholics (Fig 2, Table 1).

▶ This is an important well-conducted study by Bankole Johnson and colleagues with implications for clinical practice that go way beyond the area of addiction. In many ways, it is the model for pharmacogenetics in clinical care in that it uses genetic imprinting to decipher who among a group of patients responds to this putative antiaddiction drug. We know that not everybody responds to any given drug; our problem is we don't know (until we do the experiment) which patient will be the responder. If we knew this through pharmacogenetics, we would then target the drug up front to the patient we have identified as one likely to respond (genetically predisposed). As this study illustrates (Table 1 and Fig 2), the response determined by pharmacogenetic discrimination can be quite powerful.

P. F. Buckley, MD

The Effect of Five Smoking Cessation Pharmacotherapies on Smoking Cessation Milestones

Japuntich SJ, Piper ME, Leventhal AM, et al (Univ of Wisconsin School of Medicine and Public Health, Madison; Univ of Southern California Keck School of Medicine, Los Angeles; et al)
J Consult Clin Psychol 79:34-42, 2011

Objective.—Most smoking cessation studies have used long-term abstinence as their primary outcome measure. Recent research has suggested that long-term abstinence may be an insensitive index of important smoking cessation mechanisms. The goal of the current study was to examine the effects of 5 smoking cessation pharmacotherapies using Shiffman et al.'s (2006) approach of examining the effect of smoking cessation medications on 3 process markers of cessation or smoking cessation *milestones*: initial abstinence, lapse, and the lapse–relapse transition.

Method.—The current study ($N = 1,504$; 58.2 female and 41.8 male; 83.9 Caucasian, 13.6 African American, 2.5 other races) examined the effect of 5 smoking cessation pharmacotherapy treatments versus placebo (bupropion, nicotine lozenge, nicotine patch, bupropion + lozenge, patch + lozenge) on Shiffman et al.'s smoking cessation milestones over 8 weeks following a quit attempt.

Results.—Results show that all 5 medication conditions decreased rates of failure to achieve initial abstinence and most (with the exception of the nicotine lozenge) decreased lapse risk; however, only the nicotine patch and bupropion + lozenge conditions affected the lapse–relapse transition.

Conclusions.—These findings demonstrate that medications are effective at aiding initial abstinence and decreasing lapse risk but that they generally do not decrease relapse risk following a lapse. The analysis of cessation milestones sheds light on important impediments to long-term smoking abstinence, suggests potential mechanisms of action of smoking cessation pharmacotherapies, and identifies targets for future treatment development.

▶ This study finds a variety of replacement and reduction medications to be helpful in reducing relapse to nicotine use in the action phase of recovery. Reducing withdrawal symptoms does help reduce relapse, but if a lapse occurs, the medications are less effective at preventing relapse. Also, a substantial number of patients on placebo medication were also able to maintain abstinence consistent with the fact that a high number of former smokers went cold turkey. Given all of our available knowledge, use of medication to aid in the initial stages of recovery from smoking should be recommended by primary care givers. Efforts to increase motivation to stop smoking through motivational interviewing and self-efficacy support are behavioral strategies that also help considerably to improve results. Combining pharmacologic and behavioral treatments to aid in helping patients achieve smoking cessation leads to the best results. Many individuals make many attempts before they succeed in achieving extended abstinence, and they should be encouraged to keep trying in the face of previous failures.

R. J. Frances, MD

Addiction Treatment

A Randomized Trial of Extended Telephone-Based Continuing Care for Alcohol Dependence: Within-Treatment Substance Use Outcomes

McKay JR, Van Horn DHA, Oslin DW, et al (Univ of Pennsylvania and Philadelphia Veterans Affairs Med Ctr; Univ of Pennsylvania, Philadelphia)
J Consult Clin Psychol 78:912-923, 2010

Objective.—The study tested whether adding up to 18 months of telephone continuing care, either as monitoring and feedback (TM) or longer contacts that included counseling (TMC), to intensive outpatient programs (IOPs) improved outcomes for alcohol-dependent patients.

Method.—Participants ($N = 252$) who completed 3 weeks of IOP were randomized to up to 36 sessions of TM ($M = 11.5$ sessions), TMC ($M = 9.1$ sessions), or IOP only (treatment as usual [TAU]). Quarterly assessment of alcohol use (79.9 assessed at 18 months) was corroborated with available collateral reports ($N = 63$ at 12 months). Participants with cocaine dependence ($N = 199$) also provided urine samples.

Results.—Main effects favored TMC over TAU on any alcohol use (odds ratio [OR] = 1.88, CI [1.13, 3.14]) and any heavy alcohol use ($OR = 1.74$, CI [1.03, 2.94]). TMC produced fewer days of alcohol use during Months 10–18 and heavy alcohol use during Months 13–18 than TAU ($ds = 0.46–0.65$). TMC also produced fewer days of any alcohol use and heavy alcohol use than TM during Months 4–6 ($ds = 0.39$ and 0.43). TM produced lower percent days alcohol use than TAU during Months 10–12 and 13–15 ($ds = 0.41$ and 0.39). There were no treatment effects on rates of cocaine-positive urines.

Conclusions.—Adding telephone continuing care to IOP improved alcohol use outcomes relative to IOP alone. Conversely, shorter calls that provided monitoring and feedback but no counseling generally did not improve outcomes over IOP.

▶ The positive findings in this study point to the value of the use of the telephone with longer phone contacts, including counseling in the treatment and follow-up of patients with addictive disorders (Fig 5). Historically, clinicians were always among the first to use newly developed technologies such as cars, telephones, computers, and cell phones to improve availability and accessibility of medical and psychiatric care. In my own clinical practice, I frequently do phone sessions and give patients my cell phone number with encouragement to call as needed, especially if the patient or I am traveling and in times of urgent patient need. One positive aspect of the way the phone was used in the longer contacts in this study was that it helped mediate patients' improved use of 12-step mutual-help programs. Teaching patients to rely on making phone calls to an Alcoholics Anonymous sponsor or to a friend in the program when craving occurs is of enormous value in relapse prevention. The immediacy and availability of response to any need for help that the telephone provides is a comfort, reminder, and reassurance for anyone struggling with an

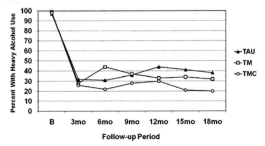

FIGURE 5.—Rates of any heavy alcohol use during follow-up. Percentage of participants who reported any heavy alcohol use within a given 3-month period of the follow-up, presented for each treatment condition. There was a trend toward a treatment condition main effect, $\chi^2(2) = 5.37, p = .068$. Telephone monitoring and counseling (TMC) produced lower rates of heavy alcohol use than treatment as usual (TAU), $\chi^2(1) = 4.29, p = .038$, and there was a trend favoring TMC over telephone monitoring (TM), $\chi^2(1) = 3.47, p = .063$. TM and TAU did not differ. B = baseline; mo = month. (Reprinted from McKay JR, Van Horn DHA, Oslin DW, et al. A randomized trial of extended telephone-based continuing care for alcohol dependence: within-treatment substance use outcomes. *J Consult Clin Psychol.* 2010;78:912-923, with permission from American Psychological Association.)

addiction. The issues to be faced in the implementation of follow-up telephone longer-contact treatment programs based on this study are confidentiality, especially with computer-based communications; reimbursement; and cost of phone services, especially when costly counseling by skilled therapists is included. The authors mention that they will be doing cost-effectiveness and contingency studies to check this out and improve compliance.

R. J. Frances, MD

Counselors' Knowledge of the Adoption of Tobacco Cessation Medications in Substance Abuse Treatment Programs

Rothrauff TC, Eby LT (Univ of Georgia, Athens)
Am J Addict 20:56-62, 2010

This study assessed counselors' knowledge of the adoption of evidence-based tobacco cessation medications (TCMs)—varenicline, bupropion, and five nicotine replacement therapies (NRTs)—and predictors of adoption in diverse substance abuse treatment settings. We used Managing Effective Relationships in Treatment Services (MERITS I) data from 658 counselors working in 26 programs. Adoption of varenicline was reported by 16% of counselors, bupropion by 11%, and NRTs by 27%. Knowledge of the adoption of all types of TCMs was more likely to be reported by counselors who worked in treatment programs that adhered less to a 12-step orientation and restricted outdoor smoking for employees. Several additional unique predictors of varenicline and NRTs were identified.

▶ This study finds low buy-in of evidence-based nicotine replacement by counselors in general, and especially low for those working in 12-step abstinence-oriented programs. The need to better train counselors in evidence-based

TABLE 1.—Counselor's Knowledge of Adoption of Tobacco Cessation Medications (TCMs) in Substance Abuse Treatment Programs

	TCM Adopted	
	Yes	No
Varenicline (N, %)	103 (16)	555 (84)
Bupropion (N, %)	71 (11)	587 (89)
Nicotine replacement therapy (N, %)	176 (27)	482 (73)

psychotherapy and pharmacotherapy approaches in general is huge. To be fair about this, physicians have not been much better at using evidence-based treatments, an example being the low use of naltrexone nationally for alcoholism compared with widespread National Institute on Alcohol Abuse and Alcoholism and National Institute on Drug Abuse recommendations. Counselors should be reminded that, although some in Alcoholics Anonymous (AA) may be prejudiced against medications, AA officially recommends that the recommendations of doctors be followed. The founder of AA, Bill Wilson, was an innovative thinker and would have welcomed effective pharmacotherapy of addictions. Leadership is also needed in bringing together the craft and the scientific aspects of the field to bring effective and innovative evidence-based treatments into general acceptance. Also, it is possible that some counselors may get fairly good results recommending smokers. Recommending that smokers try going cold turkey can also sometimes be effective. However, nicotine replacement and other strategies do work better, and counselors need to have as much zeal in treating nicotine as they do for other addictions (Table 1).

R. J. Frances, MD

Electronic Medical Records to Increase the Clinical Treatment of Tobacco Dependence: A Systematic Review
Boyle RG, Solberg LI, Fiore MC (ClearWay Minnesota[SM], Minneapolis; HealthPartners Res Foundation, Minneapolis, MN; Univ of Wisconsin Ctr for Tobacco Res and Intervention, Madison)
Am J Prev Med 39:S77-S82, 2010

Context.—The expanded use of electronic medical records (EMRs) may provide an opportunity to increase the use and impact of clinical guidelines to promote tobacco-cessation treatment in primary care settings. The objective of this systematic review is to evaluate the evidence for such an effect.

Evidence Acquisition.—After a systematic search of the English-language literature regarding an EMR effect on either smoking cessation or clinician behavior, relevant articles were abstracted and findings summarized from both observational studies and RCTs.

Evidence Synthesis.—Of ten identified studies of EMRs and tobacco, only two RCTs were found. Adding tobacco status as a vital sign resulted

TABLE 2.—RCTs of EMR-Based Interventions for Smoking Cessation

Study	Number of Clinics/ Providers	Study Period	Methods	Outcome Measures	Results
Bentz (2007)[11]	19 primary care 10 intervention/57 MDs 9 comparison/55 MDs	12 months	Cluster randomized clinical trial EMR-generated feedback vs no feedback Changes to the EMR: 1. Clinical guideline 5A's added 2. Direct fax referral to quitline	Ask, Advise, Assess, Assist calculated monthly	Higher use of Ask, Advise, Assess, Assist in feedback compared to control No difference in referral to quitline (3.6% control vs 3.9% feedback)
Linder (2009)[13]	26 primary care clinics 12 intervention/14 control	9 months	Cluster randomized clinical trial Primary outcome: smokers connecting with cessation counselor Changes to the EMR: 1. EMR enhancement of smoking status icons 2. Tobacco treatment reminders 3. Smart form to facilitate ordering meds and fax/e-mail counseling referrals	Documentation of smoking status Contact with a quitline counselor	Higher percentages of documented smoking in the intervention clinics (+17%) compared to control (+11%) Quitline contact was higher among intervention clinic patients than control (3.9% vs 0.3%)

EMR, electronic medical record.
Editor's Note: Please refer to original journal article for full references.

in an increase in some clinical guideline recommended actions, particularly documentation of smoking status. There was insufficient evidence to quantify the effect of an EMR on changes in patient smoking behaviors.

Conclusions.—While the use of EMRs to prompt or provide feedback on the clinical treatment of tobacco dependence demonstrates some promising results, substantial additional research is needed to understand the effects of EMRs on provider and patient behavior.

▶ This review does not find enough data in the studies reviewed to determine whether the increase in the use of electronic medical records (EMRs) would increase the clinical treatment of tobacco dependence (Table 2). What is important here is that research on the effects of an EMR on the effective identification, treatment, and prevention of tobacco and other substance use is needed because it seems obvious that when well done, it is reasonable to expect that this will be one of the positive outcomes of a well-designed EMR. The Department of Veterans Affairs hospitals, with their excellent use of EMRs, would be a good place to look into this vital question and other positive uses of EMRs. The deficiency of research efforts on the prevention of substance abuse as a general issue is also clearly demonstrated by the results found here.

R. J. Frances, MD

Genetics and Progression

Alcohol Consumption Indices of Genetic Risk for Alcohol Dependence
Grant JD, Agrawal A, Bucholz KK, et al (Washington Univ School of Medicine, St Louis, MO; et al)
Biol Psychiatry 66:795-800, 2009

Background.—Previous research has reported a significant genetic correlation between heaviness of alcohol consumption and alcohol dependence (AD), but this association might be driven by the influence of AD on consumption rather than the reverse. We test the genetic overlap between AD symptoms and a heaviness of consumption measure among individuals who do not have AD. A high genetic correlation between these measures would suggest that a continuous measure of consumption may have a useful role in the discovery of genes contributing to dependence risk.

Methods.—Factor analysis of five alcohol use measures was used to create a measure of heaviness of alcohol consumption. Quantitative genetic analyses of interview data from the 1989 Australian Twin Panel ($n = 6257$ individuals; $M = 29.9$ years) assessed the genetic overlap between heaviness of consumption, DSM-IV AD symptoms, DSM-IV AD symptom clustering, and DSM-IV alcohol abuse.

Results.—Genetic influences accounted for 30%–51% of the variance in the alcohol measures and genetic correlations were .90 or higher for all measures, with the correlation between consumption and dependence symptoms among nondependent individuals estimated at .97 (95% confidence interval: .80–1.00).

TABLE 4.—Point Estimates and 95% Confidence Intervals for Genetic Correlations (Above Diagonal) and Nonshared Environmental Correlations (Below Diagonal) of Heaviness of Alcohol Use and Alcohol Abuse/Dependence Variables in the Australian Young Adult Twin Panel (1989 Cohort)

	AD Symptom Count	Consumption	AD Symptom Clustering	Alcohol Abuse Diagnosis
AD Symptom Count		$.97^c$ (.91−1.00)	$.99^c$ (.80−1.00)	$.96^c$ (.73−.99)
Consumption[a]	$.53^c$ (.45−.59)		$.99^c$ (.78−1.00)	$.90^c$ (.74−1.00)
AD Symptom Clustering[b]	$.79^c$ (.69−.90)	.60 (−.26−.99)		$.95^c$ (.56−1.00)
Alcohol Abuse Diagnosis[a]	$.44^c$ (.32−.46)	$.39^c$ (.30−.51)	.68 (−.42−.98)	

AD, alcohol dependence.
[a]Undefined in those with three or more AD symptoms.
[b]Undefined in those with between zero and two AD symptoms.
$^c p < .05$.

Conclusions.—Heaviness of consumption and AD symptoms have a high degree of genetic overlap even among nondependent individuals in the general population, implying that genetic influences on dependence risk in the general population are acting to a considerable degree through heaviness of use and that quantitative measures of consumption will likely have a useful role in the identification of genes contributing to AD.

▶ The importance of a strong genetic component of a 40% to 60% contribution to alcohol dependence has led to better public acceptance of a disease model of addiction. It has also been valuable in reducing stigma and has led to research on treatments that may affect gene expression. This study finds high genetic overlap between both alcohol dependence/alcohol abuse and the quantity of consumption in individuals without alcohol dependence in an Australian sample of twins (Table 4). In addition to underlining the importance of quantitative measures of consumption in the identification of genes contributing to alcohol dependence, this study supports the value of alcohol abuse as a diagnostic construct. It is hoped that the framers of the fifth edition of the *Diagnostic and Statistical Manual of Mental Disorders,* who have planned on eliminating the alcohol abuse category in favor of severity criteria, will take note of this. Clinicians can also use these results in aiming for prevention and early case finding by watching for heavy drinking in the close relatives of those who have problems with alcohol.

R. J. Frances, MD

Gene X Disease Interaction on Orbitofrontal Gray Matter in Cocaine Addiction
Alia-Klein N, Parvaz MA, Woicik PA, et al (Brookhaven Natl Laboratory, Upton, NY; et al)
Arch Gen Psychiatry 68:283-294, 2011

Context.—Long-term cocaine use has been associated with structural deficits in brain regions having dopamine-receptive neurons. However, the concomitant use of other drugs and common genetic variability in monoamine regulation present additional structural variability.

Objective.—To examine variations in gray matter volume (GMV) as a function of lifetime drug use and the genotype of the monoamine oxidase A gene, *MAOA*, in men with cocaine use disorders (CUD) and healthy male controls.

Design.—Cross-sectional comparison.

Setting.—Clinical Research Center at Brookhaven National Laboratory.

Patients.—Forty individuals with CUD and 42 controls who underwent magnetic resonance imaging to assess GMV and were genotyped for the *MAOA* polymorphism (categorized as high- and low-repeat alleles).

Main Outcome Measures.—The impact of cocaine addiction on GMV, tested by (1) comparing the CUD group with controls, (2) testing diagnosis X *MAOA* interactions, and (3) correlating GMV with lifetime cocaine, alcohol, and cigarette smoking, and testing their unique contribution to GMV beyond other factors.

Results.—(1) Individuals with CUD had reductions in GMV in the orbitofrontal, dorsolateral prefrontal, and temporal cortex and the hippocampus compared with controls. (2) The orbitofrontal cortex reductions were uniquely driven by CUD with low-*MAOA* genotype and by lifetime cocaine use. (3) The GMV in the dorsolateral prefrontal cortex and hippocampus was driven by lifetime alcohol use beyond the genotype and other pertinent variables.

Conclusions.—Long-term cocaine users with the low-repeat *MAOA* allele have enhanced sensitivity to gray matter loss, specifically in the orbitofrontal cortex, indicating that this genotype may exacerbate the deleterious effects of cocaine in the brain. In addition, long-term alcohol use is a major contributor to gray matter loss in the dorsolateral prefrontal cortex and hippocampus, and is likely to further impair executive function and learning in cocaine addiction.

▶ This study found that chronic use of cocaine can cause greater long-term orbitofrontal, dorsolateral prefrontal, temporal cortex, and hippocampus damage observable with magnetic resonance imaging, especially when genotype XMAOA is present (Fig 3 in the original article). Chronic heavy alcohol use combined with long-term cocaine use can contribute to further gray matter loss and further impair executive function and learning. These findings and the scans themselves can be shown to patients and their families to help motivate earlier efforts to treat the addiction. This also provides an area for future personalized prevention and care if patients with vulnerable genotypes were warned early about the particularly severe brain problems they will face with chronic cocaine use. This sophisticated methodology is one of the most powerful recent advances in addiction studies. At this point, there are no treatments other than abstinence to stop or reverse the damage done, and that is an important area for further study.

R. J. Frances, MD

4 Psychiatry and the Law

Introduction

America remains a nation where domestic violence, violence, and too-great availability of guns are sources of great public concern. With unemployment rates high, especially among veterans returning from war, the dangers of an increase in these problems are great. The role of mental illness in violence is also an increasing area of public concern.

Richard J. Frances, MD

Assessment and Treatment

Anxiety Disorders Among Offenders With Antisocial Personality Disorders: A Distinct Subtype?

Hodgins S, De Brito SA, Chhabra P, et al (King's College London, England, UK; Univ of London, England, UK; West London Mental Health Trust, England, UK; et al)

Can J Psychiatry 55:784-791, 2010

Objectives.—About 50% of men with antisocial personality disorder (APD) present a comorbid anxiety disorder. Historically, it was thought that anxiety limited criminal activity and the development of APD, but recent evidence suggests that heightened responsiveness to threat may lead to persistent violent behaviour. Our study aimed to determine the prevalence of APD comorbid with anxiety disorders among offenders and the association of these comorbid disorders with violent offending.

Method.—A random sample of 495 male penitentiary inmates completed an interview using the Diagnostic Interview Schedule. After excluding men with psychotic disorders, 279 with APD were retained. All authorized access to their criminal records.

Results.—Two-thirds of the prisoners with APD presented a lifetime anxiety disorder. Among them, one-half had the onset of their anxiety disorder before they were aged 16 years. Among the offenders with APD, those with, compared with those without, anxiety disorders presented significantly more symptoms of APD, were more likely to have begun their criminal

TABLE 1.—Prevalence of Lifetime Anxiety Disorders among Incarcerated Offenders with APD

Variable	Lifetime,[a] %	Anxiety Disorders $n = 279$ Only Past,[b] %	Only Last 6 Months,[c] %
Total	68.5	45.9	20.4
OCD	6.8	2.9	3.9
Phobia	31.9	18.3	11.1
Simple phobia	21.5		
Social phobia	10.0		
Agoraphobia	9.3		
Panic disorder	1.1	0.7	0.4
GAD	48.4	29.7	18.6
PTSD	15.0	7.2	7.5

[a]Diagnostic criteria for an anxiety disorder met at any time; lifetime prevalence does not exactly equal the sum of only past and past 6 months.
[b]Diagnostic criteria for an anxiety disorder met any time before the last 6 months.
[c]No anxiety disorder before the 6 months preceding the interview, when diagnostic criteria for an anxiety disorder were met.

careers before they were aged 15 years, to have diagnoses of alcohol and (or) drug abuse and (or) dependence, and to have experienced suicidal ideas and attempts. While there were no differences in the mean number of convictions for violent offences between APD prisoners with and without anxiety disorders, more of those with anxiety disorders had been convicted of serious crimes involving interpersonal violence.

Conclusions.—Among men with APD, a substantial subgroup present life-long anxiety disorders. This pattern of comorbidity may reflect a distinct mechanism underlying violent behaviour and signalling the need for specific treatments.

▶ The very high prevalence of anxiety disorders in a criminal population might surprise anyone except for forensic psychiatrists, prison guards, or anyone spending time in jail with prisoners, who are by and large a very anxious lot (Table 1). Very often these are people who had experienced severe childhood trauma and neglect; had parents with criminal records and substance abuse; feared the consequences of their cases and their prison environment; and heavily used substances, perhaps to self-medicate, but often leading to substance-induced panic and other anxiety disorders. Initially, many prisoners also suffer from untreated withdrawal syndromes and the anxiety associated with early abstinence. Treatment of anxiety in prison is also complicated by the dangers of using dependence-producing benzodiazepines and sleep medications that can lead to abuse and may be diverted and used as currency in jail. The point that an anxious, frightened sociopath is more likely to be physically violent in jail is well taken, and the education of prison personnel on tension-reduction techniques is a good idea.

R. J. Frances, MD

Disrupted Reinforcement Signaling in the Orbitofrontal Cortex and Caudate in Youths With Conduct Disorder or Oppositional Defiant Disorder and a High Level of Psychopathic Traits

Finger EC, Marsh AA, Blair KS, et al (Univ of Western Ontario, London Canada; NIMH, Bethesda, MD; Georgetown Univ, Washington, DC)
Am J Psychiatry 168:152-162, 2011

Objective.—Dysfunction in the amygdala and orbitofrontal cortex has been reported in youths and adults with psychopathic traits. The specific nature of the functional irregularities within these structures remains poorly understood. The authors used a passive avoidance task to examine the responsiveness of these systems to early stimulus-reinforcement exposure, when prediction errors are greatest and learning maximized, and to reward in youths with psychopathic traits and comparison youths.

Method.—While performing the passive avoidance learning task, 15 youths with conduct disorder or oppositional defiant disorder plus a high level of psychopathic traits and 15 healthy subjects completed a 3.0-T fMRI scan.

Results.—Relative to the comparison youths, the youths with a disruptive behavior disorder plus psychopathic traits showed less orbitofrontal responsiveness both to early stimulus-reinforcement exposure and to rewards, as well as less caudate response to early stimulus-reinforcement exposure. There were no group differences in amygdala responsiveness to these two task measures, but amygdala responsiveness throughout the task was lower in the youths with psychopathic traits.

Conclusions.—Compromised sensitivity to early reinforcement information in the orbitofrontal cortex and caudate and to reward outcome information in the orbitofrontal cortex of youths with conduct disorder or oppositional defiant disorder plus psychopathic traits suggests that the integrated functioning of the amygdala, caudate, and orbitofrontal cortex may be disrupted. This provides a functional neural basis for why such youths are more likely to repeat disadvantageous decisions. New treatment possibilities are raised, as pharmacologic modulations of serotonin and dopamine can affect this form of learning.

▶ This shows how lack of integration of functioning and deficits in responsiveness in the amygdala, caudatate, and orbital frontal cortex bring about conduct disorder or oppositional defiant disorder plus psychopathic traits. These findings have visual support with results seen on brain imaging (Fig 3 in original article). The implications of this study for pharmacologic and other therapeutic interventions targeted at these disruptions are important and point to new possible treatments modulating serotonin and dopamine to help these youths make better decisions. There are also interesting implications as to how the increasing awareness of brain disturbances and specific brain abnormalities in conduct disorder will affect the criminal justice system and the views of juries about youths with conduct disorders as to free will versus biological determinism. Perhaps more treatment and less incarceration in the future will be tolerated and will be deemed to be cost effective as more effective prevention programs and treatments are developed.

R. J. Frances, MD

Domestic Violence

Adulthood Stressors, History of Childhood Adversity, and Risk of Perpetration of Intimate Partner Violence
Roberts AL, McLaughlin KA, Conron KJ, et al (Harvard School of Public Health, Boston, MA)
Am J Prev Med 40:128-138, 2011

Background.—More than half a million U.S. women and more than 100,000 men are treated for injuries from intimate partner violence (IPV) annually, making IPV perpetration a major public health problem. However, little is known about causes of perpetration across the life course.

Purpose.—This paper examines the role of "stress sensitization," whereby adult stressors increase risk for IPV perpetration most strongly in people with a history of childhood adversity.

Methods.—The study investigated a possible interaction effect between adulthood stressors and childhood adversities in risk of IPV perpetration, specifically, whether the difference in risk of IPV perpetration associated with past-year stressors varied by history of exposure to childhood adversity. Analyses were conducted in 2010 using de-identified data from 34 653 U.S. adults from the 2004–2005 follow-up wave of the National Epidemiologic Survey on Alcohol and Related Conditions.

Results.—There was a significant stress sensitization effect. For men with high-level childhood adversity, past-year stressors were associated with an 8.8 percentage point (pp) increased risk of perpetrating compared to a 2.3 pp increased risk among men with low-level adversity. Women with high-level childhood adversity had a 14.3 pp increased risk compared with a 2.5 pp increased risk in the low-level adversity group.

Conclusions.—Individuals with recent stressors and histories of childhood adversity are at particularly elevated risk of IPV perpetration; therefore, prevention efforts should target this population. Treatment programs for IPV perpetrators, which have not been effective in reducing risk of perpetrating, may benefit from further investigating the role of stress and stress reactivity in perpetration.

▶ Intimate partner violence is a huge public health problem that tends to pass from one generation to the next. A good argument could be made that shifting some funding from law enforcement and treatment of intimate partner violence to prevention efforts might lead to better public health in this area, especially as improved understanding of the antecedents of intimate partner violence are better understood and better prevention methods develop. That childhood and recent stressors both play a role in contributing to intimate partner violence is not a surprise (Table 4). Having parents with substance abuse and criminality,

TABLE 4.—Risk of Perpetrating Intimate Partner Violence by Level of Childhood Adversity and Adulthood Stressors

	Adulthood Past–12-Month Stressors							
	Men (%) (n=14,564)				Women (%) (n=20,089)			
Childhood Adversity	Lowest Stressors	Low-Middle Stressors	Middle-High Stressors	Highest Stressors	Lowest Stressors	Low-Middle Stressors	Middle-High Stressors	Highest Stressors
Lowest adversity	0.9 (1674)	1.1 (1144)	2.3 (741)	3.5 (322)	0.6 (2268)	1.7 (1334)	1.9 (943)	2.9 (464)
Low-middle adversity	1.4 (1076)	1.6 (1035)	3.3 (811)	5.8 (561)	1.8 (1349)	2.3 (1401)	2.6 (1394)	6.7 (1015)
Middle-high adversity	2.6 (480)	3.5 (785)	3.3 (1052)	5.0 (1237)	1.9 (1003)	5.0 (1353)	5.2 (1327)	10.4 (1234)
Highest adversity	2.9 (420)	3.1 (670)	6.8 (1035)	13.6 (1521)	3.3 (402)	2.9 (934)	10.0 (1358)	16.9 (2310)

Note: Sample included U.S. men and women aged ≥20 years (N=34,653). Values are % (*n*). Adjusted for race/ethnicity and age at interview.

early experiences of physical violence trauma, neglect, and sexual abuse will predispose to later vulnerability, perhaps in those who also have greater genetic predisposition to be vulnerable. Distinguishing the resilient from the vulnerable and finding better ways to cope with life stressors when they occur would both be helpful in detecting and preventing vulnerability to intimate partner violence.

R. J. Frances, MD

Analyzing Offense Patterns as a Function of Mental Illness to Test the Criminalization Hypothesis
Peterson J, Skeem JL, Hart E, et al (Univ of California, Irvine; et al)
Psychiatr Serv 61:1217-1222, 2010

Objective.—Programs for offenders with mental illness seem to be based on a hypothesis that untreated symptoms are the main source of criminal behavior and that linkage with psychiatric services is the solution. This study tested this criminalization hypothesis, which implies that these individuals have unique patterns of offending.

Methods.—Participants were 220 parolees; 111 had a serious mental illness, and 109 did not. Interview data and records were used to reliably classify offenders into one of five groups, based on their lifetime pattern of offending: psychotic, disadvantaged, reactive, instrumental, or gang- or drug-related affiliation. The distributions of those with and without serious mental illness were compared.

Results.—A small but important minority of offenders with a mental illness (7%, N=8) fit the criminalization hypothesis, in that their criminal behavior was a direct result of psychosis (5%, N=6) or comprised minor "survival" crimes related to poverty (2%, N=2). However, the reactive group contained virtually all offenders with a mental illness (90%, N=100) and the vast majority of offenders without a mental illness (68%, N=74), suggesting that criminal behavior for both groups chiefly was driven by hostility, disinhibition, and emotional reactivity. For most offenders with a mental illness in the reactive group, crime was also driven by substance dependence.

Conclusions.—Offenders with serious mental illness manifested heterogeneous patterns of offending that may stem from a variety of sources. Although psychiatric service linkage may reduce recidivism for a visible minority, treatment that targets impulsivity and other common criminogenic needs may be needed to prevent recidivism for the larger group (Table 4).

▶ The principal finding here is that only a small percentage of the mentally ill prisoners are likely to have a reduction of recidivism with treatment of their mental illness. There are people with severe mental illness who are prone to repeat crimes just as there are people without mental illness who are career criminals (Table 4). One flaw in this study is that it does not treat addiction

TABLE 4.—Offenders Returned to Custody Within 12 Months, by Typology and Mental Illness Status

Offender Type	With Mental Illness			Without Mental Illness			Total		
	Total N	N	%	Total N	N	%	Total N	N	%
Psychotic	6	1	17	0	0	0	6	1	17
Disadvantaged	2	0	—	4	0	—	6	0	—
Reactive	99[a]	30	30	74	15	20	173	45	26
Instrumental	3	1	33	12	2	17	15	3	20
Gang or drug related	0	0	—	19	3	16	19	3	16

[a]One participant was lost to follow-up.

as a mental illness. Therefore, there may be a significant part of what is considered or not considered a mentally ill population with addiction, who could all get reduction in recidivism if the addiction were properly treated. Also, even those prisoners who might be prone to recidivism should be given humane care in prisons. In my experience, few people suffer more emotional pain than the untreated severely mentally ill addicted prison population, especially when they are not treated for the mental illness including addiction.

R. J. Frances, MD

Barriers and facilitators of disclosures of domestic violence by mental health service users: qualitative study

Rose D, Trevillion K, Woodall A, et al (King's College London, UK; et al)
Br J Psychiatry 198:189-194, 2011

Background.—Mental health service users are at high risk of domestic violence but this is often not detected by mental health services.

Aims.—To explore the facilitators and barriers to disclosure of domestic violence from a service user and professional perspective.

Method.—A qualitative study in a socioeconomically deprived south London borough, UK, with 18 mental health service users and 20 mental health professionals. Purposive sampling of community mental health service users and mental healthcare professionals was used to recruit participants for individual interviews. Thematic analysis was used to determine dominant and subthemes. These were transformed into conceptual maps with accompanying illustrative quotations.

Results.—Service users described barriers to disclosure of domestic violence to professionals including: fear of the consequences, including fear of Social Services involvement and consequent child protection proceedings, fear that disclosure would not be believed, and fear that disclosure would lead to further violence; the hidden nature of the violence; actions of the perpetrator; and feelings of shame. The main themes for professionals concerned role boundaries, competency and confidence. Service users and professionals

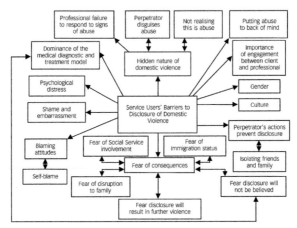

FIGURE 1.—Service users' barriers to disclosure of domestic violence. (Reprinted from Rose D, Trevillion K, Woodall A, et al. Barriers and facilitators of disclosures of domestic violence by mental health service users: qualitative study. *Br J Psychiatry*. 2011;198:189-194, with permission from Royal College of Psychiatrists.)

reported that the medical diagnostic and treatment model with its emphasis on symptoms could act as a barrier to enquiry and disclosure. Both groups reported that enquiry and disclosure were facilitated by a supportive and trusting relationship between the individual and professional.

Conclusions.—Mental health services are not currently conducive to the disclosure of domestic violence. Training of professionals in how to address domestic violence to increase their confidence and expertise is recommended.

▶ In Britain, as in many other places worldwide, 20% to 25% of women report physical sexual and emotional forms of abuse, and these numbers are likely to be higher if the barriers to seeking care described in this study were reduced. This is the first study that looks at facilitators and barriers to disclosure of domestic violence by studying both clients and providers in a poor area of London's community health clinic. Not surprisingly, stigma, fear of reprisal, of social services and child protective interference, and that their complaints would not be believed were major barriers to seeking help and reporting abuse on the consumer side (Fig 1). Treaters' lack of training, low confidence in their own ability to deal with the problem effectively, and fear of crossing boundaries were factors that contributed to barriers to effective action. An empathic supportive relationship and trust building helps reduce fear and stigma, and education of staff and patients about skills, attitudes, and knowledge helps build trust. This worldwide problem needs to be addressed with more resources and attention.

R. J. Frances, MD

Child Abuse Experts Disagree About the Threshold for Mandated Reporting

Levi BH, Crowell K (Penn State College of Medicine, Hershey, PA; Penn State Children's Hosp, Hershey, PA)
Clin Pediatr 50:321-329, 2011

Context.—Though reasonable suspicion serves as the standard threshold for when to report suspected child abuse, there is little guidance how to interpret the term.

Objective.—To examine how experts on child abuse interpret reasonable suspicion using 2 probability frameworks.

Participants.—Anonymous survey of clinical and research experts on child abuse.

Main Outcome Measures.—Responses on ordinal and visual analog scales quantifying the probability needed for "suspicion of child abuse" to rise to reasonable suspicion.

Results.—A total of 81 of 117 experts completed the survey (69% response rate, mean age 47 years, 69% female). On both the ordinal probability scale (rank order on a differential diagnosis) and the estimated probability scale (1% to 99% likelihood), experts demonstrated wide variability in defining reasonable suspicion, with no statistically significant differences found for age, race, gender, professional training, seniority, or prior education on reasonable suspicion.

Conclusions.—This study found no consensus in how experts on child abuse interpret reasonable suspicion.

▶ The lack of clarity about a threshold for mandated reporting found in this study points to a need for developing clearer standards of what constitutes abuse and then improved training for professionals regarding the standard. Surprisingly, this study did not find specific factors including training, gender, seniority, or poor education on reasonable suspicion to account for this wide variability in reporting. There are definitely situations in which appropriate interventions, ranging from evaluation to removal of a child from a dangerous environment, make an enormous difference in a child's life and can be lifesaving. Figuring out the reasons for the wide variability in what constitutes how experts on child abuse interpret reasonable suspicion is clearly the next step.

R. J. Frances, MD

Chronic conditions in children increase the risk for physical abuse — but vary with socio-economic circumstances

Svensson B, Bornehag C-G, Janson S (Karlstad Univ, Sweden)
Acta Paediatr 100:407-412, 2011

Aim.—To explore whether children (age 10, 12 and 15 years) with self-reported chronic conditions are at higher risk of physical abuse and/or exposure to intimate-partner violence than other children, while considering the importance of demographic factors.

Methods.—A national cross-sectional study of 2771 pupils in grades 4, 6 and 9 from 44 schools in Sweden (91% response rate). Conflict Tactic Scales were used to measure physical abuse and separate questions measured exposure to intimate-partner violence. A list of 13 diagnoses was used to estimate chronic conditions.

Results.—Children with chronic conditions had an increased risk for physical abuse (CPA) only (OR 1.67) as well as in combination with exposure to intimate-partner violence (IPV) (OR 2.54), but not to IPV only, compared to children without chronic conditions. Furthermore, when chronic conditions were combined with country of birth other than Sweden and living in low-income areas, the risk for CPA increased even more, indicating interactive effects.

Conclusions.—A wide range of chronic health conditions in children increased the risk for physical abuse. This indicates that certain factors unite this group of children, irrespective of the type of disability or degree of severity, but where a combination with socio-economic circumstances is of importance.

▶ Increase in physical abuse in children with chronic conditions had previously been found. This Swedish study confirms the problem and found that intimate partner violence is also more frequently witnessed by these children. What makes this study especially interesting is the finding that sociocultural factors such as economic status and country of origin and differences in culture as well as the challenges of acculturation in Swedish society for immigrants may also contribute to greater problems as risks escalated for these disadvantaged groups (Fig 1). Swedish society has gone through dramatic change in urban

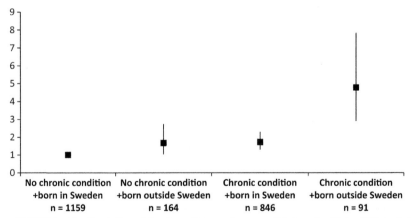

| No chronic condition +born in Sweden n = 1159 | No chronic condition +born outside Sweden n = 164 | Chronic condition +born in Sweden n = 846 | Chronic condition +born outside Sweden n = 91 |

FIGURE 1.—Combined effect of chronic conditions and country of birth on the risk for child physical abuse (CPA) when compared with referents expressed as adjusted odds ratios with 95% CI. (Reprinted from Svensson B, Bornehag C-G, Janson S. Chronic conditions in children increase the risk for physical abuse – but vary with socio-economic circumstances. *Acta Paediatr.* 2011;100:407-412, with permission from The Author(s)/Acta Pædiatrica and John Wiley and Sons (www.interscience.wiley.com).)

areas as a liberal social system and immigration have led to new challenges and opportunities for what previously had been a homogeneous population. Clearly the issue of cultural sensitivity and cultural competence are increasingly required of all service providers, especially when countries undergo multicultural adjustments. In addition to risk, it may be valuable to study which factors lead to resilience in children with chronic conditions and may improve quality of life for these children and their families. In the United States, provision of basic health care and social services are often lacking for disadvantaged populations, including in particular illegal immigrants. The cost-effectiveness of addressing these issues in all countries is vital to demonstrate a need and to increase public support for necessary resources in the current era in which all health care expenses come under increasing scrutiny.

R. J. Frances, MD

Longitudinal Risk Factors for Intimate Partner Violence Among Men in Treatment for Alcohol Use Disorders

Taft CT, O'Farrell TJ, Doron-Lamarca S, et al (Boston Univ School of Medicine, MA; Harvard Med School; et al)
J Consult Clin Psychol 78:924-935, 2010

Objective.—This study examined static and time-varying risk factors for perpetration of intimate partner violence (IPV) among men in treatment for alcohol use disorders.

Method.—Participants were 178 men diagnosed with alcohol abuse or dependence and their partners. Most (85) of the men were European American; their average age was 41.0 years. Participants completed measures assessing initial alcohol problem severity, baseline beliefs related to alcohol use, antisocial personality characteristics, alcohol and drug use, relationship adjustment, and IPV.

Results.—According to couples' reconciled reports, 42 of participants perpetrated IPV at baseline. Among this group, the IPV recurrence rate was 43 at 6-month follow-up and 36 at 12-month follow-up. For participants without IPV perpetration at baseline, new incidence of IPV was 15 and 7 at the 6-month and 12-month follow-up points, respectively. Fixed marker predictors of IPV rates included baseline alcohol problem severity variables, baseline beliefs related to alcohol use, and antisocial personality characteristics. Variable risk factor predictors included alcohol and drug use variables, relationship adjustment factors, and anger. Alcohol use variables and anger were associated with new incidents of IPV among those without reported IPV at baseline only.

Conclusions.—Findings suggest that assessing and monitoring IPV occurrence by both partners is important for men in treatment for alcohol use disorders. Results indicate vulnerability factors that may identify individuals at risk for IPV and provide targets for IPV prevention among those with alcohol use disorders. These findings can aid in the development of more comprehensive models that more precisely predict IPV.

▶ Intimate partner violence (IVP) occurs very frequently with male alcoholics, far more than in the general population and, together with child abuse, is one of the great tragedies of addiction. This study has the advantage of looking at both partners and following progress after treatment is initiated, which was found to be very significant, with massive reductions in IVP seen and recurrences or new occurrences in controls of IVP occurring more frequently with relapse. I have seen also that IVP can persist in instances in which abstinence is achieved and addiction is often only part of the problems of the family. Screening for IVP in the population of patients with addiction and providing targeted treatments that help reduce IVP, in addition to achieving and maintaining abstinence, are important components of treatment programs. As a result of denial, fear of loss of relationships, and fear of legal action and reporting, most alcoholic men will not readily admit to spousal or child abuse, and staff needs to be trained in observing patterns and diagnosing problems. Involving spouses in gathering information and treatment is essential, although they are also often codependent and frightened to reveal problems.

R. J. Frances, MD

Violence

Guns don't kill crowds, people with semi-automatics do
Kamerow D (RTI International)
BMJ 342:d477, 2011

Why can't we do a better job of protecting society from this type of attack?

Once again in the United States a seriously mentally ill man is suspected of mowing down a crowd before he can be wrestled to the ground.

This time the victims included a Congresswoman and a federal judge. A wave of shock spread across the country and around the world. Liberals blamed the mood of the country and violent rhetoric from conservative leaders. Conservatives howled with injustice and attacked the liberals for attacking them.

The handgun used for the attack was a Glock 19, a lightweight, compact, semi-automatic pistol that comes with a standard magazine holding 15 bullets of 9 mm calibre. Glock pistols have become the overwhelming choice of police departments around the world because of their light polymer construction and their ease of firing. They are called "semi-automatic" guns because, unlike revolvers that have one bullet per chamber, all the bullets can be fired by simply squeezing and re-squeezing the trigger. Jared Loughner, the alleged gunman, had legally purchased such a weapon in November, along with an extended capacity magazine that allowed him to fire 33 times without stopping to reload.

Loughner, 22, was clearly mentally ill. Press reports after the event have documented a mind unravelling and descending into madness over the previous year. He lost his friends. He had repeated run-ins with school authorities. He disrupted his college classes, and classmates sat next to the door, fearing that he might get violent. He posted bizarre theories and claims on internet sites, leading one regular poster to label him as having schizophrenia and to plead with him to get help or start taking his medications again. He had several encounters with the police, including one on the day of the shooting. But no one made a formal complaint, and Loughner never received a psychiatric evaluation.

Ever responsive, the US Congress immediately sprang into action to fix the problem. One Congressman introduced legislation making it a crime to carry a gun within 1000 feet (300 m) of a member of Congress. Laughably unenforceable, patently self protectionist, and just plain silly, it seemed the perfect response to the tragedy. In fact no legislation is likely to be passed in response to this event.

The second amendment to the US Constitution states that "the right of the people to keep and bear arms shall not be infringed." Americans, with the exception of some pockets of opposition on the two coasts, believe that citizens have a right to own and carry guns. Apparently most of us like having guns around, and there is no chance that any laws will be passed to limit access to them significantly. No amount of handgun related violence and no high profile killings will change this.

Three years ago a similarly deranged young man, Seung-Hui Cho, killed 32 fellow students at a Virginia university. He used a Glock 19 as well. His rampage did lead to changes in state and national laws to make it more difficult for mentally ill people to buy guns. Unfortunately such restrictions work only if a person is in the mental health system, and Loughner never made it that far.

We are told that guns don't kill people, that people kill people, and that what we have here is a failure of the mental health treatment system, not the legal system. But in order to kill a lot of people fast, before being stopped, people need access to guns that are easy to fire and have lots of bullets in them.

I don't think the problem is the mood of the country or who was placed in Sarah Palin's cross-hairs in her campaign literature. There will always be seriously disturbed individuals out there who, because of our country's history and experience, will have a chance to access guns. Given that we have no realistic chance of banning handguns, if we have any hope of preventing future such tragedies there are only two things we can do.

Firstly, we need to prevent the sale of equipment that facilitates such easy carnage: high capacity magazines for easily concealed guns. What is the purpose of a 33 shot magazine for a Glock? Who needs to fire 33 times without reloading? If Loughner had had a revolver instead of a 33 shot Glock he would have succeeded in shooting his target but probably not many more people. Cho would have had to stop to reload more often and likely could have been stopped short of killing 32 others.

Secondly, it must be made clear that it is everyone's job to report obviously disturbed people and get them into treatment. Neither Loughner nor Cho was a close call. Many people sensed that they were dangers to themselves and others. If someone had stepped up and reported Loughner, he might have had a paper trail that would have prevented him from buying his gun.

Guns don't kill crowds, but mentally disturbed people with high capacity semi-automatic pistols do.

▶ Even after repeated mass shootings in the United States, including the shooting of a congresswoman, judge, children, and others in Arizona, little is likely to be done to prevent this. This is the most important point made in this article. Why can't Congress pass better gun control laws? At the very least, why can't our leaders ban automatic concealed weapons that can quickly kill many innocent victims in a crowd? More careful screening for mental illness and criminality before allowing individuals to purchase a gun would also help, but only modestly because these guns can also be easily obtained illegally. The time has come for a greater push against the gun lobby Wild West culture that contributes to a level of violence that should not be tolerated in a civilized society. Interestingly, this article appeared in the *British Journal of Medicine*. People in the United States should look to Britain and Canada for better models of gun control.

R. J. Frances, MD

Homicide of Strangers by People With a Psychotic Illness
Nielssen O, Bourget D, Laajasalo T, et al (St Vincent's Hosp, Sydney, New South Wales, Australia; Univ of Ottawa, Ontario, Canada; Univ of Helsinki, Finland; et al)
Schizophr Bull 37:572-579, 2011

Background.—The homicide of strangers by people with psychosis, referred to here as "stranger homicides," are rare and tragic events that generate adverse publicity for mental health services and have resulted in significant changes in mental health policy and law.

Aim.—To estimate the incidence of stranger homicides, using data from previously published studies, and to compare the characteristics of psychotic offenders who killed strangers with the characteristics of those who killed a close relative.

Method.—Meta-analysis of the population-based studies of homicide by persons suffering from a psychosis in which the number of subjects who killed strangers was also reported. Characteristics of stranger homicide and family homicide offenders were examined in a multicenter case-control study of homicide during psychotic illness in four high-income countries.

Results.—A pooled estimate of 1 stranger homicide per 14.3 million people per year (95% confidence interval, 1 in 18.9 million to 1 in 11.5

TABLE 3.—Details of the Stranger-Homicide Offences Committed by People with Psychosis

	Stranger-Homicides, n (%)	Family-Homicides, n (%)	Odds Ratio or t Statistic	95% Confidence Interval of the Odds Ratio, P Value
Total	42	42		
Homicide at victims home or workplace	8 (19)	20 (48)	0.26	0.10–0.67[a]
Multiple victims	8 (19)	11 (26)	0.66	0.24–1.86
Knife or firearm use	23 (55)	18 (43)	1.61	0.68–3.82
Excessive force used	12 (29)	19 (45)	0.48	0.20–1.20
Intoxicated with drugs or alcohol	7 (17)	5 (12)	1.48	0.43–5.10
Age of victim (SD)	36.7 (19.1)	42.6 (23.9)	T = 1.13	P = 0.10
Male victim	27 (64)	15 (36)	3.60	1.46–8.85[a]
Legal finding of full criminal responsibility	3 (7)	2 (5)	0.65	0.10–4.10

[a]Significant at <0.05.

million people per year) was calculated by meta-analysis of 7 studies. The characteristics of the 42 stranger homicide offenders from New South Wales [NSW], Quebec and Eastern Ontario, Finland, and the Netherlands were identified. Twenty seven (64%) of these had never previously received treatment with antipsychotic medication. The stranger homicide offenders were more likely to be homeless, have exhibited antisocial conduct, and had fewer negative symptoms than those who killed family members. The victims of stranger homicide were mostly adult males and the homicides rarely occurred in the victim's home or workplace.

Conclusions.—Stranger homicide in psychosis is extremely rare and is even rarer for a patient who has received treatment with antipsychotic medication. A lack of distinguishing characteristics of stranger homicide offenders and an extremely low base rate of stranger-homicide suggests that risk assessment of patients known to have a psychotic illness will be of little assistance in the prevention of stranger homicides (Table 3).

▶ This multinational study finds homicides of strangers by people with a psychotic illness to be extremely rare and therefore unpredictable (Table 3). The finding that in 64% of these rare cases the perpetrator had not been treated with antipsychotics raises a glimmer of hope that wider dissemination of treatment might reduce risk of homicides by psychotic individuals. When these events occur, they are widely publicized and add significantly to the stigma and fears that are engendered in the general public of severe mental illness, which are mostly irrational. Stranger homicides have also been associated with addiction, homelessness, and antisocial behavior in combination with severe mental illness.

R. J. Frances, MD

Homicide, Suicide, and Unintentional Firearm Fatality: Comparing the United States With Other High-Income Countries, 2003
Richardson EG, Hemenway D (UCLA School of Public Health; Harvard School of Public Health, Boston, MA)
J Trauma 70:238-243, 2011

Background.—Violent death is a major public health problem in the United States and throughout the world.

Methods.—A cross-sectional analysis of the World Health Organization Mortality Database analyzes homicides and suicides (both disaggregated as firearm related and non-firearm related) and unintentional and undetermined firearm deaths from 23 populous high-income Organization for Economic Co-Operation and Development countries that provided data to the World Health Organization for 2003.

TABLE 3.—Ratio of US Death Rates to Death Rates in Other High Income Countries, Overall and by Gender, 2003, and Statistical Tests Showing the Significance of Each Fatality Occurrence in the US vs. Non-US Countries

	0−4 yr	5−14 y	15−24 yr	25−34 yr	35−64 yr	65+ yr	Totals
Overall							
Gun homicide rate	7.8	13.4	42.7	23.2	11.9	8.0	19.5
Nongun homicide	4.3	1.8	3.4	2.9	2.8	2.5	2.9
Total homicide rate	4.4	3.6	14.2	9.4	5.1	3.3	6.9
Gun suicide rate	—	8.0	8.8	8.9	5.8	5.9	5.8
Nongun suicide rate	—	1.2	0.6	0.5	0.4	0.2	0.4
Total suicide rate	—	1.6	1.2	0.9	0.7	0.7	0.7
Unintentional gun death	—	10.6	11.6	6.9	4.0	4.7	5.5
Undetermined gun death	0.5*	4.5	2.0	1.0*	0.6*	0.3	0.8
Firearm death rates	6.8	10.6	17.3	12.8	6.3	5.6	7.5
Firearm deaths	68	368	7,408	7,040	16,301	6,239	37,424
Males							
Gun homicide rate	5.7	20.3	46.7	25.1	12.8	8.8	22.0
Nongun homicide	4.8	1.7	3.4	2.8	2.8	3.0	2.9
Total homicide rate	4.8	4.2	17.0	11.1	5.6	3.8	8.2
Gun suicide rate	0.0	7.9	8.7	8.5	5.3	5.5	5.3
Nongun suicide rate	0.0	1.4	0.6	0.5	0.4	0.2	0.3
Total suicide rate	0.0	2.0	1.3	1.0	0.8	0.8	0.8
Unintentional gun death	0.0	9.9	10.8	6.9	3.7	4.2	5.2
Undetermined gun death	0.7*	4.5	2.1	1.0*	0.5*	0.3*	0.7*
Firearm death rates	5.7	11.7	17.6	12.8	5.8	5.3	7.2
Firearm deaths	44	288	6,674	6,211	13,845	5,701	32,763
Females							
Gun homicide rate	15.3	7.3	23.6	14.7	9.6	7.1	11.6
Nongun homicide	3.8	1.8	3.5	3.1	2.7	2.1	2.8
Total homicide rate	4.0	2.9	6.9	5.4	4.2	2.7	4.4
Gun suicide rate	0.0	8.3	9.5	12.7	16.4	19.0	14.4
Nongun suicide rate	0.0	0.9	0.5	0.5	0.5	0.2	0.4
Total suicide rate	0.0	1.1	0.7	0.7	0.7	0.3	0.6
Unintentional gun death	0.0	0.0	30.4	6.7	10.0	17.3	12.0
Undetermined gun death	0.0	0.0	1.4*	0.8*	1.7	0.3*	1.2*
Firearm death rates	10.2*	7.8	14.2	12.3	11.8	11.1	11.5
Firearm deaths	24	80	734	829	2,456	538	4,661

*All associations testing significant differences between US and non-US countries are significant at the $p < 0.05$ level except for those denoted by asterisk.

Results.—The US homicide rates were 6.9 times higher than rates in the other high-income countries, driven by firearm homicide rates that were 19.5 times higher. For 15-year olds to 24-year olds, firearm homicide rates in the United States were 42.7 times higher than in the other countries. For US males, firearm homicide rates were 22.0 times higher, and for US females, firearm homicide rates were 11.4 times higher. The US firearm suicide rates were 5.8 times higher than in the other countries, though overall suicide rates were 30% lower. The US unintentional firearm deaths were 5.2 times higher than in the other countries. Among these 23 countries, 80% of all firearm deaths occurred in the United States, 86% of women killed by firearms were US women, and 87% of all children aged 0 to 14 killed by firearms were US children.

Conclusions.—The United States has far higher rates of firearm deaths— firearm homicides, firearm suicides, and unintentional firearm deaths compared with other high-income countries. The US overall suicide rate is not out of line with these countries, but the United States is an outlier in terms of our overall homicide rate (Table 3).

▶ This study analyzes a World Health Organization database relating firearm fatalities of suicide and homicide with astounding and alarming statistical findings. The United States, having a 42.7-fold higher youth homicide rate compared with similar high-income countries, indicates a severe neglect of a critically serious need for gun control and the need to look for means of reducing violence in our culture (Table 3). The public health implications of the findings of this study are obvious, and these findings clearly need public dissemination and should lead to public outcry for policy reform. When will the shooting of a public figure or reports of a gun-related suicide or accidental death in a young person result in efforts to make the needed changes to reduce gun-related violence? What role should psychiatrists play in publicly speaking out and leading this fight? Any delay just increases the loss of life in America, a toll most heavily and tragically directed at young Americans.

R. J. Frances, MD

Overcrowding in psychiatric wards and physical assaults on staff: data-linked longitudinal study
Virtanen M, Vahtera J, Batty GD, et al (Finnish Inst of Occupational Health, Helsinki, Finland; Univ of Turku and Turku Univ Hosp, Finland; Univ College London, UK; et al)
Br J Psychiatry 198:149-155, 2011

Background.—Patient overcrowding and violent assaults by patients are two major problems in psychiatric healthcare. However, evidence of an association between overcrowding and aggressive behaviour among patients is mixed and limited to small-scale studies.

Aims.—This study examined the association between ward overcrowding and violent physical assaults in acute-care psychiatric in-patient hospital wards.

Method.—Longitudinal study using ward-level monthly records of bed occupancy and staff reports of the timing of violent acts during a 5-month period in 90 in-patient wards in 13 acute psychiatric hospitals in Finland. In total 1098 employees (physicians, ward head nurses, registered nurses, licensed practical nurses) participated in the study. The outcome measure was staff reports of the timing of physical assaults on both themselves and ward property.

Results.—We found that 46% of hospital staff were working in over-crowded wards, as indicated by >10 percentage units of excess bed occupancy, whereas only 30% of hospital personnel were working in a ward with no excess occupancy. An excess bed occupancy rate of >10 percentage

TABLE 2.—Univariate Associations of Individual Staff Characteristics and Organisational Characteristics with the Onset of Violent Physical Assaults Reported by Ward Staff (For a More Detailed Version See Online Table DS2)

Characteristic	n	Assaults on an Employee Events, n (%)	OR (95% CI)	n	Assaults on ward Property Events, n (%)	OR (95% CI)
All	1098	178 (16)		1089	264 (24)	
Gender						
Female	755	114 (15)	1.00	748	154 (21)	1.00
Male	343	64 (19)	1.24 (0.93–1.65)	341	110 (32)	1.57 (1.26–1.96)
Age						
20–29	152	31 (20)	1.00	151	51 (34)	1.00
30–39	274	59 (22)	1.04 (0.69–1.57)	273	78 (29)	0.82 (0.60–1.11)
40–49	374	53 (14)	0.66 (0.44–1.01)	369	85 (23)	0.64 (0.47–0.87)
50–63	298	35 (12)	0.54 (0.34–0.86)	296	50 (17)	0.46 (0.32–0.65)
Occupation						
Physician/head nurse	136	11 (8)	1.00	133	21 (16)	1.00
Registered psychiatric nurse	500	83 (17)	1.96 (1.07–3.61)	498	131 (26)	1.62 (1.05–2.50)
Licensed practical psychiatric nurse	462	84 (18)	2.19 (1.19–4.02)	458	112 (24)	1.51 (0.98–2.35)
Type of job contract						
Permanent	907	144 (16)	1.00	899	210 (23)	1.00
Temporary	191	34 (18)	1.15 (0.81–1.64)	190	54 (28)	1.26 (0.96–1.64)
Length of job contract (years)						
<1	381	68 (18)	1.00	379	98 (26)	1.00
1–4	463	70 (15)	0.81 (0.59–1.11)	458	103 (22)	0.83 (0.64–1.07)
>4	254	40 (16)	0.84 (0.58–1.21)	252	63 (25)	0.92 (0.69–1.23)
Specialty						
Adults	856	129 (15)	1.00	847	189 (22)	1.00
Children/adolescents	242	49 (20)	1.31 (0.96–1.79)	242	75 (31)	1.36 (1.07–1.73)
Ward size (Sum of patient days)[a]						
≤300	321	35 (11)	1.00	319	53 (17)	1.00
301–500	393	69 (18)	1.51 (1.01–2.25)	390	126 (32)	1.85 (1.36–2.51)
<500	384	74 (19)	2.11 (1.43–3.11)	380	85 (22)	1.64 (1.19–2.27)

OR, odds ratio.
[a]As indicated by the sum of patient days during the month at the beginning of follow-up.

units at the time of an event was associated with violent assaults towards employees (odds ratio (OR) = 1.72, 95% CI 1.05—2.80; OR = 3.04, 95% CI 1.51—6.13 in adult wards) after adjustment for confounding factors. No association was found with assaults on ward property (OR = 1.06, 95% CI 0.75—1.50).

Conclusions.—These findings suggest that patient overcrowding is highly prevalent in psychiatric hospitals and, importantly, may increase the risk of violence directed at staff.

▶ This is the first study of its kind demonstrating an increase in violent assaults in inpatient psychiatric units that are overcrowded, with excess bed occupancy (Table 2). The findings are not surprising in light of animal studies indicating overcrowding as a risk factor for aggressive behavior. This is not a controlled study and is based on staff reports; it does not indicate staffing patterns or whether there may be more violent-prone patients in the hospital at times when overcrowding becomes a necessity. Also, diagnosis of substance abuse or psychotic problems is not controlled for in this study. However, if replicated, which I would find likely, this study indicates the need to provide adequate space, staffing, and staff training to help reduce violent behavior in hospital and emergency room settings. The setting of care, attitude of staff, and appropriate use of medication are all factors that can help prevent and reduce violence in a hospital setting.

R. J. Frances, MD

Rates of Homicide During the First Episode of Psychosis and After Treatment: A Systematic Review and Meta-analysis
Nielssen O, Large M (UNSW at St Vincent's Hosp, Darlinghurst, Australia; Private Practice, Sydney, Australia)
Schizophr Bull 36:702-712, 2010

The observation that almost half of the homicides committed by people with a psychotic illness occur before initial treatment suggests an increased risk of homicide during the first episode of psychosis. The aim of this study was to estimate the rates of homicide during the first episode of psychosis and after treatment. A systematic search located 10 studies that reported details of all the homicide offenders with a psychotic illness within a known population during a specified period and reported the number of people who had received treatment prior to the offense. Meta-analysis of these studies showed that 38.5% (95% confidence interval [CI] = 31.1%— 46.5%) of homicides occurred during the first episode of psychosis, prior to initial treatment. Homicides during first-episode psychosis occurred at a rate of 1.59 homicides per 1000 (95% CI = 1.06—2.40), equivalent to 1 in 629 presentations. The annual rate of homicide after treatment for psychosis was 0.11 homicides per 1000 patients (95% CI = 0.07—0.16), equivalent to 1 homicide in 9090 patients with schizophrenia per year. The rate ratio of

TABLE 5.—Meta-analysis of the Rate Ratio of Homicide in First-Episode Psychosis and the Annual Rate After Treatment

First Author	Rate Ratio	Lower 95% Confidence Interval Limit	Upper 95% Confidence Interval Limit	Z Value	P Value
Appleby[2]	14.20	10.09	19.98	15.23	.000
Bourget[12]	18.94	10.88	32.69	10.40	.000
Erb[13]	11.24	5.11	24.70	6.02	.000
Grunberg[14]	11.56	2.89	46.22	3.46	.000
Häfner[15]	17.18	13.56	21.78	23.53	.000
Laajasalo[16]	4.81	2.54	7.36	4.66	.000
Meehan[1]	19.17	12.41	29.61	13.31	.000
Nielssen[3]	40.91	25.53	63.08	16.80	.000
Simpson[17]	16.63	10.13	27.31	11.11	.000
Valevski[18]	16.26	8.09	32.68	7.83	.000
Pooled estimate (random-effects model)	15.48	11.04	21.71	15.88	.000

Editor's Note: Please refer to original journal article for full references.

homicide in the first episode of psychosis in these studies was 15.5 (95% CI = 11.0−21.7) times the annual rate of homicide after treatment for psychosis. Hence, the rate of homicide in the first episode of psychosis appears to be higher than previously recognized, whereas the annual rate of homicide by patients with schizophrenia after treatment is lower than previous estimates. Earlier treatment of first-episode psychosis might prevent some homicides (Table 5).

▶ Because homicide is a rare event, perhaps society expects too much of psychiatrists in terms of attributing responsibility to them to try to predict, control, and prevent homicidal behavior in the mentally ill. Substance abuse and psychosis have higher representation related to homicides, and we can try to divine risk; however, there is also the danger of committing some people to hospital stays who would not actually act on violent impulses. Having said this, the current study provides evidence that first-episode psychotic episodes increase risk for homicide and that patients who have been treated for psychosis probably present a much lower risk (Table 5). This would argue for a value in early detection, case finding, and treatment initiation earlier in the course of a psychotic illness, possibly having the potential to reduce the number of homicides caused by mental illness. There may be a danger of overdiagnosis if we do this, which could lead to overuse of medications with their attendant side effects. We need to study the risks and benefits of any public efforts at prevention.

R. J. Frances, MD

Euthanasia

Assisted suicide: why psychiatrists should engage in the debate
Hotopf M, Lee W, Price A (King's College London, UK)
Br J Psychiatry 198:83-84, 2011

There is an increasing appetite for a change in the law to allow assisted suicide. This editorial suggests that psychiatrists should engage in the debate because the issues at stake will affect us, and we are likely to have a significant part to play were the law to be changed. We suggest that there are three main areas where psychiatrists' expertise may be informative: (a) the extent to which safeguards to limit the availability of assisted dying to target groups can be applied safely and fairly, including to individuals with psychiatric disorders; (b) the complexities inherent in assessing mental capacity; and (c) the degree to which individuals adapt or change their desires, particularly in relation to suicidal behaviours.

▶ This British commentary encouraging psychiatrists to weigh in on the debate on assisted suicide makes important points. Psychiatrists have a great deal of experience in evaluating parasuicidal potential and mental capacity, and they would have a role if assisted suicide were allowed. There is significant danger that a poorly designed law could endanger patients who lack the mental capacity to decide for themselves to end their lives, as well as patients with treatable psychiatric disorders or pain problems that could be manageable with treatment but who are desperate for relief and may not be getting adequate care. The motivation to die may wax and wane, as it does with all suicidal patients, and it takes some people time to adjust to facing a life-threatening illnesses. Psychiatrists have knowledge and skills that can be useful in many areas of public policy and perhaps too often remain quiet or are not asked for their opinions when they may be of great benefit to all.

R. J. Frances, MD

Legal Issues

Involuntary Civil Commitments After the Implementation of California's Mental Health Services Act
Bruckner TA, Yoon J, Brown TT, et al (Univ of California, Irvine; Georgia Southern Univ, Statesboro; Univ of California, Berkeley; et al)
Psychiatr Serv 61:1006-1011, 2010

Objective.—As of fiscal year 2008–2009, California's Mental Health Services Act (MHSA) has distributed $3.2 billion in new tax revenues to county mental health systems. This voter-approved act attempts to address the needs of unserved and underserved consumers with severe mental illness by implementing a "whatever it takes" approach. The research literature indicates that the incidence of involuntary treatment may gauge the overall functioning of the public mental health system. Consistent with the notion that the MHSA may facilitate effective treatment of severe mental illness, the authors tested the hypothesis that the incidence of two types of involuntary treatment—72-hour holds and 14-day psychiatric civil commitments—declines as the enhancement of service access and quality is supported by MHSA funds.

Methods.—The investigators obtained quarterly counts of involuntary 72-hour holds (N=593,751) and 14-day psychiatric hospitalizations (N=202,554) for 28 counties, with over 22 million inhabitants, from July 2000 to June 2007. A fixed-effects regression approach adjusted for temporal patterns in treatment.

Results.—The petitions for involuntary 14-day hospitalizations, but not involuntary 72-hour holds, fell below expected values after disbursement of MHSA funds. In these counties, 3,073 fewer involuntary 14-day treatments—approximately 10% below expected levels—could be attributed to disbursement of MHSA funds. Results remained robust to alternative regression specifications.

Conclusions.—Fewer than expected involuntary 14-day holds for continued hospitalization may indicate an important shift in service delivery. MHSA funds may have facilitated the discharge of clients from the hospital by providing enhanced resources and access to a range of less-restrictive community-based treatment alternatives (Fig 2).

▶ This article reports on a large survey of over 28 counties serving 22 million people in California that found a significant 10% reduction in petitions for involuntary hospitalizations, a result, the authors believe, of improved funding and provision of psychiatric services to the severely mentally ill in California (Fig 2). It stands to reason that providing better outpatient treatment would not only reduce involuntary commitment but lead to many other benefits, including improved function of these individuals, fewer prison incarcerations, relief for families struggling with the effects of their relatives' severe mental illness, and considerable reduction in suffering. This study also indicates that greater use of less restrictive alternatives is likely to occur when there are

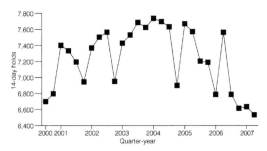

FIGURE 2.—Count of involuntary 14-day psychiatric holds (code 5250) in 28 California counties, by quarter-year, July 2000 to June 2007. (Reprinted with permission from Psychiatric Services, Bruckner TA, Yoon J, Brown TT, et al. Involuntary civil commitments after the implementation of California's mental health services act. *Psychiatr Serv.* 2010;61:1006-1011 © American Psychiatric Association, Inc.)

more quality treatment alternatives available. One concern I have is that as California liberalizes drug laws, there may be more substance-induced severe psychiatric problems that will emerge in costly ways to both the mental health and prison systems.

R. J. Frances, MD

Postdisaster Course of Alcohol Use Disorders in Systematically Studied Survivors of 10 Disasters

North CS, Ringwalt CL, Downs D, et al (Univ of Texas Southwestern Med Ctr, Dallas; Pacific Inst for Res and Evaluation, Chapel Hill, NC; et al)

Arch Gen Psychiatry 68:173-180, 2011

Context.—Although several studies have suggested that alcohol use may increase after disasters, it is unclear whether any apparent postdisaster increases regularly translate into new cases of alcohol use disorders.

Objective.—To determine the relationship of predisaster and postdisaster prevalence of alcohol use disorders and to examine the incidence of alcohol use disorders in relation to disasters.

Design.—Data from 10 disasters, studied within the first few postdisaster months and at 1 to 3 years postdisaster, were merged and examined.

Participants.—Six hundred ninety-seven directly exposed survivors of 10 disasters.

Measures.—The Diagnostic Interview Schedule for DSM-III-R provided lifetime diagnoses of alcohol abuse and dependence, and onset and recency questions allowed a determination of whether the disorder had been present either prior to or following the event, or both.

Results.—While the postdisaster prevalence of alcohol use disorders was 19%, only 0.3% of the sample developed an acute new postdisaster alcohol use disorder. Most of those in recovery, however, consumed alcohol after the disaster (83%) and coped with their emotions by drinking alcohol (22%). Those with a postdisaster alcohol use disorder were more than 4 times as likely as those without to cope with their disaster-related emotions by drinking alcohol (40% vs 9%).

Conclusions.—The vast majority of postdisaster alcohol use disorders represented the continuation or recurrence of preexisting problems. Findings suggest that those in recovery as well as those who drink to cope with their emotions represent groups warranting potential concern for postdisaster mental health intervention. Further research is needed to clarify the clinical significance of changes in alcohol use after disasters.

▶ At the time of writing this, Japan is reeling from an 8.8 earthquake and tsunami and fears related to meltdowns of nuclear reactors in the country that was first to experience a nuclear attack. Disasters have always been part of life, and with the increasing availability of media coverage, they have a greater impact on people's minds and actions. Those most immediately affected and exposed to a disaster feel the effects most immediately and are more likely to have posttraumatic stress disorder symptoms. This article finds only a small increase in new substance abuse disorders after disasters but high recurrence, relapse, and increase in use among those who drink to cope with their emotions (Fig 2 in the original article). Public health measures should target those people with a history that would suggest risk for addiction problems. Twelve-step programs and mutual-help efforts to bring people together in their communities offer an alternative coping approach of mutual help and should be encouraged in community efforts in planning for disaster response. This study has implications for forensic cases where there was preexisting alcoholism with a relapse after a disaster. In such cases, attributing and parceling out degree of causation by the new trauma and stress versus vulnerability because of a preexisting condition may affect jury awards of damages and degree of responsibility of those who may be sued or held accountable for not preventing or for ensuring a disaster.

R. J. Frances, MD

Miscellaneous

Association of Socioeconomic Position With Health Behaviors and Mortality
Stringhini S, Sabia S, Shipley M, et al (Centre for Res in Epidemiology and Population Health, Villejuif, France; Univ College London, England)
JAMA 303:1159-1166, 2010

Context.—Previous studies may have underestimated the contribution of health behaviors to social inequalities in mortality because health behaviors were assessed only at the baseline of the study.

Objective.—To examine the role of health behaviors in the association between socioeconomic position and mortality and compare whether their contribution differs when assessed at only 1 point in time with that assessed longitudinally through the follow-up period.

Design, Setting, and Participants.—Established in 1985, the British Whitehall II longitudinal cohort study includes 10 308 civil servants, aged 35 to 55 years, living in London, England. Analyses are based on 9590 men and women followed up for mortality until April 30, 2009. Socioeconomic position was derived from civil service employment grade (high, intermediate, and low) at baseline. Smoking, alcohol consumption, diet, and physical activity were assessed 4 times during the follow-up period.

Main Outcome Measures.—All-cause and cause-specific mortality.

Results.—A total of 654 participants died during the follow-up period. In the analyses adjusted for sex and year of birth, those with the lowest socioeconomic position had 1.60 times higher risk of death from all causes than those with the highest socioeconomic position (a rate difference of 1.94/1000 person-years). This association was attenuated by 42% (95% confidence interval [CI], 21%-94%) when health behaviors assessed at baseline were entered into the model and by 72% (95% CI, 42%-154%) when they were entered as time-dependent covariates. The corresponding attenuations were 29% (95% CI, 11%-54%) and 45% (95% CI, 24%-79%) for cardiovascular mortality and 61% (95% CI, 16%-425%) and 94% (95% CI, 35%-595%) for noncancer and noncardiovascular mortality. The difference between the baseline only and repeated assessments of health behaviors was mostly due to an increased explanatory power of diet (from 7% to 17% for all-cause mortality, respectively), physical activity (from 5% to 21% for all-cause mortality), and alcohol consumption (from 3% to 12% for all-cause mortality). The role of smoking, the strongest mediator in these analyses, did not change when using baseline or repeat assessments (from 32% to 35% for all-cause mortality).

Conclusion.—In a civil service population in London, England, there was an association between socioeconomic position and mortality that was substantially accounted for by adjustment for health behaviors, particularly when the behaviors were assessed repeatedly.

▶ This British longitudinal study of contributions of health behaviors in relation to social inequalities in mortality has important public policy implications. The finding over time that lower socioeconomic position predicts a 1.6-fold increased chance of mortality, which can be mitigated by improving health behaviors, implies that fostering of prosperity for the disadvantaged and programs aiding the poor and providing good health care, including prevention services, will save lives. This study was done in a country that provides national health care and availability of services to the poor, and policy makers and the public in the United States should be aware of the benefits of reducing suffering, morbidity, and death by making care affordable and available. Those who are opposed to taxing the rich in favor of recommending trimming governmental budgets by reducing spending for health care, reducing spending on education, and reducing subsidies to the poor in the United States need to be aware of the increased death toll that such policies cause. Companies also need to be aware of how supporting programs for their workers aimed at changing health-related behaviors can both reduce costs and save lives. Psychiatrists play an important role at many levels in promoting efforts to help motivate patients to make the necessary lifestyle changes that can improve health and reduce mortality, especially in relation to diet, substance misuse, and early identification and treatment of psychiatric problems.

R. J. Frances, MD

5 Hospital and Community Psychiatry

Economic Issues

Economic Costs of Neuroticism: A Population-Based Study

Cuijpers P, Smit F, Penninx BWJH, et al (VU Univ and VU Univ Med Ctr, Amsterdam, the Netherlands; et al)
Arch Gen Psychiatry 67:1086-1093, 2010

Context.—The importance of neuroticism for mental health care use and public health is well established. However, most research has focused on the association between neuroticism and a single specific disorder or health outcome, and the overall effect of neuroticism on use of somatic and mental health care and on society is not clear.

Objective.—To examine the economic costs of neuroticism to get an impression of the overall effect of neuroticism on mental health care and on society in general.

Design.—Cross-sectional population-based study.

Setting.—General population.

Participants.—A large representative sample (N = 5504) of the Dutch general population.

Main Outcome Measures.—The costs (health service uptake in primary and secondary mental health care, out-of-pocket costs, and production losses) associated with neuroticism.

Results.—The total per capita excess costs were $12 362 per year for the reference year 2007 in the 5% highest scorers of neuroticism, $8243 in the 10% highest scorers, and $5572 in the 25% highest scorers. The per capita excess costs of neuroticism are considerably higher than those of mental disorders. The total excess costs of neuroticism per 1 million inhabitants resulting from the 25% highest scorers ($1.393 billion) were approximately 2.5 times as high as the excess costs of common mental disorders ($585 million).

Conclusions.—The economic costs of neuroticism are enormous and exceed those of common mental disorders. We should start thinking about interventions that focus not on each of the specific negative outcomes of neuroticism but rather on the starting point itself.

▶ The opening paragraph pulled me up short. "It is well established that neurotic people are more vulnerable to mental disorders, including depression, anxiety disorders, schizophrenia, eating disorders, and personality disorders. Furthermore, neuroticism is related to higher levels of comorbidity, to the onset of comorbidity, and to greater use of mental health services. Neurotic patients more often express medically unfounded somatic complaints, and several studies suggest that neuroticism is associated with general health problems, including cardiovascular disease, asthma, and irritable bowel syndrome, even after controlling for depression and other risk factors."

Wow! In America the term neurosis has been taboo for years, and these Dutch scientists are now showing how pervasive and expensive it is. Amazing! Read that conclusion again, "The economic costs of neuroticism are enormous and exceed those of common mental disorders." Enormous. So what do we do about it? Well, the authors suggest we use neuroticism "as a starting point for the development of new interventions for prevention and treatment? Because neuroticism is a personality characteristic, it is relatively stable, although there are indications that personality can change to a certain extent during the life course." They state that "selective serotonin reuptake inhibitors may reduce the level of neuroticism in depressed patients. However, it should not be expected that current treatments can cure or substantially reduce neuroticism. Given the stability of this personality trait, the high heritability, and the likely gene-environment correlations operating for this trait, it is unlikely that treatment will be achieved easily. On the other hand, we should not be too pessimistic about interventions to reduce mental health problems associated with neuroticism." If these guys are right, we've got some work to do. Fascinating stuff!

J. A. Talbott, MD

Mental Health and Substance Use Disorder Spending in the Department of Veterans Affairs, Fiscal Years 2000–2007
Wagner TH, Sinnott P, Siroka AM (Dept of Veterans Affairs Palo Alto Healthcare System, Menlo Park, CA)
Psychiatr Serv 62:389-395, 2011

Objective.—This study analyzed spending for treatment of mental health and substance use disorders in the Department of Veterans Affairs (VA) in fiscal years (FYs) 2000 through 2007.

Methods.—VA spending as reported in the VA Decision Support System was linked to patient utilization data as reported in the Patient Treatment Files, the National Patient Care Database, and the VA Fee Basis files. All care and costs from FY 2000 to FY 2007 were analyzed.

TABLE 4.—Prevalence of Chronic General Medical Conditions and Mental and Substance Use Disorders Among Users of Department of Veterans Affairs Health Care, Fiscal Years (FY) 2000–2007[a]

Condition	Rank[b]	FY 2000	FY 2001	FY 2002	FY 2003	FY 2004	FY 2005	FY 2006	FY 2007	Per-Year Change (%)
Hypertension	1	39,901	43,337	45,910	48,335	50,379	51,499	52,377	52,847	4.1
Ischemic heart disease	2	17,410	18,458	19,037	19,090	19,162	19,210	18,970	18,612	1.0
Diabetes	3	16,814	18,083	19,239	20,095	20,837	21,504	22,172	22,666	4.4
Arthritis	4	16,282	16,692	16,936	17,232	17,682	17,729	17,588	17,166	.8
Lower back pain	5	10,955	11,171	11,351	11,880	12,916	13,688	14,327	15,205	4.8
Depression	6	10,950	11,235	11,727	12,484	13,062	13,206	13,510	14,187	3.8
Tobacco-nicotine dependence	11	7,422	8,460	9,245	10,030	11,190	12,016	12,205	13,024	8.4
Alcohol use disorder or alcohol-related disorder	13	5,302	4,924	4,630	4,487	4,668	4,734	4,744	4,917	-1.1
Posttraumatic stress	14	4,992	4,875	4,945	5,202	5,659	6,360	6,838	7,702	6.4
Schizophrenia	20	3,048	2,628	2,325	2,150	2,010	1,928	1,853	1,809	-7.2
Drug use disorder[c]	21	3,020	2,808	2,653	2,606	2,702	2,743	2,804	2,953	-.3
Other psychosis	28	1,278	1,189	1,210	1,344	1,553	1,561	1,204	1,076	-2.4
Other personality disorder	29	996	864	759	707	684	687	660	660	-5.7
Borderline personality disorder	44	211	189	168	161	159	163	158	167	-3.3
Antisocial personality disorder	45	169	144	141	130	128	127	121	120	-4.7

[a]Authors' analysis of Department of Veterans Affairs (VA) Patient Treatment Files and National Patient Care Database. Prevalence per 100,000 veterans who used VA health care in the fiscal year. An individual may be counted twice.
[b]Rank is based on the prevalence in FY 2000 and is relative to the 56 conditions tracked.
[c]Excludes alcohol and tobacco.

Results.—Over the study period the number of veterans treated at the VA increased from 3.7 million to over 5.1 million (an average increase of 4.9% per year), and costs increased .7% per person per year. For mental health and substance use disorder treatment, the volume of inpatient care decreased markedly, residential care increased, and spending decreased on average 2% per year (from $668 in FY 2000 to $578 per person in FY 2007). FY 2007 saw large increases in mental health spending, bucking the trend from FY 2000 through FY 2006.

Conclusions.—VA's continued emphasis on outpatient and residential care was evident through 2007. This trend in spending might be unimpressive if VA were enrolling healthier Veterans, but the opposite seems to be true: over this time period the prevalence of most chronic conditions, including depression and posttraumatic stress disorder, increased. VA spending on mental health care grew rapidly in 2007, and given current military activities, this trend is likely to increase (Table 4).

▶ As the largest health care system in the United States, the Department of Veterans Affairs (VA or Veterans Administration) system is a fascinating model to study. It is one left out of many experts' thinking, calculations, and ken. It is much more in line with a socialized medical system than Medicare, which conservative seniors want preserved in their famous battle cry, "Keep government out of our lives, but don't touch our Medicare." Doctors are salaried, budgets are fixed, decisions are centralized, care is often free, there is unlimited access, and so on. For the most part, it delivers excellent care. There are several lessons to be learned here. First, although the United States' non-VA "per capita [mental health] spending increased from $104.25 to $148.56" an almost 50% increase between 2000 and 2006, in the VA it decreased by about 10% (Fig 1 in the original article). Second, the VA saw more patients who were increasingly sicker, and its total budget was still manageable. Finally (Table 4), despite the lore that the VA only treats substance abusers and victims of posttraumatic stress disorder, the most prevalent mental illness is depression. The VA has a lot to teach legislators about health care reform if some can just get past the socialized medicine phobia.

J. A. Talbott, MD

Association Between Prior Authorization for Medications and Health Service Use by Medicaid Patients With Bipolar Disorder

Lu CY, Adams AS, Ross-Degnan D, et al (Harvard Med School, Boston, MA)
Psychiatr Serv 62:186-193, 2011

Objective.—This study examined the association between a Medicaid prior-authorization policy for second-generation antipsychotic and anticonvulsant agents and medication discontinuation and health service use by patients with bipolar disorder.

Methods.—A pre-post design with a historical comparison group was used to analyze Maine Medicaid and Medicare claims data. A total of 946 newly treated patients were identified during the eight-month policy (July 2003—February 2004), and a comparison group of 1,014 was identified from the prepolicy period (July 2002—February 2003). Patients were stratified by number of visits to community mental health centers (CMHCs) before medication initiation (proxy for illness severity): CMHC attenders, at least two visits; nonattenders, fewer than two. Changes in rates of medication discontinuation and outpatient, emergency room, and hospital visits were estimated.

Results.—Compared with nonattenders, at baseline CMHC attenders had substantially higher rates of comorbid mental disorders and use of medications and health services. The policy was associated with increased medication discontinuation among attenders and nonattenders, reductions in mental health visits after discontinuation among attenders ($-.64$ per patient per month; $p<.05$), and increases in emergency room visits after discontinuation among nonattenders (.16 per patient per month; $p<.05$). During the eight-month policy period, the policy had no detectable impact on hospitalization risk.

Conclusions.—The prior-authorization policy was associated with increased medication discontinuation and subsequent changes in health service use. Although small, these unintended effects raise concerns about quality of care for a group of vulnerable patients. Long-term consequences of prior-authorization policies on patient outcomes warrant further investigation.

▶ Disclosure and rationale for my comments: the day I wrote this, I had just been told by my university hospital pharmacy that the pharmacy benefit company managing university faculty members' drugs required prior authorization of a prescription written for an antifungal medication of which I had taken 2 of the 3 months' course. As a consequence I visited the pharmacy 3 times, called the company twice, and bugged the attending physician and resident once each. At one point, I almost caved in and said, "screw it, 2 months may have worked" and quit the full course; at another point, I almost paid the "retail" price just to avoid the hassle. Now, I am not psychotic or bipolar, toenail fungus is not life-threatening nor quality-of-life impairing, and I am educated, privileged, and know how to work the system. However, this is not the case for those who are mentally impaired and reliant on Medicare or Medicaid; for them, such hoops may be too much to jump through.

So returning to the article at hand, is it any wonder that prior authorization results in an "increased medication discontinuation and subsequent changes in health service use" and that "Although small, these unintended effects raise concerns about quality of care for a group of vulnerable patients"?

J. A. Talbott, MD

Capitation of Public Mental Health Services in Colorado: A Five-Year Follow-Up of System-Level Effects
Bloom JR, Wang H, Kang SH, et al (Univ of California, Berkeley; Kaiser Permanente, Oakland, CA; et al)
Psychiatr Serv 62:179-185, 2011

Objective.—Capitated Medicaid mental health programs have reduced costs over the short term by lowering the utilization of high-cost inpatient services. This study examined the five-year effects of capitated financing in community mental health centers (CMHCs) by comparing not-for-profit with for-profit programs.

Methods.—Data were from the Medicaid billing system in Colorado for the precapitation year (1994) and a shadow billing system for the postcapitation years (1995–1999). In a panel design, a random-effect approach estimated the impact of two financing systems on service utilization and cost while adjusting for all the covariates.

Results.—Consistent with predictions, in both the for-profit and the not-for-profit CMHCs, relative to the precapitation year, there were significant reductions in each postcapitation year in high-cost treatments (inpatient treatment) for all but one comparison (not-for-profit CMHCs in 1999). Also consistent with predictions, the for-profit programs realized significant reductions in cost per user for both outpatient services and total services. In the not-for-profit programs, there were no significant changes in cost per user for total services; a significant reduction in cost per user for outpatient services was found only in the first two years, 1995 and 1996).

Conclusions.—The evidence suggests that different strategies were used by the not-for-profit and for-profit programs to control expenditures and utilization and that the for-profit programs were more successful in reducing cost per user.

▶ I have a visceral reaction to seeing the conclusion of studies such as these: it is disbelief tainted with disgust. Why? Well, I think our public system is much maligned, that for-profit outfits are callous and uncaring, and that comparisons are difficult. I think the public guys are the white hats and the private guys the bad folks. But maybe I've got it all wrong. I mean look here: the for-profit bunch had a 66% "reduction in the cost per person by the second postcapitation year." How can this be without horrendous denial of care? But there's no evidence of such. No, it takes one a long time, nearly to the end of the article, to read a small piece of ammunition supporting one's visceral response. The statement that "the drop attenuated over time in for-profit programs, suggesting that initial cost savings may overstate long-term effects." Aha. That confirms the stereotype. The greedy bunch show they can reduce costs drastically but, having squeezed all the juice out initially, have no more to get. Indeed, the field seems to agree that managed care, capitation, and other entities jolted the system, but its effect was 1 time only and unsustainable.

J. A. Talbott, MD

Epidemiology, Diagnosis, and Trends

Understanding Excess Mortality in Persons With Mental Illness: 17-Year Follow Up of a Nationally Representative US Survey
Druss BG, Zhao L, Von Esenwein S, et al (Emory Univ, Atlanta, GA; et al)
Med Care 49:599-604, 2011

Background.—Although growing concern has been expressed about premature medical mortality in persons with mental illness, limited data are available quantifying the extent and correlates of this problem using population-based, nationally representative samples.

Methods.—The study used data from the 1989 National Health Interview Survey mental health supplement, with mortality data through 2006 linked through the National Death Index (80,850 participants, 16,435 deaths). Multivariable models adjusting for demographic factors assessed the increased hazard of mortality adding socioeconomic status, healthcare variables, clinical factors first separately, and then together.

Results.—Persons with mental disorders died an average of 8.2 years younger than the rest of the population ($P < 0.001$). Adjusting for demographic factors, presence of a mental illness was associated with a significant risk of excess mortality, (hazard ratio = 2.06, 95% confidence interval = 1.71-2.40), with 95.4% of deaths owing to medical rather than unnatural causes. Adding socioeconomic variables to the model, the hazard ratio was 1.77 ($P < 0.001$); adding health system factors, it was 1.80 ($P < 0.001$)); adding baseline clinical characteristics, the hazard ratio was 1.32 ($P < 0.001$). After adding all the 3 groups of variables simultaneously, the association was reduced by 82% from baseline and became statistically nonsignificant (hazard ratio = 1.19, $P = 0.053$).

Conclusions.—The results of the study underscore the complex causes and high burden of medical mortality among persons with mental disorders in the United States. Efforts to address this public health problem will need to address the socioeconomic, healthcare, and clinical risk factors that underlie it.

▶ The fact that the mentally ill have shorter life spans and have 2 times the mortality rates of non—mentally ill persons has been known for many years. What has not been so clear is what the contributing factors are. This careful 17-year study by the Druss group sheds a great deal of light on these factors. As they state boldly:

- Individuals with mental illnesses die younger than individuals without those disorders, largely owing to medical causes rather than accidents and suicides.

- Nearly all of the excess mortality in this sample was due to medical rather than mental health causes,

- The largest contributing factor to excess mortality was the group of clinical factors, which alone accounted for 70% of the excess mortality.

- Together, these 3 groups of variables (socioeconomic status, health care variables, clinical factors) explained 82% of the excess mortality.

In brief, then, the reasons for the mentally ill dying earlier are several, lying in different domains, and eliminating excess mortality will take approaches that address these several issues (that is, socioeconomic, health care, and clinical risk factors).
Not an easy analysis, and there are no easy solutions.

J. A. Talbott, MD

Violent crime runs in families: a total population study of 12.5 million individuals
Frisell T, Lichtenstein P, Långström N (Karolinska Institutet, Stockholm, Sweden)
Psychol Med 41:97-105, 2011

Background.—Etiological theory and prior research with small or selected samples suggest that interpersonal violence clusters in families. However, the strength and pattern of this aggregation remains mostly unknown.

Method.—We investigated all convictions for violent crime in Sweden 1973–2004 among more than 12.5 million individuals in the nationwide Multi-Generation Register, and compared rates of violent convictions among relatives of violent individuals with relatives of matched, non-violent controls, using a nested case–control design.

Results.—We found strong familial aggregation of interpersonal violence among first-degree relatives [e.g. odds ratio (OR)$_{sibling}$ 4.3, 95% confidence interval (CI) 4.2–4.3], lower for more distant relatives (e.g. OR$_{cousin}$ 1.9, 95% CI 1.9–1.9). Risk patterns across biological and adoptive relations provided evidence for both genetic and environmental influences on the development of violent behavior. Familial risks were stronger among women, in higher socio-economic strata, and for early onset interpersonal violence. There were crime-specific effects (e.g. OR$_{sibling}$ for arson 22.4, 95% CI 12.2–41.2), suggesting both general and subtype-specific familial risk factors for violent behavior.

Conclusions.—The observed familiality should be accounted for in criminological research, applied violence risk assessment, and prevention efforts (Fig 3).

▶ This is a fascinating study about which there may be no clinical implications or interventions. What do I mean? Let's start with the prior research that, according to the authors, shows that "Intergenerational transmission, that is a correlation between parent and offspring behavior, has been reported for

- criminal convictions
- serious violent offending

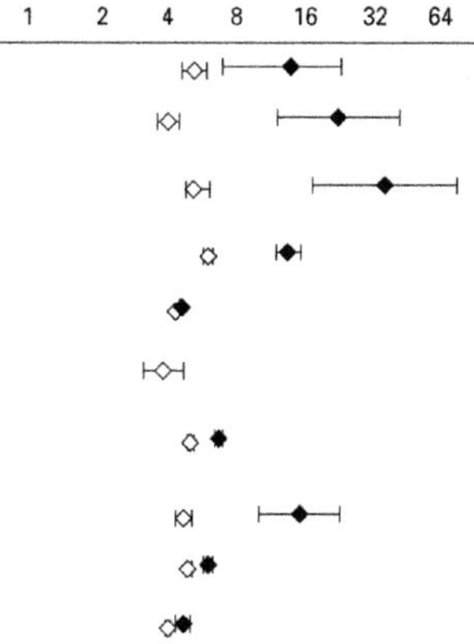

Violence subtype	Sibling risk: Odds ratio (95% CI)							Violence of same subtype	Any violence
	1	2	4	8	16	32	64		
Homicide								12.8 (7.1–23.0)	5.3 (4.7–6.0)
Arson								22.4 (12.2–41.2)	4.1 (3.7–4.6)
Kidnapping or illegal confinement								35.7 (17.4–73.0)	5.3 (4.9–6.2)
Robbery								13.5 (12.0–15.3)	6.1 (5.8–6.4)
Assault								4.7 (4.6–4.7)	4.4 (4.4–4.5)
Violation of a person's/ woman's integrity								–	3.9 (3.2–4.8)
Threats and violence against an officer								6.8 (6.5–7.1)	5.1 (5.0–5.3)
Unlawful coercion								15.2 (10.1–22.8)	4.8 (4.4–5.2)
Unlawful threat								6.1 (5.8–6.4)	5.0 (4.9–5.2)
Intimidation								4.8 (4.4–5.1)	4.1 (4.0–4.2)

FIGURE 3.—Relative risk for crime among siblings of violent index persons in the Swedish total population 1973–2004, divided by subtype of violent crime. Graph shows odds ratios (ORs) and 95% confidence intervals (CIs) for siblings' conviction for crime of the same subtype (◆) and any violent crime (◇). (Reprinted from Frisell T, Lichtenstein P, Långström N. Violent crime runs in families: a total population study of 12.5 million individuals. *Psychol Med.* 2011;41:97-105, copyright 2011 Cambridge University Press. Reprinted with the permission of Cambridge University Press.)

- criminal careers
- partner violence
- aggressive behavior
- inconsistent or hostile parenting
- child abuse
- substance use."

Incredible, but because all but one of the prior studies establishing these findings were small, these researchers tapped into a much larger database of more than 12 million Swedish citizens and got robust results. The running in families result can be accounted for both by genes (starting with the fact that 40% of antisocial behavior is genetically determined) and environmental causes, and the behavior includes a host of crimes (Fig 3), including violation of a person's integrity, robbery, arson, unlawful coercion, robbery, lethal violence, kidnapping, and illegal confinement. But what can we physicians do about these facts? Precious little, I fear, except encourage further work on the possible environmental causes as well as endorse what the authors call, "... prevention and intervention efforts that involve the families of violent individuals."

J. A. Talbott, MD

Prospective cohort study of mental health during imprisonment

Hassan L, Birmingham L, Harty MA, et al (Lancashire Care NHS Foundation Trust and The Univ of Manchester, UK; Hampshire Partnership Foundation NHS Trust and Univ of Southampton, Knowle, UK; King's College London, UK; et al)

Br J Psychiatry 198:37-42, 2011

Background.—Mental illness is common among prisoners, but little evidence exists regarding changes in symptoms in custody over time.

Aims.—To investigate the prevalence and predictors of psychiatric symptoms among prisoners during early custody.

Method.—In a prospective cohort study, 3079 prisoners were screened for mental illness within 3 days of reception. To establish baseline diagnoses and symptoms, 980 prisoners were interviewed; all remaining in custody were followed up 1 month and 2 months later.

Results.—Symptom prevalence was highest during the first week of custody. Prevalence showed a linear decline among men and convicted prisoners, but not women or remand prisoners. It decreased among prisoners with depression, but not among prisoners with other mental illnesses.

Conclusions.—Overall, imprisonment did not exacerbate psychiatric symptoms, although differences in group responses were observed. Continued discussion regarding non-custodial alternatives for vulnerable groups and increased support for all during early custody are recommended.

▶ A group I am part of has been examining letters written by people and family members of people incarcerated in the penal system in the United States suffering from mental illness, and these letters are horrific. The letters detail jailings for trivial or clearly psychiatric reasons, stoppage of medication, inability to get appropriate care or diagnostic workups, lack of planning for discharge, lack of community placements, and slippage of communication and coordination at almost every step of the way. A member of this group, Mark Munetz, has written a clever article[1] that clearly demonstrates these problems. So it is with surprise that I read the conclusions of the authors of this study from the United Kingdom that shows that overall, "imprisonment did not exacerbate psychiatric symptoms"; indeed, they found "significant linear decreases in symptom intensity in three groups: men, convicted prisoners and individuals with major depressive disorder." This leads me to wonder if the United Kingdom treats its patients with mental illness in the correctional system better than we do, if our respondents complain more or if our letters came from only those people who suffered adversely. I do not know which.

J. A. Talbott, MD

Reference

1. Munetz MR, Griffin PA. Use of the Sequential Intercept Model as an approach to decriminalization of people with serious mental illness. *Psychiatr Serv.* 2006;57: 544-549.

Mental health of the non-heterosexual population of England

Chakraborty A, McManus S, Brugha TS, et al (Univ College London, UK; Natl Centre for Social Res, London, UK; Univ of Leicester, UK; et al)
Br J Psychiatry 198:143-148, 2011

Background.—There has been little research into the prevalence of mental health problems in lesbian, gay and bisexual (LGB) people in the UK with most work conducted in the USA.

Aims.—To relate the prevalence of mental disorder, self-harm and suicide attempts to sexual orientation in England, and to test whether psychiatric problems were associated with discrimination on grounds of sexuality.

Method.—The Adult Psychiatric Morbidity Survey 2007 ($n=7403$) was representative of the population living in private UK households. Standardised questions provided demographic information. Neurotic symptoms, common mental disorders, probable psychosis, suicidality, alcohol and drug dependence and service utilisation were assessed. In addition, detailed information was obtained about aspects of sexual identity and perceived discrimination on these grounds.

Results.—Self-reported identification as non-heterosexual (determined by both orientation and sexual partnership, separately) was associated with unhappiness, neurotic disorders overall, depressive episodes, generalised anxiety disorder, obsessive-compulsive disorder, phobic disorder, probable psychosis, suicidal thoughts and acts, self-harm and alcohol and drug dependence. Mental health-related general practitioner consultations and community care service use over the previous year were also elevated. In the non-heterosexual group, discrimination on the grounds of sexual orientation predicted certain neurotic disorder outcomes, even after adjustment for potentially confounding demographic variables.

Conclusions.—This study corroborates international findings that people of non-heterosexual orientation report elevated levels of mental health problems and service usage, and it lends further support to the suggestion that perceived discrimination may act as a social stressor in the genesis of mental health problems in this population.

▶ While the authors say that most of the publications of most of the research on mental health issues in nonheterosexual populations has been done in the United States, because these articles are visible to people all over the world, I thought this one should be included. It is useful to remind ourselves of several things:

There's a lot of discrimination out there, and it affects one's mental health.

Physicians aren't always free of such attitudes, to say the least.

Nonheterosexual populations have (Table 1 in original article) a lot of bad things going on:

They have double the incidence of drug and alcohol dependence.

30% to 40% of people have more suicidal thoughts and attempts and self-harmful behavior.

Depending on the disorder, these populations have about 1.5 to 3.5 times more diagnosable mental illnesses.

The one thing in this contribution that I found simplistic was its recommendation that the results "call not only for a response by professionals in primary care and mental health services but also efforts at prevention." How exactly? The only thing I think will prevent such elevated figures would be a total end to discrimination, and I don't see that happening overnight.

J. A. Talbott, MD

Mental Health Services in 42 Low- and Middle-Income Countries: A WHO-AIMS Cross-National Analysis
Saxena S, Lora A, Morris J, et al (World Health Organization (WHO), Geneva, Switzerland; et al)
Psychiatr Serv 62:123-125, 2011

Objective.—The authors describe characteristics and capacities of mental health systems in low- and middle-income countries.

Methods.—The World Health Organization Assessment Instrument for Mental Health Systems was used to assess services in 42 countries (13 low-, 24 lower-middle, and five upper-middle income).

Results.—Of 36 countries with a mental health plan, 90% include the goal of developing community services. However, inpatient facilities are the main service providers, with less than one community contact (.70) for each inpatient day. Mental hospitals consume 80% of mental health budgets, and outpatient care is limited.

Conclusions.—Mental health services in participating countries are limited and often hospital based.

▶ I think there are several notable points to be made about this survey undertaken by the World Health Organization, led by Dr Shekhar Saxena, director of its Department of Mental Health and Substance Abuse. First, one cannot undertake any initiative unless you know what the situation now is. (Even the European Union's Mental Health Committee didn't have the data on basic numbers of beds, services, etc, in its constituent well-developed countries when the Union was formed in 1993.) So collecting information like this is necessary before formulating or implementing any plan or reform. Second, it might be easy to conclude from the findings that low- and middle-income countries have few community services and rely too heavily on expensive hospital treatment, but we know that some high-income countries (Japan springs to mind) also have such a pattern. Finally, there is an unstated bias in this survey, which is that hospitals are bad and expensive and community services good and less costly, which drives policy makers to leap toward deinstitutionalization before boosting community care. One has to read nearly to the end of this contribution to realize a strange paradox: that although there is a paucity of day treatment and residential care throughout these 42 countries, those at the top of the scale (upper middle income) in fact used their hospitals as residential treatment programs as well as to deliver acute care rather than primarily delivering acute care as did the low-income countries.

J. A. Talbott, MD

Trends in the Duration of Emergency Department Visits, 2001–2006
Slade EP, Dixon LB, Semmel S (Univ of Maryland, Baltimore)
Psychiatr Serv 61:878-884, 2010

Objective.—This study estimated trends in the duration of emergency department visits from 2001 to 2006 and compared duration by presenting complaint—mental health related or non—mental health related.

Methods.—Data on visits (N=193,077) were from the National Hospital Ambulatory Medical Care Survey Emergency Department databases. Visits were classified as mental health visits if the primary reason for the visit was a common mental health symptom or disorder, a problem related to substance use, suicidal behaviors, or a need for counseling. Regression models were adjusted for year, diagnosis type, discharge status, payment source, demographic characteristics, receipt of medical care during the visit, mode of arrival, and immediacy of need for treatment.

Results.—The duration of all emergency department visits increased at an annual rate of 2.3%. Trends were similar for mental health visits and non—mental health visits. Throughout the period the average duration of mental health visits exceeded the average duration of non—mental health visits by 42% (p<.001). This difference was related to the longer durations of mental health visits ending in transfer and visits by persons with serious mental illness or substance use disorders.

Conclusions.—From 2001 to 2006, the duration of emergency department visits made by patients presenting with mental health complaints and visits made by all other patients increased at similar rates. However, the longer visits for certain groups of mental health patients suggest that emergency departments incur higher costs in connection with the delivery of services to persons in need of acute stabilization.

▶ For as long as I can recall, both emergency room (ER) psychiatrists and administrators have complained about increasing use of ERs. Indeed, I became involved in organized psychiatry (that is, the American Psychiatric Association) because of this occurring in New York City in 1968. This is not to diminish the significance of the authors' findings (who are members of the same department where I work) but to say that this feeling is not new. In their first paragraph, the authors state that stakeholders are concerned about increasing backlogs and the total volume of ER visits has been increasing as well. Their finding of a 2.3% increase a year in duration of ER visits over their study period is daunting. In addition, their finding that those awaiting transfer to a different facility were kept even longer is logical but also dismaying and costly. All 3 recommendations they make to alleviate this situation—"expansion of capacity to provide services, increased reimbursement of services, or improved communication with clinical care programs"—cost more and, in these times of cost-cutting, are hard to achieve. The increasing use of ERs to acutely stabilize patients has been going on for years, and I'm not sure what would halt it.

J. A. Talbott, MD

Serious Psychological Distress and Mental Health Service Use Among Community-Dwelling Older U.S. Adults

Han B, Gfroerer JC, Colpe LJ, et al (U.S. Dept of Health and Human Services, Rockville, MD)
Psychiatr Serv 62:291-298, 2011

Objectives.—This study examined the prevalence and predictors of past-year serious psychological distress and receipt of mental health services among community-dwelling older adults in the United States.

Methods.—The sample included 9,957 adults aged 65 or older from the 2004–2007 National Survey on Drug Use and Health. Serious psychological distress was defined as having a score of 13 or higher on the K6 scale of nonspecific psychological distress. Descriptive analyses and logistic regression modeling were applied.

Results.—Among community-dwelling older adults, 4.7% had serious psychological distress in the past year. Among those with past-year serious psychological distress, 37.7% received mental health services in the past year (4.8% received inpatient services, 15.8% received outpatient services, and 32.1% received prescription medications) (weighted percentages). Logistic regression results suggested that among older adults with serious psychological distress, receipt of mental health services was more likely among women, non-Hispanic whites, those who were married, those who were highly educated, Medicare-Medicaid dual beneficiaries, those with a major depressive episode, and those with more general medical conditions.

Conclusions.—These results suggest the need to screen for mental health problems among older adults and to improve the use and the quality of their mental health services. Since 2008 significant changes have revolutionized payment for mental health care and may promote access to mental health care in this population. Further studies are needed to assess trends in mental health service utilization among older adults and in the quality of their mental health care over time.

▶ I selected this contribution for several reasons.

It seems to me that despite the graying of America, the literature in geriatric psychiatry in general psychiatric journals is not growing at a similar pace; there is an explosion in the number of geriatric people in this group, and I do not think we're studying it nor equipped to care for it. When the authors state that "the number of older adults with major psychiatric illnesses is expected to more than double, from seven million to 15 million ... between 2000 and 2030," that's pretty scary. Now, the percentage of older Americans with serious psychological distress may not seem high at 4.7%, but considering the finding that 62.3% did not receive mental health services, there is a serious disconnect between symptoms/illnesses and diagnosis/treatment. (It's interesting to note that I arrived at this number by subtracting from 100 the percentage that do receive services, which was written in the abstract [37.7%] as though it were a positive finding but struck me as not so great; it was only on digging into the discussion that I saw that they too noted the 62.3% who did not receive care.)

Finally, the fact that clinicians rely so much on prescription drugs in this population reflects a distressing but inevitable trend to blitz older people with more medications rather than use equally effective talk therapy.

J. A. Talbott, MD

Schizophrenia

Exercise Therapy for Schizophrenia

Gorczynski P, Faulkner G (Univ of Toronto, Ontario, Canada)
Schizophr Bull 36:665-666, 2010

Background.—The health benefits of physical activity and exercise are well documented, and these effects could help people with schizophrenia.

Objectives.—To determine the mental health effects of exercise/physical activity programs for people with schizophrenia or schizophrenia-like illnesses.

Search Methods.—We searched the Cochrane Schizophrenia Group Trials Register (December 2008), which is based on regular searches of CINAHL, EMBASE, MEDLINE, and PsycINFO. We also inspected references within relevant papers.

Selection Criteria.—We included all randomized controlled trials comparing any intervention where physical activity or exercise was considered to be the main or active ingredient with standard care or other treatments for people with schizophrenia or schizophrenia-like illnesses.

Data Collection and Analysis.—We independently inspected citations and abstracts, ordered papers, quality assessed, and data extracted. For binary outcomes, we calculated a fixed-effect risk ratio and its 95% CI. Where possible, the weighted number needed to treat/harm statistic (NNT/H) and its 95% CI was also calculated. For continuous outcomes, endpoint data were preferred to change data. We synthesized nonskewed data from valid scales using a weighted mean difference.

Results.—Three randomized controlled trials met the inclusion criteria. Trials assessed the effects of exercise on physical and mental health. Overall numbers leaving the trials were similar. Two trials compared exercise with standard care and both found exercise to significantly improve negative symptoms of mental state (Mental Health Inventory Depression: 1 RCT, $n = 10$, Mean Difference [MD] 17.50 CI 6.70—28.30, Positive and Negative Syndrome Scale [PANSS] negative: 1 RCT, $n = 10$, MD -8.50 CI -11.11 to -5.89; figure 1). No absolute effects were found for positive

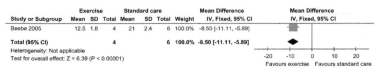

FIGURE 1.—Comparison 1: Exercise vs Standard Care; Outcome: Mental state PANSS Negative endpoint score (low score 5 good). (Reprinted from Gorczynski P, Faulkner G. Exercise therapy for schizophrenia. *Schizophr Bull.* 2010;36:665-666, by permission of the Oxford University Press on behalf of the Maryland Psychiatric Research Center.)

symptoms of mental state. Physical health improved significantly in the exercise group compared with those in standard care (1 RCT, $n = 13$, MD 79.50 CI 33.82–125.18; figure 2), but no effect on peoples' weight/BMI was apparent. One study compared exercise with yoga and found that yoga had a better outcome for mental state (PANSS total: 1 RCT, $n = 41$, MD 14.95 CI 2.60–27.30). The same trial also found that those in the yoga group had significantly better quality of life scores (World Health Organization Quality of Life physical: 1 RCT, $n = 41$, MD −9.22 CI −18.86 to 0.42). Adverse effects (Abnormal Voluntary Movements Scale total scores) were, however, similar.

Authors' Conclusions.—Although studies included in this review are small and used various measures of physical and mental health, results indicated that regular exercise programs are possible in this population and that they can have healthful effects on both the physical and mental health and well being of individuals with schizophrenia. Larger randomized studies are required before any definitive conclusions can be drawn (Fig 1).

▶ I think this tiny article speaks volumes. Wow. Now, most of us are familiar with the multiple studies showing the positive effects of exercise on depression; a commonly cited one is the study by Babyak et al.[1] But I daresay not much is talked about regarding persons suffering from schizophrenia (a Google search shows 17 million hits for exercise and depression and only 1.77 million for schizophrenia). While the numbers of studies are low, the results are not (Fig 1), and one might well think next of how we incorporate exercise into our treatment plans. The obstacles are many: I recall a passionate runner who was a friend-colleague in New York and whom I literally ran into one morning running in Central Park and later asked him how he got really depressed patients off their duffs. "It's hard work," he said. Indeed, but maybe worth it.

J. A. Talbott, MD

Reference

1. Babyak M, Blumenthal JA, Herman S, et al. Exercise treatment for major depression: maintenance of therapeutic benefit at 10 months. *Psychosom Med.* 2000;62:633-638.

Barriers to Care

Trends in Behavioral Health Care Service Provision by Community Health Centers, 1998–2007
Wells R, Morrissey JP, Lee I-H, et al (Univ of North Carolina, Chapel Hill)
Psychiatr Serv 61:759-764, 2010

Objective.—The federal government boosted support for community health centers in medically underserved areas in 2002–2007. This investigation compared trends in behavioral health services provided by community health centers nationwide during the first several years of that initiative with immediately prior trends.

Methods.—Data were extracted from the Health Resources and Services Administration's Uniform Data System on community health centers for 1998–2007 (2007, N=1,067). Regression analyses revealed trends in individual community health centers' likelihood of providing on-site specialty mental health care, crisis services, and substance abuse treatment. Aggregate data were used to show national trends in numbers of behavioral health encounters, patients, and encounters per patient.

Results.—The number of federally funded community health centers increased 43% between 2001 and 2007, from 748 to 1,067, over twice the annual growth rate between 1998 and 2001. However, trends in individual community health centers' likelihood of providing different types of behavioral health care were generally consistent across the two time periods. In 2007, 77% of community health centers offered specialty mental health services, 20% offered 24-hour crisis intervention services, and 51% offered substance abuse treatment. The mean number of mental health encounters per mental health patient at community health centers in 2007 was 2.9.

Conclusions.—The behavioral health care safety net has widened through rapid recent growth in the number of community health centers as well as a continuing increase in the proportion offering specialty mental health services.

▶ I make a mistake and I make it repeatedly—I misread Community Health Center (CMH) as Community Mental Health Center (CMHC). In any case, if I am reading this correctly, the increased provision of specialty mental health care to the poor in America in CMHs was the result of a 43% increase in their numbers rather than in the amount of such care being provided by individual CMHs. As heartening as this is, as is the fact that an increasing proportion of the population is now being reached, maybe the next step is increasing the percentage of behavioral health care provided from 77% to 100% for specialty mental health care services, from 51% to 100% for substance abuse treatment, and from 20% to 100% for 24-hour crisis intervention. Again, if I'm reading it correctly, it appears that Bush's investment of $1 billion paid off in the development of new CMHCs, but the addition of $7.2 million for expanding mental health services did not.

J. A. Talbott, MD

Continuity of Care After Inpatient Discharge of Patients With Schizophrenia in the Medicaid Program: A Retrospective Longitudinal Cohort Analysis
Olfson M, Marcus SC, Doshi JA (Columbia Univ and New York State Psychiatric Inst; Univ of Pennsylvania, Philadelphia; Univ of Pennsylvania School of Medicine, Philadelphia)
J Clin Psychiatry 71:831-838, 2010

Objective.—This study seeks to identify patient, facility, county, and state policy factors associated with timely schizophrenia-related outpatient treatment following hospital discharge.

Method.—A retrospective longitudinal cohort analysis was performed of 2003 national Medicaid claims data supplemented with the American Hospital Association facility survey, the Area Resource File, and a Substance Abuse and Mental Health Services Administration Medicaid policy report. The analysis focuses on treatment episodes of adults, aged 20 to 63 years, who received inpatient care for *ICD-9-CM*—diagnosed schizophrenia (59,567 total treatment episodes). Rate and adjusted odds ratio (AOR) of schizophrenia-related outpatient visits within 7 days and 30 days following hospital discharge are assessed.

Results.—Of the 59,567 hospital discharges, 41.7% received schizophrenia-related outpatient visits in 7 days and 59.3% in 30 days following hospital discharge. The adjusted odds of 30-day follow-up outpatient visits were significantly related to preadmission outpatient mental health visits (AOR = 3.72; 99% CI, 3.44−4.03), depot (AOR = 2.83; 99% CI, 2.53−3.18) or oral (AOR = 1.73; 99% CI, 1.62−1.84) antipsychotics as compared with no antipsychotics, and absence of a substance use disorder diagnosis (AOR = 1.35; 99% CI, 1.25−1.45). General hospital as compared with a psychiatric hospital treatment (AOR = 1.32; 99% CI, 1.14−1.54) and patient residence in a county with a larger number of psychiatrists per capita (AOR = 1.27; 99% CI, 1.08−1.50) were related to receiving follow-up out-patient visits. By contrast, residence in a county with a high poverty rate (AOR = 0.60; 99% CI, 0.54−0.67) and treatment in a state with prior authorization requirements for < 12 annual outpatient visits (AOR = 0.69; 99% CI, 0.63−0.75) reduced the odds of follow-up care.

Conclusions.—Patient characteristics, clinical management, geographical resource availability, and the mental health policy environment all appear to shape access to care following hospital discharge in the community treatment of adult schizophrenia.

▶ Many years ago, I took a look at what was then called the revolving door in state hospitals and concluded that with 100 admissions, "readmissions compris[ed] 60% of all admissions, ... [and] 84 might have been prevented and that almost half of these might have been prevented with minor improvements of existing services necessitating no additional expenditure of money."[1] From there, it was but a short hop to suggest that something new was needed to link patients with services, especially on discharge, which we called a continuity agent.[2] Over 30 years later, the issue of lack of continuity of care still bedevils our system and our patients. The authors have done a magnificent job at detailing the factors associated with the disconnect between inpatient and outpatient care. They grouped them in 4 categories; I stopped counting after about a dozen. What does this mean? To me it means that there is no single simple reason for discontinuity and no simple single fix for the situation. But who will have the scope and wisdom as well as power at whatever levels of government, management, and service provision to remedy each factor? Even if we had universal, single-payer, sectorized mental health care, is there one locus or authority that could make change happen? I'm afraid not.

J. A. Talbott, MD

References

1. Talbott JA. Stopping the revolving door: a study of readmissions to a state hospital. *Psychiatr Q.* 1974;48:159-168.
2. Granet RB, Talbott JA. The continuity agent: Creating a new role to bridge the gaps in the mental health system. *Hosp Community Psychiatry.* 1978;29:132-133.

Using Medicaid Claims Data to Identify Service Gaps for High-Need Clients: The NYC Mental Health Care Monitoring Initiative

Smith TE, Appel A, Donahue SA, et al (New York State Office of Mental Health, Albany; New York City Dept of Health and Mental Hygiene)
Psychiatr Serv 62:9-11, 2011

Public mental health authorities have access to large administrative databases. Advances in information technology now make it possible to use secondary analyses of these data to inform policy and clinical interventions. New York City and State mental health authorities developed an initiative using Medicaid claims and other administrative data to identify individuals with serious mental illness living in New York City (NYC) who are at risk of lapses in care. The NYC Mental Health Care Monitoring Initiative represents one of the first efforts to create "evidence-based policy." The authors describe the initiative's background, development, and key collaborations.

▶ Back when I was superintendent (director) of a state mental hospital in New York City, I and my fellow administrators would groan when the IT/IS people in Albany would announce new initiatives to collect and report data from our facilities. In brief, like the drunk looking for a lost item under a street light because the light was better there than where he dropped it, these technical wizards would collect and disseminate data they could easily collect and was important to them, but not to us or our patients. With that in mind, I was heartened to see that only 40 years later, the information gurus have identified data from Medicaid service use or lack of such that will actually help patients and administrators meet patients' unmet needs. I only hope that even with New York City and State budget problems there will be follow-up research demonstrating the clinical and economic benefits of this new tool.

J. A. Talbott, MD

Mental Health—Related Beliefs as a Barrier to Service Use for Military Personnel and Veterans: A Review

Vogt D (U.S. Dept of Veterans Affairs Boston Healthcare System, MA)
Psychiatr Serv 62:135-142, 2011

Objective.—Although military personnel are at high risk of mental health problems, research findings indicate that many military personnel and veterans do not seek needed mental health care. Thus it is critical to identify factors that interfere with the use of mental health services for this population, and where possible, intervene to reduce barriers to care. The overarching goal of this review was to examine what is known with regard to concerns about public stigma and personal beliefs about mental illness and mental health treatment as potential barriers to service use in military and veteran populations and to provide recommendations for future research on this topic.

Methods.—Fifteen empirical articles on mental health beliefs and service use were identified via a review of the military and veteran literature included in PsycINFO and PubMed databases.

Results.—Although results suggest that mental health beliefs may be an important predictor of service use for this population, several gaps were identified in the current literature. Limitations include a lack of attention to the association between mental health beliefs and service use, a limited focus on personal beliefs about mental illness and mental health treatment, and the application of measures of mental health beliefs with questionable or undocumented psychometric properties.

Conclusions.—Studies that attend to these important issues and that examine mental health beliefs in the broader context within which decisions about seeking health care are made can be used to best target resources to engage military personnel and veterans in health care.

▶ There is a great deal of concern expressed by the military and the Veterans' Administration personnel about the high rate of suicide, depression, and post-traumatic stress disorder in discharged or post-combat-zone members of the military. The author has taken a careful look at the research (albeit sparse) that exists to ascertain what some of the personal barriers to help-seeking are and concludes that "both concerns about public stigma and personal beliefs about mental illness and mental health treatment may serve as important barriers to service use." I would add another factor that she doesn't highlight: the macho/warrior/keep-it-to-yourself attitude of the military. There was a subtle shift in terminology a few years ago when we were getting farther into the wars in Iraq and Afghanistan to call members of the military "warriors." It has a cinematographic ring to it, but carries an unwelcome halo of strength and machismo and assumes anything wrong is a weakness. We already knew from veterans returning from Vietnam that they felt a need to keep problems to themselves, work them out alone, and not express anything that could be seen as a "weakness." Well, things have only gotten worse, despite greater exposure of average citizens to patients because of deinstitutionalization, media campaigns, and the general public's more accepting attitudes toward mental illness. We also know from the literature that everything from pain to help-seeking is culturally influenced, and we know that many of the people entering military service now are immigrants or new arrivals to the United States; so it's no surprise that they may be more reluctant to seek help as well.

J. A. Talbott, MD

Community Care

The Effect of Community Mental Health Services on Hospitalization Rates in Virginia

Wanchek TN, McGarvey EL, Leon-Verdin M, et al (Univ of Virginia, Charlottesville)
Psychiatr Serv 62:194-199, 2011

Objective.—This study examined the relationship between the availability of mental health outpatient services provided by 40 publicly funded community service boards (CSBs) and the use of inpatient mental health treatment among Medicaid recipients.

Methods.—Three-year data were obtained for Medicaid recipients aged 18–64 from the Medicaid claims database for the Commonwealth of Virginia. Medicaid recipients who had a mental disorder diagnosis and who had received at least one community mental health service were included in the sample. A multivariate regression model was used for the analyses.

Results.—Of the 11,107 individuals included, 27% had schizophrenia-related disorders and 32% had affective psychoses; 60% were white and 37% were black; and the average age was 40.1 ± 13.1 years. In this sample, greater use of outpatient mental health services, but not greater variety of services available, was correlated with fewer inpatient hospital days for mental health treatment ($-1.0 \pm .2$ days of hospitalization).

Conclusions.—Virginia's CSBs provide a range of outpatient mental health services that are designed to enable individuals to remain in their community. The availability of community-based mental health services was correlated with lower rates of inpatient hospitalization for mental illness. More research, however, is needed to establish causality and to determine which services are most effective at reducing the need for inpatient care.

▶ At a time when the nation's economy is in the toilet and the daily news brings word of new cuts in mental health services across the country, it is heartening to read that good community mental health services do result in reductions, although not huge, of more expensive hospitalization, saving some money. Now, this is not the first time such a finding has been reported, and it should not lead to the misguided conclusion that we no longer need hospitals if we have good community care, a road we went down in the heyday of community mental health. Nonetheless, it is good news. The authors state nicely that community care is good not just because it saves money but because "People deserve care that provides the best clinical and functional outcomes." They are wise to say that "More research ... is needed ... to determine which services are most effective at reducing the need for inpatient care." After decades of mental health services research, we still do not know which services work for which people at what cost with what outcomes, but we're getting there.

J. A. Talbott, MD

Who Terminates From ACT and Why? Data From the National VA Mental Health Intensive Case Management Program

Mohamed S, Rosenheck R, Cuerdon T (Dept of Veterans Affairs (VA) Northeast Program Evaluation Ctr, West Haven, CT; VA New England Mental Illness Res, West Haven, CT; Office of Mental Health Services, Washington, DC)
Psychiatr Serv 61:675-683, 2010

Objective.—One of the original principles of assertive community treatment (ACT) is that treatment should be time unlimited. Although termination is not uncommon in ACT, it has not been empirically studied. This study examined termination from a large program based on ACT.

Methods.—This study used national data from the Department of Veterans Affairs Mental Health Intensive Case Management program modeled on ACT to compare veteran characteristics, patterns of service delivery, and early clinical changes among veterans who terminated early (less than one year) and later (one to three years) with those of veterans had not terminated after three years. Bivariate comparisons and multinomial logistic regression analyses were used to identify factors associated with early and later termination.

Results.—Among 1,402 veterans enrolled in fiscal years (FY) 2002–2004, 16% terminated early, 26% terminated later, and 57% had not terminated after three years. Compared with those who had not terminated, those who terminated early showed higher suicidality scores, and participants who terminated early and those who terminated later were less likely to have a diagnosis of schizophrenia and were more likely to have lower quality of life at entry. Stronger differentiating effects were observed for program participation. Those who terminated received less intensive services during the first six months of participation and had a weaker therapeutic alliance. Although participants who terminated early showed more violent behavior at follow-up than the other two groups, there were no other differences in early clinical changes.

Conclusions.—Rates of both early and later termination were substantial, and less active participation was a stronger predictor of termination than either patient characteristics or clinical changes. A diagnosis of schizophrenia was associated with continued treatment. Further research is needed to determine the impact of termination on longer-term outcomes.

▶ Well, here we go into semantics—what does substantial mean, as in the authors' statement that "Rates of both early and later termination were substantial..."? Their findings are that of those enrolled in the Veterans Administration's (VA's) version of Assertive Community Treatment "16% terminated before one year (early), 26% terminated from one to three years (later), and 57% had not terminated after three years." Sounds pretty good to me compared with a lot of standard treatments.

Other thoughts I had about this contribution to the literature concern the fact that patients suffering from schizophrenia, patients who received more intensive services, and patients with higher qualities of life, less drug use, and less suicidality have a better chance of sticking with these programs. This led the authors to postulate that those suffering from dual diagnoses require a different form of treatment known as integrated treatment. I agree, and the data are compelling about the effectiveness of such programs, leading one to wonder why the VA doesn't follow suit.

J. A. Talbott, MD

Introduction to the Special Section on Assisted Outpatient Treatment in New York State

Swartz MS (Duke Univ Med Ctr, Durham, NC)
Psychiatr Serv 61:967-969, 2010

Background.—"Kendra's Law" was enacted by New York State in 1999 to provide for involuntary outpatient commitment. The statute authorizes preventive court-ordered treatment before illness exacerbation likely to trigger involuntary inpatient commitment. The thresholds for inpatient and outpatient commitment are identical, so clinicians must judge whether an individual is ill enough for commitment while recommending outpatient treatment. Kendra's Law authorizes court-ordered community treatment and provides the resources and oversight needed for a viable, less restrictive alternative to involuntary hospitalization. Appropriations are provided for assisted outpatient treatment (AOT) program administration and permanent increases in service dollars for both AOT and non-AOT consumers. Debate as to the effectiveness of Kendra's Law and the AOT program continues. This law is the only involuntary outpatient commitment statute that is not yet permanent legislation, being authorized thus far on two, 5-year statutory renewals governed by internal evaluation by New York's Office of Mental Health (OMH). The results of the latest evaluation were reported.

Methods.—The assessment team analyzed AOT administrative records and clinical services data covering 1999 through 2007 as well as new data from key informant interviews throughout the state and voluntary service recipients in six selected counties.

Results.—The implementation of Kendra's Law differs across the state, with clear regional differences in the use of AOT First and Enhanced Voluntary Services First, two models of AOT. These differences question how fairly the statute is being applied.

Medicaid claims and state records reveal that AOT participants have lower rates of hospitalization, improved receipt of psychotropic medications, and improved receipt of intensive case management services compared to their pre-AOT experience. Case manager reports confirm these findings. When court orders are in place for more than 6 months, improved rates of medication possession and decreased hospitalizations were likely to persist even after the involuntary outpatient commitment is over. Receiving intensive case coordination services after AOT improved hospitalization and medication possession outcomes. Also, persons who had previous long-term court orders have these positive outcomes even without receiving ongoing intensive case coordination services. Once the court order is lifted, former AOT recipients are not hindered from voluntarily seeking and receiving intensive services.

Concern was raised over "queue jumping" through the AOT program. After the first 3 years of the program, increased service capacity funded during program commencement also expanded services for those not having court-ordered treatment.

An important measure of the effectiveness of community treatment programs that serve consumers at high risk for incarceration is involvement in the criminal justice system. Arrest rates for AOT consumers were relatively lower than those for consumers receiving voluntary treatment.

Regional levels of guideline-recommended medication possession were improved in persons with severe mental illness after undergoing the AOT program. The trajectories of the improvement differed by region, revealing a need for policy makers to monitor changes in treatment quality regionally and among enrollees who need different levels of treatment.

Conclusions.—The report suggests that the New York AOT program can improve several important outcomes for consumers without negative consequences. A carefully conducted randomized controlled trial is needed to assess whether voluntary agreements are effective alternatives to the AOT approach. The experience of New York may not be generalizable to other states or countries, and budgetary constraints have hobbled AOT's operations, effectiveness, and equitable allocation of services. Kendra's Law was once again renewed for a limited 5-year period.

▶ New York State in 1999 passed a law, Kendra's Law, establishing a new form of outpatient commitment called Assisted Outpatient Treatment. In a special section in the October issue of *Psychiatric Services*, Marvin Swartz and colleagues published 5 articles on various aspects of the law's outcome. I chose to highlight Dr Swartz's introduction to the series because I think that taken together, rather than individually, they show how thoughtful, well-resourced programs can "add value" to a state's array of services rather than compromise any one. Each article in the section has some interesting twists. The first, by Robbins and colleagues,[1] showed large differences in the way the law was applied, which they attributed to a "lack of guidance." I'm not so sure; given the extraordinary differences in the way states and counties handle legal and educational issues, this may be a similar regional difference. Then, the second article[2] showed decreased rates of hospitalization, etc, but as the authors are careful to point out, is not the result of a "carefully conducted randomized trial." Third is the issue of outcomes after the involuntary commitment court order was over,[3] which showed that the idea of a "booster shot" or jump start to ensure medication and treatment continuance worked. Then comes the answer to a critical question—does the innovative program compromise existing ones—and the answer[4] is yes, in the beginning, but no, over the long term. And finally, the authors looked at whether arrests went down, and they did.[5] So what's the downside in this approach? If everything's hunky-dory, why aren't all states doing it? Well, as the authors point out, states may not be willing or able to put up new resources (even New York may find itself in a bind soon) and think a bit outside the box, and they may be reluctanct to abandon efforts to have patients agree voluntarily to special services.

J. A. Talbott, MD

References

1. Robbins PC, Keator KJ, Steadman HJ, Swanson JW, Wilder CM, Swartz MS. Assisted outpatient treatment in New York: regional differences in New York's assisted outpatient treatment program. *Psychiatr Serv.* 2010;61:970-975.
2. Swartz MS, Wilder CM, Swanson JW, et al. Assessing outcomes for consumers in New York's assisted outpatient treatment program. *Psychiatr Serv.* 2010;61: 976-981.
3. Van Dorn RA, Swanson JW, Swartz MS, et al. Continuing medication and hospitalization outcomes after assisted outpatient treatment in New York. *Psychiatr Serv.* 2010;61:982-987.
4. Swanson JW, Van Dorn RA, Swartz MS, et al. Robbing Peter to pay Paul: did New York State's outpatient commitment program crowd out voluntary service recipients? *Psychiatr Serv.* 2010;61:988-995.
5. Gilbert AR, Moser LL, Van Dorn RA, et al. Reductions in arrest under assisted outpatient treatment in New York. *Psychiatr Serv.* 2010;61:996-999.

Assessing Outcomes for Consumers in New York's Assisted Outpatient Treatment Program
Swartz MS, Wilder CM, Swanson JW, et al (Duke Univ Med Ctr, Durham, NC; et al)
Psychiatr Serv 61:976-981, 2010

Objective.—This study examined whether New York State's assisted outpatient treatment (AOT) program, a form of involuntary outpatient commitment, improves a range of policy-relevant outcomes for court-ordered individuals.

Methods.—Administrative data from New York State's Office of Mental Health and Medicaid claims between 1999 and 2007 were linked to examine whether consumers under a court order for AOT experienced reduced rates of hospitalization, shorter hospital stays, and improvements in other outcomes. Multivariable analyses controlling for relevant covariates were used to examine the likelihood that AOT produced these effects.

Results.—On the basis of Medicaid claims and state reports for 3,576 AOT consumers, the likelihood of psychiatric hospital admission was significantly reduced by approximately 25% during the initial six-month court order (odds ratio [OR]=.77, 95% confidence interval [CI]=.72−.82) and by over one-third during a subsequent six-month renewal of the order (OR=.59, CI=.54−.65) compared with the period before initiation of the court order. Similar significant reductions in days of hospitalization were evident during initial court orders and subsequent renewals (OR=.80, CI=.78−.82, and OR=.84, CI=.81−.86, respectively). Improvements were also evident in receipt of psychotropic medications and intensive case management services. Analysis of data from case manager reports showed similar reductions in hospital admissions and improved engagement in services.

Conclusions.—Consumers who received court orders for AOT appeared to experience a number of improved outcomes: reduced hospitalization and length of stay, increased receipt of psychotropic medication and intensive case management services, and greater engagement in outpatient services.

▶ The study found "reductions in psychiatric hospitalizations, improved rates of psychotropic medication possession, enhanced case management services, and improvements in related outcomes" for people in involuntary outpatient commitment. So what's not to like? Unless you're a rabid American Civil Liberties Union member or extreme patients' rights person, everything points in the right direction.

I had two thoughts: first, I recall a study published by George Vaillant[1] that showed that addicts forced to go to the Lexington Kentucky Addiction Service had good outcomes. Second, as part of a Group for the Advancement of Psychiatry Committee on Community Psychiatry, we solicited letters through the good graces of "Dear Abby" from mentally ill persons and their family members in the correctional system. Two letters were striking in saying that their relatives received better treatment of their psychiatric illnesses in the correctional system than in the community.

Words and phrases such as "forced," "coercive," and "against one's will" all color the issue; in many ways I prefer New York State's terminology of "assisted outpatient treatment." As is clear from my points above, I think these sorts of efforts succeed.

J. A. Talbott, MD

Reference

1. Vaillant GE. A 20-year follow-up of New York narcotic addicts. *Arch Gen Psychiatry.* 1973;29:237-241.

Initiation of Primary Care—Mental Health Integration Programs in the VA Health System: Associations With Psychiatric Diagnoses in Primary Care
Zivin K, Pfeiffer PN, Szymanski BR, et al (Natl Serious Mental Illness Treatment Res and Evaluation Ctr and Health Services Res and Development (HSR&D) Ctr for Clinical Management Res, Ann Arbor, MI; et al)
Med Care 48:843-851, 2010

Background.—Providing collaborative mental health treatment within primary care settings improves depression outcomes and may improve detection of mental disorders. Few studies have assessed the effect of collaborative mental health treatment programs on diagnosis of mental disorders in primary care populations. In 2008, many Department of Veterans Affairs (VA) facilities implemented collaborative care programs, as part of the VA's Primary Care—Mental Health Integration (PC-MHI) program.

Objectives.—To assess the prevalence of diagnosed mental health conditions among primary care patient populations in association with PC-MHI programs, overall and for patient subpopulations that may be less likely to receive mental health treatment.

Research Design.—Using a difference-in-differences analysis, we evaluated whether the rates of psychiatric diagnoses among primary care patient populations at 294 VA facilities changed from fiscal year (FY)07 to FY08, and whether trends differed at facilities with PC-MHI encounters in FY08. Subgroup analyses examined whether trends differed by patient age and race/ethnicity.

Subjects, Measures, and Results.—From FY07 to FY08, the prevalence of diagnosed depression, anxiety, post-traumatic stress disorder, and alcohol abuse increased more in the 137 facilities with PC-MHI program encounters than in the 157 facilities without these encounters. Increases were more likely among patients who were younger (18–64) and white.

Conclusions.—Initiation of PC-MHI programs was associated with elevated diagnosis patterns, which may enhance recognition of mental health needs among primary care patients. Increases in diagnosis prevalence were not uniform across patient subgroups. Further research is needed on treatment processes and outcomes for individuals receiving services in PC-MHI programs.

▶ A number of years ago, our university practice plan established satellite clinics in several community locations. The model was to have one-sixth of the medical staff be psychiatric and have the psychiatrist work shoulder to shoulder with primary care physicians and share problems and insights, do consultations, and essentially avoid the dropped calls of patients referred to specialists who never show up. I thought the model was brilliant and efficient and couldn't imagine how the primary care physicians came up with it. Which was all moot since after things were up and running, it was clear to the administrators that the psychiatrists weren't economical in a fee for service environment. On the other hand, our Veterans Administration Hospital, which operates on a more black box funding model, soon after declared that it would integrate psychiatric and primary care and its fate is quite different.

The authors of this contribution start by flatly stating that, "Numerous studies indicate that integration of mental health services into primary care settings improves outcomes for depression and may improve screening and detection of mental health conditions more broadly" and then went on to show that, "From FY07 to FY08, the prevalence of diagnosed depression, anxiety, post-traumatic stress disorder, and alcohol abuse increased more in the 137 facilities with PC-MHI program encounters than in the 157 facilities without these encounters." It is a logical jump from diagnosis to recognition of need to treatment itself to better outcomes, so the model should have an enormous impact on everything from the economy to workforce strength to lessened need for other medical care.

J. A. Talbott, MD

Alternatives to standard acute in-patient care in England: readmissions, service use and cost after discharge
Byford S, Sharac J, Lloyd-Evans B, et al (King's College London, UK; Univ College London, UK)
Br J Psychiatry 197:s20-s25, 2010

Background.—Residential alternatives to standard psychiatric admissions are associated with shorter lengths of stay, but little is known about the impact on readmissions.

Aims.—To explore readmissions, use of community mental health services and costs after discharge from alternative and standard services.

Method.—Data on use of hospital and community mental health services were collected from clinical records for participants in six alternative and six standard services for 12 months from the date of index admission.

Results.—After discharge, the mean number and length of readmissions, use of community mental health services and costs did not differ significantly between standard and alternative services. Cost of index admission and total 12-month cost per participant were significantly higher for standard services.

Conclusions.—Shorter lengths of stay in residential alternatives are not associated with greater frequency or length of readmissions or greater use of community mental health services after discharge.

▶ This area of community alternatives to inpatient hospitalization has fascinated me for years and confirmation that readmissions are not more common when using them is very reassuring. In 1994, one of my 10 lessons learned about the chronic mentally ill since 1955 was "...that: Lesson #9: Alternatives To Hospitals Are Better."[1] However, in fairness, while I very much believe community care is better for many people, it is not for all, and indeed my Lesson #1 was Different

Strokes For Different Folks, that is, that "any system of care for persons suffering from schizophrenia must not be unifocal; that is, it cannot focus only on hospital treatment or only on community care. Instead, it must accommodate persons who have sudden onsets of illness (eg, with emergency and crisis services), chronic onsets (eg, with monitoring and periodic reassessment); undulating courses (eg, with acute crisis, hospital, and outpatient services), simple courses (outpatient, partial hospital, supervised housing, community care teams, residential care, case management, etc.); poorer outcomes (ongoing long-term care) and better outcomes." I still believe in both lessons and in nations where there is a balance rather than a crusade for one or the other, things work better for people I'm convinced.

J. A. Talbott, MD

Reference

1. Talbott JA. Lessons learned about the chronic mentally ill since 1955. In: Ancill RJ, Holliday S, Higenbottam J, eds. *Schizophrenia 1994: Exploring the Spectrum of Psychosis.* London: Wiley & Sons; 1994. Reprinted in Psychiatr Serv 55:1152-1159. October 2004:1-20.

Residential alternatives to acute in-patient care in England: satisfaction, ward atmosphere and service user experiences
Osborn DPJ, Lloyd-Evans B, Johnson S, et al (Univ College London, UK; et al)
Br J Psychiatry 197:s41-s45, 2010

Background.—Alternatives to traditional in-patient services may be associated with a better experience of admission.

Aims.—To compare patient satisfaction, ward atmosphere and perceived coercion in the two types of service, using validated measures.

Method.—The experience of 314 patients in four residential alternatives and four standard services were compared using the Client Satisfaction Questionnaire (CSQ), the Service Satisfaction Scale — Residential form (SSS—Res), the Ward Atmosphere Scale (WAS) and the Admission Experience Scale (AES).

Results.—Compared with standard wards, service users from alternative services reported greater levels of satisfaction (mean difference CSQ 3.3, 95% CI 1.8 to 4.9; SSS—Res 11.4, 95% CI 5.0 to 17.7). On the AES, service users in alternatives perceived less coercion (mean difference −1.3, 95% CI −1.8 to −0.8) and having more 'voice' (mean difference 0.9, 95% CI 0.6 to 1.2). Greater autonomy, more support and less anger and aggression were revealed by WAS scores. Differences in CSQ and AES scores remained significant after multivariable adjustment, but SSS—Res results were attenuated, mainly by detention status.

Conclusions.—Community alternatives were associated with greater service user satisfaction and less negative experiences. Some but not all of these differences were explained by differences in the two populations, particularly in involuntary admission.

▶ For the past several decades, it has become clear to most people that alternatives to hospitals or traditional care result in outcomes that are as favorable as traditional care and better liked by patients. So why another study?

Well, here the authors were looking at several quite different types of residential facilities: "a clinical crisis house; crisis team beds; a non-clinical (Black minority ethnic) crisis house; and a general therapeutic ward, implementing the Tidal Model of care." (I must admit I had to look up the latter, being unfamiliar with the Tidal Model of care. That great resource, Wikipedia, defines it as using "a recovery model for the promotion of mental health…[which] focuses on the continuous process of change inherent in all people. It seeks to reveal the meaning of people's experiences, emphasizing the importance of their own voice and wisdom through the power of metaphor. It aims to empower people to lead their own recovery rather than being directed by professionals.")

Interestingly, despite the loopy-sounding nontraditional description of its care model, the Tidal Model didn't perform better than a comparison traditional ward while there was definitely "greater satisfaction with the alternative services than with their comparison." Score 1 for traditional alternatives.

J. A. Talbott, MD

A Controlled Before-and-After Evaluation of a Mobile Crisis Partnership Between Mental Health and Police Services in Nova Scotia

Kisely S, Campbell LA, Peddle S, et al (Univ of Queensland, Brisbane, Australia; Dalhousie Univ, Halifax, Nova Scotia, Canada; et al)
Can J Psychiatry 55:662-668, 2010

Objectives.—Police are often the front-line response to people experiencing mental health crises. This study examined the impact of an integrated mobile crisis team formed in partnership between mental health services, municipal police, and emergency health services. The service offered short-term crisis management, with mobile interventions being attended by a plainclothes police officer and a mental health professional.

Methods.—We used a mixed-methods design encompassing: a controlled before-and-after quantitative comparison of the intervention area with a control area without access to such a service, for 1 year before and 2 years after program implementation; and qualitative assessments of the views of service recipients, families, police officers, and health staff at baseline and 2 years afterward.

Results.—The integrated service resulted in increased use by people in crisis, families, and service partners (for example, from 464 to 1666 service recipients per year). Despite increased service use, time spent on-scene and call-to-door time were reduced. At year 2, the time spent on-scene by police (136 minutes) was significantly lower than in the control area (165 minutes) (Student t test $= 3.4$, $df = 1649$, $P < 0.001$). After adjusting for confounders, people seen by the integrated team ($n = 295$) showed greater engagement than control subjects as measured by outpatient contacts (b $= 1.3$, $\chi^2 = 92.7$, $df = 1$, $P < 0.001$). The service data findings were supported by the qualitative results of focus groups and interviews.

Conclusions.—Partnerships between the police department and mental health system can improve collaboration, efficiency, and the treatment of people with mental illness.

▶ In the heyday of the Community Mental Health movement, psychiatrists were encouraged to become involved with all sorts of community resources and agencies, from schools to social agencies to police forces. Many of us in the late 1960s and early 1970s were involved in training police about community relations[1] and identification and handling of seriously mentally ill persons, often prematurely discharged from state hospitals. Others found riding around in patrol cars more exciting than treating the chronically mentally ill. The literature in those days was rich with examples of programs and efforts.

Then came an inevitable switch away from community consultation to a return to treatment of the severely and chronically mentally ill. Now that, however, especially in the United States, the mentally ill are housed and dealt with in the correctional system rather than the mental health system there is new focus on training the police and others. This article is an example of this new look at an old situation and, even though it occurred in Canada, is an example of improved patient care through coordinating disparate systems.

J. A. Talbott, MD

Reference

1. Talbott JA, Talbott SW. Training police in community relations and urban problems. *Am J Psychiatry*. 1971;127:894-900.

Outreach and Support in South London (OASIS). Outcomes of non-attenders to a service for people at high risk of psychosis: the case for a more assertive approach to assessment
Green CEL, McGuire PK, Ashworth M, et al (King's College London, UK)
Psychol Med 41:243-250, 2011

Background.—International agreement dictates that clients must be help-seeking before any assessment or intervention can be implemented by an 'at-risk service'. Little is known about individuals who decline input. This study aimed to define the size of the unengaged population of an 'at-risk service', to compare this group to those who did engage in terms of sociodemographic and clinical features and to assess the clinical outcomes of those who did not engage with the service.

Method.—Groups were compared using data collected routinely as part of the service's clinical protocol. Data on service use and psychopathology since referral to Outreach and Support in South London (OASIS) were collected indirectly from clients' general practitioners (GPs) and by screening electronic patient notes held by the local Mental Health Trust.

Results.—Over one-fifth ($n = 91$, 21.2%) of those referred did not attend or engage with the service. Approximately half of this group subsequently received a diagnosis of mental illness. A diagnosis of psychosis was given to 22.6%. Nearly 70% presented to other mental health services. There were no demographic differences, except that those who engaged with the service were more likely to be employed.

Conclusions.—Over one-fifth of those referred to services for people at high risk of psychosis do not attend or engage. However, many of this group require mental health care, and a substantial proportion has, or will later develop, psychosis. A more assertive approach to assessing individuals who are at high risk of psychosis but fail to engage may be indicated.

▶ Let me see if I understand this:

1. People who are at high risk for developing psychosis can be identified, even in a deprived inner-city area.

2. More than a fifth of those so identified do not get involved right away.

3. But half have a mental illness and almost a quarter has psychosis.

4. And many require mental health care.

5. And many later develop psychosis.

6. But because of an "international agreement and practice [that] dictates that clients themselves must be help-seeking before any formal assessment or intervention can be implemented" formulated by a body known as the International Early Psychosis Association Writing Group in 2005, people like the authors are reluctant to pursue "a more assertive approach to assessing individuals who are at high risk of psychosis but fail to engage,"[1] instead rather weakly suggesting that such an assertive approach may be indicated. What business are we in here, political correctness or fighting disease?

J. A. Talbott, MD

Reference

1. Green CE, McGuire PK, Ashworth M, Valmaggia LR. Outreach and Support in South London (OASIS). Outcomes of non-attenders to a service for people at high risk of psychosis: the case for a more assertive approach to assessment. *Psychol Med.* 2011;41:243-250.

Hospital Costs and Length of Stay Among Homeless Patients Admitted to Medical, Surgical, and Psychiatric Services

Hwang SW, Weaver J, Aubry T, et al (St Michael's Hosp, Toronto, Ontario, Canada; Univ of Ottawa, Ontario, Canada)
Med Care 49:350-354, 2011

Background.—Homeless individuals often suffer from serious health conditions and are frequently hospitalized. This study compares hospitalization costs for homeless and housed patients, with and without adjustment for patient and service characteristics.

Methods.—Administrative data on 93,426 admissions at an academic teaching hospital in Toronto, Canada, were collected over a 5-year period. These data included an identifier for patients who were homeless. Each admission was allocated a cost in Canadian dollars based on Ontario Case Costing methodology. Associations between homeless status and cost were examined for the entire sample and stratified by medical, surgical, and psychiatric services.

Results.—Data were analyzed for 90,345 housed patient admissions (mean cost, $12,555) and 3081 homeless patient admissions (mean cost, $13,516). After adjustment for age, gender, and resource intensity weight, homeless patient admissions cost $2559 more than housed patient admissions (95% CI, $2053, $3066). For patients on medical and surgical services, much of this difference was explained by more alternate level of care days spent in the hospital, during which patients did not require the level of services provided in an acute care facility. Homeless patient admissions on the psychiatric service cost $1058 more than housed patient admissions (95% CI, $480, $1635) even after adjustment for length of stay.

Conclusions.—Homeless patients on medical and surgical services remain hospitalized longer than housed patients, resulting in substantial excess costs. Homeless patients admitted for psychiatric conditions have higher costs not explained by prolonged length of stay. These observations may help guide development of community-based interventions for homeless individuals and reduce their use of inpatient care.

▶ Homeless persons with or without severe mental illnesses rack up more expensive hospital bills than nonhomeless ones. Is this surprising? Not at all. Then why did I select this article for abstraction and comment? For several reasons. First, it illustrates once again the fact that society is more willing to pay for treatment than prevention, that decision makers have an extraordinary inability to implement long-term solutions and instead focus on quick fixes, and that unless we figure out how to think globally about expenses, we will be doomed to keep repeating our failures. Second, although I am a great admirer of one-payer systems and especially those in Canada's provinces, a rational, national health care system does not solve every problem. Third, because the quantification of the difference of cost incurred by homeless persons in general hospitals versus nonhomeless ones is really quite significant—about 20%—and seen that way represents a potential for significant savings, not to mention doing the right thing: providing better care and getting better outcomes.

J. A. Talbott, MD

Trial of an Electronic Decision Support System to Facilitate Shared Decision Making in Community Mental Health

Woltmann EM, Wilkniss SM, Teachout A, et al (Univ of Michigan, Ann Arbor; Thresholds Psychiatric Rehabilitation Ctrs, Chicago, IL; et al)
Psychiatr Serv 62:54-60, 2011

Objectives.—Involvement of community mental health consumers in mental health decision making has been consistently associated with improvements in health outcomes. Electronic decision support systems (EDSSs) that support both consumer and provider decision making may be a sustainable way to improve dyadic communication in a field with approximately 50% workforce turnover per year. This study examined the feasibility of such a system and investigated proximal outcomes of the system's performance.

Methods.—A cluster randomized design was used to evaluate an EDSS at three urban community mental health sites. Case managers (N = 20) were randomly assigned to the EDSS-supported planning group or to the usual care planning group. Consumers (N = 80) were assigned to the same group as their case managers. User satisfaction with the care planning process was assessed for consumers and case managers (possible scores range from 1 to 5, with higher summary scores indicating more satisfaction). Recall of the care plan was assessed for consumers. Linear regression with adjustment for grouping by worker was used to assess satisfaction scores. A Wilcoxon rank-sum test was used to examine knowledge of the care plan.

Results.—Compared with case managers in the control group, those in the intervention group were significantly more satisfied with the care planning process (mean ± SD score = 4.0 ± .5 versus 3.3 ± .5; adjusted p = .01). Compared with consumers in the control group, those in the intervention group had significantly greater recall of their care plans three days after the planning session (mean proportion of plan goals recalled = 75% ± 28% versus 57% ± 32%; p = .02). There were no differences between the clients in the intervention and control groups regarding satisfaction.

Conclusions.—This study demonstrated that clients can build their own care plans and negotiate and revise them with their case managers using an EDSS.

▶ This is fascinating. When I read the title and abstract I thought, "What a neat idea; I'll bet the patients in the study group were much more satisfied than those in the control group with the care planning process." But no, they were no more satisfied. Now why did I think that? First, because patients are more honest, forthcoming, and revealing on the Internet or to a third party—just look at

"Dear Abby." Second, because it seemed logical that patients could have both the first and last word—the first in their statement of what they wanted and the last in that they didn't need to do anything they didn't want to. In fact, however, both groups are pretty negative, and the authors surmise this is because of dissatisfaction with the services they get rather than the planning that goes into it. Maybe. But maybe it also has to do with dissatisfaction with having a chronic illness that can for the most part be managed but not cured and to the illness itself. At the end of the day, however, like asking patients in a primary care physician's office to fill out a history and review of systems, I think asking patients first will have positive effects.

J. A. Talbott, MD

Self-Help and Community Mental Health Agency Outcomes: A Recovery-Focused Randomized Controlled Trial

Segal SP, Silverman CJ, Temkin TL (Univ of California, Berkeley; Kaiser Permanente of Northern California, Oakland, CA)
Psychiatr Serv 61:905-910, 2010

Objective.—Self-help agencies (SHAs) are consumer-operated service organizations managed as participatory democracies. Members are involved in all aspects of organizational management, because a premise of SHAs is that organizationally empowered individuals become more empowered in their own lives, which promotes recovery. The study sought to determine the effectiveness of combined SHA and community mental health agency (CMHA) services in assisting recovery for persons with serious mental illness.

Methods.—A weighted sample of new clients seeking CMHA services was randomly assigned to regular CMHA services or to combined SHA-CMHA services at five proximally located pairs of SHA drop-in centers and county CMHAs. Member-clients (N=505) were assessed at baseline and at one, three, and eight months on five recovery-focused outcome measures: personal empowerment, self-efficacy, social integration, hope, and psychological functioning. Scales had high levels of reliability and independently established validity. Outcomes were evaluated with a repeated-measures multivariate analysis of covariance.

Results.—Overall results indicated that combined SHA-CMHA services were significantly better able to promote recovery of client-members than CMHA services alone. The sample with combined services showed greater improvements in personal empowerment (F=3.99, df=3 and 491, p<.008), self-efficacy (F=11.20, df=3 and 491, p<.001), and independent social integration (F=12.13, df=3 and 491, p<.001). Hopelessness (F=4.36, df=3 and 491, p<.005) and symptoms (F=4.49, df=3 and 491, p<.004) dissipated more quickly and to a greater extent in the combined condition than in the CMHA-only condition.

Conclusions.—Member-empowering SHAs run as participatory democracies in combination with CMHA services produced more positive recovery-focused results than CMHA services alone.

▶ I have been a great believer in self-help and peer-support groups ever since I saw how effective they are in helping patients with everything from amputations to "-ostomies" recover. However, I was vigorously attacked by one self-help advocate on a TV program in the 1960s because he believed that they should function instead of, not alongside, mainstream therapeutic efforts. So it was with pleasure and relief that I read this article's conclusion that "Member-empowering SHAs...in combination with CMHA [community mental health agency] services produced more positive recovery-focused results than CMHA services alone." I'd be willing to bet that both are more effective than self-help agencies (SHAs) alone. Another area that the authors investigate but I am less informed about relates to the type of governance or attitude SHAs have, particularly "participatory democracy—like organizations." Certainly we know that involving mentally ill persons in treatment decisions greatly enhances joint treatment planning, compliance/adherence and, I am convinced, outcomes. So I guess this is one more tool to promote self-esteem, self-sufficiency, and recovery.

J. A. Talbott, MD

Hospital Care

Predicting Time to Readmission in Patients With Recent Histories of Recurrent Psychiatric Hospitalization: A Matched-Control Survival Analysis
Schmutte T, Dunn CL, Sledge WH (Yale Univ School of Medicine, New Haven, CT)
J Nerv Ment Dis 198:860-863, 2010

The most robust predictor of future psychiatric hospitalization is the number of previous admissions. About half of psychiatric inpatients with histories of repeated hospitalizations are readmitted within 12 months. This study sought to determine which patient characteristics predicted time-to-readmission within 12 months after controlling for the number of previous hospitalizations in 75 adults with recent histories of recurrent admissions and 75 matched controls. Results revealed multiple clinical and demographic between-group differences at index hospitalization. However, the only predictors of shorter time-to-readmission in multivariate Cox proportional hazards were unemployment (hazards ratio = 9.26) and residential living status (hazards ratio = 2.05) after controlling for prior hospitalizations (hazard ratio = 1.24). Unemployment and residential living status were not proxies of psychosis or moderated by illness severity or comorbid substance use. Results suggest that early psychiatric readmission may be more influenced by residential and employment status than by severe mental illness.

▶ A very wise mentor/teacher/colleague of mine once said that all admissions to mental hospitals were more likely caused by social situations and not by mental disorders; in other words, persons living in precarious housing situations, in difficult economic straits, or with tumultuous families were more likely to seek admission or be admitted whatever their psychiatric condition than those otherwise housed, supported, surrounded, etc. The authors here have confirmed that bit of wisdom through a study of readmissions. For years, I was one of those who regarded readmission as a failure of the last treatment plan, which of course included housing placement/return, but it was a failure, rather than a circumstance. I think I was naive then and in search of an unattainable perfect solution. With the implementation of President Obama's Health Care plan, the issue of readmissions will take on a whole new meaning because once in place, readmissions will carry a fiscal sting to them. As explained in the Pump Handle, a public health blog, http://scienceblogs.com/thepumphandle/ 2010/05/reducing_hospital_readmissions.php "The Patient Protection and Affordable Care Act (the new healthcare law) will reduce Medicare payments to hospitals with excess hospital readmissions,..." Another friend/colleague who runs a big hospital system in New York City expressed concern that while reducing readmissions was wise, separating preventable from nonpreventable readmissions was difficult and complicated in psychiatry by patient behavior and substance abuse comorbidity. It will be interesting to see what happens and how both general and psychiatric hospitals cope with this new pressure.

J. A. Talbott, MD

Readmission: A useful indicator of the quality of inpatient psychiatric care
Byrne SL, Hooke GR, Page AC (The Univ of Western Australia, Crawley, Australia)
J Affect Disord 126:206-213, 2010

Background.—The literature is unclear regarding the relationship between hospital outcome (i.e., symptom improvement during a hospital admission) and readmission, questioning the validity of readmission as an indicator of the quality of the previous hospitalization. Thus, the present aim was to examine if hospital outcome is a predictor of readmission and identify the factors that may mask any effects.

Methods.—A naturalistic historical study compared the predictors of readmission over the 30 days, 6 months and 5 years following discharge for first-ever admitted inpatients with depression ($n = 478$) to all inpatients regardless of prior hospitalisations and current diagnoses ($n = 1177$).

Results.—Hospital outcome, as indicated by changes from admission to discharge in scores on symptom measures, during both first-ever admissions and admissions which are not the first, predicted readmissions over all time periods for all patients, not only those with depression. However, this finding was only significant when hospital outcome was assessed by improvements on a patient-reported symptom measure, and not a clinician-rated measure.

Limitations.—The sample included inpatients treated at a private psychiatric hospital and therefore it is unknown if these findings can be generalised to patients treated in a public system.

Conclusions.—These findings support that readmission may be a useful indicator of the quality of the previous hospitalization.

▶ This would seem to merely affirm the obvious—what the wife of a prominent college president used to call "Duh" research—of course readmission represents a failure in or of something. But a failure in what? In treatment where assessment of readiness for discharge, treatment planning, in discharge planning, follow-up, aggressive outpatient/community monitoring, community resources, case management, patient compliance/adherence, appropriate referral, in effective linkage between inpatient and outpatient care, physician and staff competence or a combination?

A long time ago, when deinstitutionalization was at its worst, I took a look at 100 consecutive readmissions to a state hospital and came to the not-very-surprising conclusion that "84 might have been prevented, and that almost half of these might have been prevented with minor improvements of existing services necessitating no additional expenditure of money."[1] While our patient population consisted of more than patients suffering from just depression, their needs were much more comprehensive than these authors imply and the solutions much more dependent on a better mental health system. I sincerely trust that in the 36 years between them, despite the difference in populations, national health systems, and treatment sophistication, we're doing a better job. The next task for the researchers is to do a Wennberg-type[2] look at differences between and among hospitals, states (in Australia and America), and nations.

J. A. Talbott, MD

References

1. Talbott JA. Stopping the revolving door—a study of readmissions to a state hospital. *Psychiatr Q.* 1974;48:159-168.
2. Wennberg JE, Fisher ES, eds. The Care of Patients with Severe Chronic Illness: A Report on the Medicare Program by the Dartmouth Atlas Project. Hanover, NH: The Center for the Evaluative Clinical Sciences, Dartmouth Atlas Project; 2006.

Effects of Adopting a Smoke-Free Policy in State Psychiatric Hospitals
Hollen V, Ortiz G, Schacht L, et al (Natl Association of State Mental Health Program Directors Res Inst, Inc, Alexandria, VA; et al)
Psychiatr Serv 61:899-904, 2010

Objective.—The aim of this study was to investigate how adopting a smoke-free policy in state psychiatric hospitals affected key factors, including adverse events, smoking cessation treatment options, and specialty training for clinical staff about smoking-related issues.

Methods.—Hospitals were surveyed in 2006 and 2008 about their smoking policies, smoking cessation aids, milieu management, smoking cessation treatment options, and aftercare planning and referrals for smoking education. Comparisons were made between hospitals that went smoke-free between the two time periods (N=28) and those that did not (N=42).

Results.—Among hospitals that changed to a smoke-free policy, the proportion that reported adverse events decreased by 75% or more in three areas: smoking or tobacco use as a precursor to incidents that led to seclusion or restraint, smoking-related health conditions, and coercion or threats among patients and staff. Hospitals that did not adopt a smoke-free policy cited several barriers, including resistance from staff, patients, and advocates.

Conclusions.—Although staff were concerned that implementing a smoke-free policy would have negative effects, this was not borne out. Findings indicated that adopting a smoke-free policy was associated with a positive impact on hospitals, as evidenced by a reduction in negative events related to smoking. After adoption of a smoke-free policy, fewer hospitals reported seclusion or restraint related to smoking, coercion, and smoking-related health conditions, and there was no increase in reported elopements or fires. For hospitals adopting a smoke-free policy in 2008, there was no significant difference between 2006 and 2008 in the number offering nicotine replacement therapies or clinical staff specialty training. Results suggest that smoking cessation practices are not changing in the hospital as a result of a change in policy.

▶ The surgeon general's first report on smoking was published and issued in 1964, yet many general hospitals did not institute no-smoking policies until decades thereafter. I recall 2 events that made a big impression on me. The first occurred around 1973 to 1975 when I was superintendent of a state psychiatric hospital and the idea of segregating smokers or stopping smoking was met with incredulity by the staff and patients; it would be cruel and punitive, not healthful and sensible. The second was in the 1980s when doing Boards at a Veterans' Administration Hospital where smoking was prohibited inside but cigarettes were distributed freely outside—what a mixed message. Even today at my university medical center, the hospital forbids smoking on its sidewalks, prompting smoking staff and faculty to walk across the street and smoke on the university's sidewalks—bizarre. This article's striking conclusion that not only was such a policy not impossible to implement but led to "fewer adverse consequences" should be helpful to other states and hospital administrators.

J. A. Talbott, MD

Overcrowding in psychiatric wards and physical assaults on staff: data-linked longitudinal study

Virtanen M, Vahtera J, Batty GD, et al (Finnish Inst of Occupational Health, Helsinki, Finland; Univ of Turku and Turku Univ Hosp, Finland; Univ of Edinburgh, UK; et al)
Br J Psychiatry 198:149-155, 2011

Background.—Patient overcrowding and violent assaults by patients are two major problems in psychiatric healthcare. However, evidence of an association between overcrowding and aggressive behaviour among patients is mixed and limited to small-scale studies.

Aims.—This study examined the association between ward overcrowding and violent physical assaults in acute-care psychiatric in-patient hospital wards.

Method.—Longitudinal study using ward-level monthly records of bed occupancy and staff reports of the timing of violent acts during a 5-month period in 90 in-patient wards in 13 acute psychiatric hospitals in Finland. In total 1098 employees (physicians, ward head nurses, registered nurses, licensed practical nurses) participated in the study. The outcome measure was staff reports of the timing of physical assaults on both themselves and ward property.

Results.—We found that 46% of hospital staff were working in overcrowded wards, as indicated by >10 percentage units of excess bed occupancy, whereas only 30% of hospital personnel were working in a ward with no excess occupancy. An excess bed occupancy rate of >10 percentage units at the time of an event was associated with violent assaults towards employees (odds ratio (OR) = 1.72, 95% CI 1.05−2.80; OR = 3.04, 95% CI 1.51−6.13 in adult wards) after adjustment for confounding factors. No association was found with assaults on ward property (OR = 1.06, 95% CI 0.75−1.50).

Conclusions.—These findings suggest that patient overcrowding is highly prevalent in psychiatric hospitals and, importantly, may increase the risk of violence directed at staff.

▶ Violence in hospitals has become a major problem in recent years. An oncologist at Johns Hopkins Hospital was stabbed because a family member was disappointed by the outcome of a procedure. Almost half of French physicians, both in solo practice and in hospitals, were reported to have suffered a violent attack from patients. Add to this psychosis or other severe mental disorders, and there is increased cause for concern for the safety of people working in medical settings.

Intuitively, therefore, it is logical to assume that anything that adds to stress or tension in an inpatient mental hospital unit treating acutely ill mental patients will result in increased violence. So it is surprising to read that the authors of this study state that there have been no large-scale studies on the linkage and, even more surprisingly, some studies showed a null or opposite result. But this study should lay these doubts to rest. The hitch, of course, is that at a time when internationally, health care, especially mental health care, is being squeezed economically, it is a long shot to expect policy makers to relieve crowding to reduce violence.

J. A. Talbott, MD

Adverse Events Associated With Organizational Factors of General Hospital Inpatient Psychiatric Care Environments
Hanrahan NP, Kumar A, Aiken LH (Univ of Pennsylvania, Philadelphia)
Psychiatr Serv 61:569-574, 2010

Objective.—Although general hospitals receive nearly 60% of all inpatient psychiatric admissions, little is known about the care environment and related adverse events. The purpose of this study was to determine the occurrence of adverse events and examine the extent to which organizing factors of inpatient psychiatric care environments were associated with the occurrence of these events. The events examined were wrong medication, patient falls with injuries, complaints from patients and families, work-related staff injuries, and verbal abuse directed toward nurses.

Methods.—This cross-sectional study used data from a 1999 nurse survey linked with hospital data. Nurse surveys from 353 psychiatric registered nurses working in 67 Pennsylvania general hospitals provided information on nurse characteristics, organizational factors, and the occurrence of adverse events. Linear regression models and robust clustering methods at the hospital level were used to study the relationship of organizational factors of psychiatric care environments and adverse event outcomes.

Results.—Verbal abuse toward registered nurses (79%), complaints (61%), patient falls with injuries (44%), and work-related injuries (39%) were frequent occurrences. Better management skill was associated with fewer patient falls and fewer work-related injuries to staff. In addition, fewer occurrences of staff injuries were associated with better nurse-physician relationship and lower patient-to-nurse staffing ratios.

Conclusions.—Adverse events are frequent for inpatient psychiatric care in general hospitals, and organizational factors of care environments are associated with adverse event outcomes. Further development of evidence-based quality and safety monitoring of inpatient psychiatric care in general hospitals is imperative.

▶ When I sat on my hospital's medical executive committee, I witnessed several occasions when one or more chiefs of service would complain that staffing cuts or shortages could impair patient care, and their protestations were largely not attended to. I think this was for several reasons, principal among them was that they and we all as well as the public had no data.

Now, as these authors point out, studies have shown and the Institute of Medicine has sounded off loudly that medical errors have serious consequences. But most work has concerned what they call the medical-surgical sector, and psychiatry has lagged behind.

This study reveals some interesting findings, which they call organizational factors that underpin some poor patient care outcomes. I think it's a bit more complex than what those 2 words encompass. For nursing, staffing cuts are motivated by cost cutting and right sizing and what staffs are needed for what tasks—which is a complicated explanation and combines a number of diverse pressures and social trends. In a different manner, the verbal abuse of nurses (often by physicians) also results from several different forces: medical education, natural selection, gender imbalance, power differential, and social hierarchy issues. While it is comforting to think that falls can be partly stopped by hiring more skilled managers and injuries reduced by better nursing staffing ratios, I suspect many of our problems call for much more comprehensive and differently targeted changes in society, education, funding, and human rights.

J. A. Talbott, MD

Post-Traumatic Stress Disorder (PTSD) and Stress

Greater Prevalence and Incidence of Dementia in Older Veterans with Posttraumatic Stress Disorder

Qureshi SU, Kimbrell T, Pyne JM, et al (Michael E. DeBakey Veterans Affairs Med Ctr, Houston, TX; Veterans Affairs South Central Mental Illness Res, North Little Rock, AR; Central Arkansas Veterans Healthcare System, Little Rock, AR)
J Am Geriatr Soc 58:1627-1633, 2010

Objectives.—To explore the association between posttraumatic stress disorder (PTSD) and dementia in older veterans.

Design.—Administrative database study of individuals seen within one regional division of the Veterans Affairs healthcare network.

Setting.—Veterans Integrated Service Network 16.

Participants.—Veterans aged 65 and older who had a diagnosis of PTSD or who were recipients of a Purple Heart (PH) and a comparison group of the same age with no PTSD diagnosis or PH were divided into four groups: those with PTSD and no PH (PTSD+/PH−, n = 3,660), those with PH and no PTSD (PTSD−/PH+, n = 1,503), those with PTSD and a PH (PTSD+/PH+, n = 153), and those without PTSD or a PH (PTSD-/PH−, n = 5,165).

Measurements.—Incidence and prevalence of dementia after controlling for confounding factors in multivariate logistic regression.

Results.—The PTSD+/PH− group had a significantly higher incidence and prevalence of dementia than the groups without PTSD with or without a PH. The prevalence and incidence of a dementia diagnosis remained two times as high in the PTSD+/PH− group as in the PTSD−/PH + or PTSD−/PH− group after adjusting for the confounding factors. There were no statistically significant differences between the other groups.

Conclusion.—The incidence and prevalence of dementia is greater in veterans with PTSD. It is unclear whether this is due to a common risk factor underlying PTSD and dementia or to PTSD being a risk factor for dementia. Regardless, this study suggests that veterans with PTSD should be screened more closely for dementia. Because PTSD is so common in veterans, this association has important implications for veteran care.

▶ Let me start with the bottom line here and quote the first sentence of the last paragraph: "Older veterans with PTSD had twice the incidence and prevalence of dementia diagnoses as those without, even after accounting for confounding illnesses, combat-related trauma, and number of primary care and mental health visits." Wow! The authors state they do not know whether posttraumatic stress disorder (PTSD) predisposes to dementia or whether PTSD is an early marker of dementia or they share a common risk factor. But while the authors' findings are awesome, Soo Borson in an accompanying editorial[1] extends their consequences even more, stating that "a causal link between PTSD and cognitive impairment in late life would have enormous global implications in a world facing a rising societal burden of dementia, a shrinking workforce to sustain its economies, and the difficulties of containing human violence." She goes on to remind us that the US military is but one of the groups exposed to "deeply traumatizing experiences with lifetime effect," and we must also reckon with the hundreds of thousands of civilians exposed to genocide, deprived of meaning in their lives, raped, physically abused, suffering severe mental illnesses and sudden deaths, experiencing car crashes, imprisoned, and those who are first responders.

J. A. Talbott, MD

Reference

1. Borson S. Posttraumatic stress disorder and dementia: a lifelong cost of war? *J Am Geriatr Soc.* 2010;58:1797-1798.

Is Peacekeeping Peaceful? A Systematic Review

Sareen J, Stein MB, Thoresen S, et al (Univ of Manitoba, Winnipeg; Univ of California, San Diego; Norwegian Centre for Violence and Traumatic Stress Studies, Oslo, Norway; et al)
Can J Psychiatry 55:464-472, 2010

Objective.—To systematically review the literature on the association between deployment to a peacekeeping mission and distress, mental disorders, and suicide.

Methods.—Peer-reviewed English publications were found through key word searches in MEDLINE, PsycINFO, Scopus, and Embase, and by contacting authors in the field. Sixty-eight articles were included in this review.

Results.—Some studies have found higher levels of postdeployment distress and posttraumatic stress disorder (PTSD) symptoms. Most studies have not shown an increased risk of suicide in former peacekeepers. Correlates of distress and PTSD symptoms included level of exposure to traumatic events during deployment, number of deployments, predeployment personality traits or disorder, and postdeployment stressors. Perceived meaningfulness of the mission, postdeployment social supports, and positive perception of homecoming were associated with lower likelihood of distress.

Conclusions.—Most peacekeepers do not develop high levels of distress or symptoms of PTSD. As postdeployment distress is consistently shown to be associated with high levels of exposure to combat during deployment, targeted interventions for peacekeepers who have been exposed to high levels of combat should be considered.

▶ The answer to the question posed in the title is, "Of course not." But on the other hand, it may not be as posttraumatic stress disorder producing as one might fear. Since peacekeeping became a function of multinational organizations such as the United Nations and North Atlantic Treaty Organization and the African Union starting in 1948, Wikipedia (http://en.wikipedia.org/wiki/Peacekeeping) says there have been 63 missions. Many of these have involved civil wars where massacres and genocide occurred, so one would expect troops involved to be affected. The authors constructed a nifty figure (Fig 1 in the original article) that shows all the interactions of risk and protective factors that are not limited to peacekeepers but to all who could be involved in stressful situations. One area that is almost impossible to really judge is the intercountry differences that may involve culture, motivation, training, deployment schedules, and health services available in the variety of nations whose soldiers are involved in such activities. In addition, one factor I found interesting was the perceived meaningfulness of the mission. That and the homecoming reception were of course sizeable factors in how our post-Vietnam troops were affected. The authors' final recommendation seems most suitable, that is, to provide "targeted interventions for peacekeepers who have been exposed to high levels of combat ..."

J. A. Talbott, MD

The Mental Health of Partners of Australian Vietnam Veterans Three Decades After the War and Its Relation to Veteran Military Service, Combat, and PTSD

O'Toole BI, Outram S, Catts SV, et al (Univ of Sydney ANZAC Res Inst, New South Wales, Australia; Newcastle Univ, New South Wales, Australia; Queensland Univ, Brisbane, Australia)
J Nerv Ment Dis 198:841-845, 2010

This study assessed psychiatric diagnoses in female partners of Australian Vietnam veterans, compared these with national Australian population statistics, and assessed their relationship with veterans' military service and mental health. Independent assessments of 240 veteran-partner couples used standardized physical and psychiatric diagnostic interviews that permitted comparison with Australian population data. Multivariate regression modeling examined associations of veterans' war service, combat, and psychiatric status with women's mental health. Anxiety disorders and severe recurrent depression were among 11 of 17 psychiatric diagnoses that were significantly in excess of population expectations. Veterans' combat and post-traumatic stress disorder were significant predictors of women's depressive disorder, particularly severe depression. We conclude that veterans' war service and mental health sequelae including post-traumatic stress disorder are associated with higher rates of mental disorder in their female partners 3 decades after the war.

▶ While these data and conclusions are not counterintuitive, they are of great interest. We know from US studies that marital discord and divorce rates are higher in returning veterans, especially those suffering from symptoms of post-traumatic stress disorder. I think most Americans remember the Vietnam War as an American experience/tragedy, forgetting the solidarity and contributions of others, especially the Australians and South Koreans, both of whose physicians I worked with; they were in the same boat as we were. So when a study from Australia shows that 17 diagnoses were in excess of population expectations (Table 1 in the original article), these findings have implications for us. Thirty years after the hostilities ceased, the female partners of Australian combat troops still show significant morbidity. As the authors emphasize, the increase in anxiety and depression carries with it the increased use of psychiatric medication, health service utilization, and economic burden to the country.

J. A. Talbott, MD

Acute Stress Disorder as a Predictor of Posttraumatic Stress Disorder: A Systematic Review
Bryant RA (Univ of New South Wales, Sydney, Australia)
J Clin Psychiatry 72:233-239, 2011

Objective.—The utility of the acute stress disorder diagnosis to describe acute stress reactions and predict subsequent posttraumatic stress disorder (PTSD) was evaluated.

Data Sources.—A systematic search was conducted in the PsycINFO, MEDLINE, and PubMed databases for English-language articles published between 1994 and 2009 using keywords that combined *acute stress disorder and posttraumatic stress disorder.*

Study Selection.—Studies were selected that assessed for acute stress disorder within 1 month of trauma exposure and assessed at a later time for PTSD, using established measures of acute stress disorder and PTSD.

Data Extraction.—For each study, capacity of the acute stress disorder diagnosis to predict PTSD was calculated in terms of sensitivity, specificity, and positive and negative predictive power. For studies that reported subsyndromal acute stress disorder, the same analyses were calculated for cases that initially satisfied subsyndromal acute stress disorder criteria.

Data Synthesis.—Twenty-two studies were identified as suitable for analysis (19 with adults and 3 with children). Diagnosis of acute stress disorder resulted in half the rate of distressed people in the acute phase being identified relative to including cases with subsyndromal acute stress disorder. In terms of prediction, the acute stress disorder diagnosis had reasonable positive predictive power (proportion of people with acute stress disorder who later developed PTSD). In contrast, the sensitivity (proportion of people who developed PTSD who initially met criteria for acute stress disorder) was poor.

Conclusions.—The acute stress disorder diagnosis does not adequately identify the majority of people who will eventually develop PTSD. There is a need to formally describe acute stress reactions, but this goal may be achieved more usefully by describing the broad range of initial reactions rather than by attempting to predict subsequent PTSD.

▶ The conclusions that "acute stress disorder diagnosis does not adequately identify the majority of people who will eventually develop PTSD" but that it had "a reasonable positive predictive power" albeit poorly—"sensitive"—do not surprise me. Although we did no careful studies or follow-up of soldiers who had acute stress disorders in Vietnam, it was apparent to me that clinically they were different, albeit overlapping syndromes. I was most distressed that the author needed to concern himself with how to code and diagnose such acute disorders so that victims "receive needed mental health care." What sort of a world do we live in, in America, where the tail of coding and diagnosing wag the dog of proper care and treatment? There are acute stress reactions, chronic stress reactions, delayed (sometimes for decades) ones, and a host of other sequelae—all are real and merit treatment.

J. A. Talbott, MD

Tsunami-exposed Tourist Survivors: Signs of Recovery in a 3-year Perspective
Johannesson KB, Lundin T, Fröjd T, et al (Uppsala Univ Hosp, Sweden; et al)
J Nerv Ment Dis 199:162-169, 2011

Long-term follow-up after disaster exposure indicates increased rates of psychological distress. However, trajectories and rates of recovery in large samples of disaster-exposed survivors are largely lacking. A group of 3457 Swedish survivors temporarily on vacation in Southeast Asia during the 2004 tsunami were assessed by postal questionnaire at 14 months and 3 years after the tsunami regarding post-traumatic stress reactions (IES-R) and general mental health (GHQ-12). There was a general pattern of resilience and recovery 3 years postdisaster. Severe exposure and traumatic bereavement were associated with increased post-traumatic stress reactions and heightened risk for impaired mental health. The rate of recovery was lower among respondents exposed to life threat and among bereaved. Severe trauma exposure and bereavement seem to have considerable long-term impact on psychological distress and appear to slow down the recovery process. Readiness among health agencies for identification of symptoms and provision of interventions might facilitate optimal recovery.

▶ Ironically, this article appeared in March 2011, the same month as a tsunami hit Japan and 7 years after the tsunami of 2004. Many of the findings confirm what other research on civilian disasters and indeed combat exposure has shown, specifically that: (1) Those severely exposed still had increased posttraumatic stress reactions and affected general mental health; (2) There was a decrease of symptoms in all survivors, although the rate of recovery was slower among respondents exposed to life threats and among bereaved; (3) Resilience is common in highly exposed individuals; (4) The highly exposed had approximately 3 times the IES-R scores of the less exposed; (5) Bereaved had 86% higher IES-R score than those with no loss; (6) The effect of exposure seemed to slow the process of recuperation; (7) Suicidal ideation was modest in all groups; (8) Previous psychiatric problems and previously experienced traumatic life events were associated with higher levels of long-term trauma reactions and higher risk for psychological distress; (9) A factor positively associated with recovery at both the time points was satisfaction with social support; (10) Other factors were middle age, marriage/cohabitation, male sex, and higher level of education; (11) Another positive factor could be that one-third of respondents had revisited the area, of which 90% reported this as important.

Since so many of these findings were or are already known, why did I choose this article? Mainly because, despite the differences between this year's tsunami in Japan and the 2004 tsunami in Southeast Asia, that is, the devastating coincidental earthquake and nuclear plant contamination as well as the fact that many of those affected in Japan lost their homes as well as loved ones versus the Swedish tourists being able to return home, the long-term outcome is not entirely bleak.

J. A. Talbott, MD

Effectiveness of Mental Health Screening and Coordination of In-Theater Care Prior to Deployment to Iraq: A Cohort Study
Warner CH, Appenzeller GN, Parker JR, et al (Command and General Staff College, Fort Leavenworth, KS; U.S. Army Med Activity Alaska, Fort Wainwright, AK; Winn Army Community Hosp, Fort Stewart, GA; et al)
Am J Psychiatry 168:378-385, 2011

Objective.—The authors assessed the effectiveness of a systematic method of predeployment mental health screening to determine whether screening decreased negative outcomes during deployment in Iraq's combat setting.

Method.—Primary care providers performed directed mental health screenings during standard predeployment medical screening. If indicated, on-site mental health providers assessed occupational functioning with unit leaders and coordinated in-theater care for those cleared for deployment. Mental health-related clinical encounters and evacuations during the first 6 months of deployment in 2007 were compared for 10,678 soldiers from three screened combat brigades and 10,353 soldiers from three comparable unscreened combat brigades.

Results.—Of 10,678 soldiers screened, 819 (7.7%, 95% confidence interval [CI]=7.2–8.2) received further mental health evaluation; of these, 74 (9.0%, 95% CI=7.1–11.0) were not cleared to deploy and 96 (11.7%, 95% CI=9.5–13.9) were deployed with additional requirements. After 6 months, soldiers in screened brigades had significantly lower rates of clinical contacts than did those in unscreened brigades for suicidal ideation (0.4%, 95% CI=0.3–0.5, compared with 0.9%, 95% CI=0.7–1.1), for combat stress (15.7%, 95% CI=15.0–16.4, compared with 22.0%, 95% CI=21.2–22.8), and for psychiatric disorders (2.9%, 95% CI=2.6–3.2, compared with 13.2%, 95% CI=12.5–13.8), as well as lower rates of occupational impairment (0.6%, 95% CI=0.4–0.7, compared with 1.8%, 95% CI=1.5–2.1) and air evacuation for behavioral health reasons (0.1%, 95% CI=0.1–0.2, compared with 0.3%, 95% CI=0.2–0.4).

Conclusions.—Predeployment mental health screening was associated with significant reductions in occupationally impairing mental health problems, medical evacuations from Iraq for mental health reasons, and suicidal ideation. This predeployment screening process provides a feasible system for screening soldiers and coordinating mental health support during deployment.

▶ For years, or at least since World War II, US Army lore and scientific evidence held that it was impossible to screen for those who would have problems in combat. Study after study looked at predisposing factors to developing posttraumatic stress disorder. Although there was some evidence that a troubled adolescence, school problems, and family alcoholism or trouble contributed somewhat to the incidence of posttraumatic stress disorder, there was never a silver bullet. Now comes this study. The difference between 1 in 8 and 1 in 35, that is, 14% versus 2.8%, is enormous. Now, the authors do admit that "given the study's short time frame (6 months), our data do not allow us to assess whether the screening had longer-term benefits." Therefore, what we saw following the Vietnam War, that is, ex-military personnel developing symptoms of posttraumatic stress disorder months, years and even decades afterward, cannot be ascertained at this point. We will simply have to see.

J. A. Talbott, MD

Preinjury Psychiatric Status, Injury Severity, and Postdeployment Posttraumatic Stress Disorder

Sandweiss DA, for the Millennium Cohort Study Team (Naval Health Res Ctr, San Diego, CA; et al)

Arch Gen Psychiatry 68:496-504, 2011

Context.—Physical injury has been associated with the development of posttraumatic stress disorder (PTSD). Previous studies have retrospectively examined the relationship of preinjury psychiatric status and postinjury PTSD with conflicting results, but no prospective studies regarding this subject have been conducted, to our knowledge.

Objective.—To prospectively assess the relationship of predeployment psychiatric status and injury severity with postdeployment PTSD.

Design.—Prospective, longitudinal study.

Setting.—United States military personnel deployed in support of the conflicts in Iraq and Afghanistan.

Participants.—United States service member participants in the Millennium Cohort Study who completed a baseline questionnaire (from July 1, 2001, through June 30, 2003) and at least 1 follow-up questionnaire (from June 1, 2004, through February 14, 2006, and from May 15, 2007, through December 31, 2008) and who were deployed in the intervening period. Self-reported health information was used to prospectively examine the relationship between baseline psychiatric status and follow-up PTSD in injured and uninjured deployed individuals.

Main Outcome Measures.—A positive screening result using the PTSD Checklist-Civilian Version.

Results.—Of 22 630 eligible participants, 1840 (8.1%) screened positive for PTSD at follow-up, and 183 (0.8%) sustained a deployment-related physical injury that was documented in the Joint Theater Trauma Registry or the Navy-Marine Corps Combat Trauma Registry Expeditionary Medical Encounter Database. The odds of screening positive for PTSD symptoms were 2.52 (95% confidence interval, 2.01-3.16) times greater in those with 1 or more defined baseline mental health disorder and 16.1% (odds ratio, 1.16; 95% confidence interval, 1.01-1.34) greater for every 3-unit increase in the Injury Severity Score. Irrespective of injury severity, self-reported preinjury psychiatric status was significantly associated with PTSD at follow-up.

Conclusions.—Baseline psychiatric status and deployment-related physical injuries were associated with screening positive for postdeployment PTSD. More vulnerable members of the deployed population might be identified and benefit from interventions targeted to prevent or to ensure early identification and treatment of postdeployment PTSD.

▶ "More vulnerable members of the deployed population might be identified and benefit from interventions targeted to prevent or to ensure early identification and treatment of postdeployment PTSD." OK. That's the last sentence of the authors' conclusions to this fascinating prospective study (a first) of members of the military's relationship of posttraumatic stress disorder postdeployment, postcombat, with their preinjury, precombat mental state. However, it should be the first sentence of a "White Paper" or some such document that spells out the cost and benefits of expanding screening such as that performed in the Millennium Cohort Study and what concrete steps need to be taken, at what cost, "to prevent or to ensure early identification and treatment" of posttraumatic stress disorder. The military, Veterans Administration, and civilian medical and psychiatric services are overwhelmed by the need for treatment that they face, and because we know that increasing numbers of deployments lead to increasing numbers of the military acquiring posttraumatic stress disorder, let's hope the Congress can face up to the facts revealed here.

J. A. Talbott, MD

Mental Health Service Use After the World Trade Center Disaster: Utilization Trends and Comparative Effectiveness
Boscarino JA, Adams RE, Figley CR (Geisinger Clinic, Danville, PA; Kent State Univ, OH; Tulane Univ, New Orleans, LA)
J Nerv Ment Dis 199:91-99, 2011

Previous research suggested that community-level mental health service use was low following the World Trade Center Disaster (WTCD) and that brief interventions were effective. In the current study, we assess service use during a longer follow-up period and compare the effectiveness of brief versus multisession interventions. To assess these, we conducted baseline diagnostic interviews among New York City residents 1 year after the WTCD ($N = 2368$) and follow-up interviews 2 years afterward ($N = 1681$). At follow-up, there was an increase in mental health utilization, especially for psychotropic medication use, and a decrease in use of physicians for mental health treatment. The best predictor of service use at follow-up was higher WTCD exposure. Using propensity score matching to control for selection bias, brief mental health interventions appeared more effective than multisession interventions. These intervention findings held even after matching on demographic, stress exposure, mental health history, treatment history, access to care, other key variables. Our study suggested that community-level mental health service use increased in the follow-up period and that brief interventions were more effective than conventional multisession interventions. Since this study was designed to assess treatment outcomes, our findings raise clinical questions.

▶ Many of these findings confirm existing studies: we know that exposure increases the problem and that most people did not seek care. What is interesting to me are the following:

1. the fact that while many experts predicted help seeking would hit the roof, it did not,
2. the delayed (12- to 24-month) increase in seeking help,

3. the effectiveness of brief over multisession interventions, and
4. increased psychotropic medication use.

A close friend of mine sits at a desk that faced the World Trade Center and saw the whole thing. It shocked her to her bones, but she never sought help, although she is a psychologically sophisticated person. I was watching TV in (of all places) our Shock-Trauma Center as they played the film of the first tower being hit and then saw the second one struck. I was shaken to my bones but never sought help. Now, 2 instances don't make great science, but one can be severely affected without being traumatized as it were, and I suspect many New Yorkers were like my friend.

As for the delay in seeking help until after 1 to 2 years—I wonder if, like post-traumatic combat reactions, one holds things together for a while but eventually weakens. As for brief interventions, we certainly know that cognitive behavioral therapy (CBT) beats all the other couples in head-to-head effectiveness studies with a host of disorders; we don't know if these were CBT interventions, but maybe there were. But the later medication rise is a bit puzzling to me—maybe that too is a release from someone trying to hold it together.

J. A. Talbott, MD

Long-term Posttraumatic Stress Symptoms Among 3,271 Civilian Survivors of the September 11, 2001, Terrorist Attacks on the World Trade Center
DiGrande L, Neria Y, Brackbill RM, et al (New York City Dept of Health and Mental Hygiene; Columbia Univ Med Ctr, NY; Agency for Toxic Substances and Disease Registry, Atlanta, GA; et al)
Am J Epidemiol 173:271-281, 2011

Although the September 11, 2001, terrorist attacks were the largest human-made disaster in US history, there is little extant research documenting the attacks' consequences among those most directly affected, that is, persons who were in the World Trade Center towers. Data from a cross-sectional survey conducted 2–3 years after the attacks ascertained the prevalence of long-term, disaster-related posttraumatic stress symptoms and probable posttraumatic stress disorder (PTSD) in 3,271 civilians who evacuated World Trade Center towers 1 and 2. Overall, 95.6% of survivors reported at least 1 current posttraumatic stress symptom. The authors estimated the probable rate of PTSD at 15.0% by using the PTSD Checklist. Women and minorities were at an increased risk of PTSD. A strong inverse relation with annual income was observed. Five characteristics of direct exposure to the terrorist attacks independently predicted PTSD: being on a high floor in the towers, initiating evacuation late, being caught in the dust cloud that resulted from the tower collapses, personally witnessing horror, and sustaining an injury. Working for an employer that sustained fatalities also increased risk. Each addition of an experience of direct exposure resulted in a 2-fold increase in the risk of PTSD (odds ratio = 2.09, 95% confidence interval: 1.84, 2.36).

Identification of these risk factors may be useful when screening survivors of large-scale terrorist events for long-term psychological sequelae.

▶ This is an incredible study of an unthinkable event: the September 11, 2001, World Trade Center attack. It is difficult to write a commentary about the article because there is so much detail and the authors in the text give so many findings and explain them so well. But several things caught my eye. As we know from past studies (mainly on combat trauma), the extent of exposure and cumulative exposure affect the amount of posttraumatic stress and other disorders, and these findings are confirmed here. And as we know from other September 11, 2001, studies, women and poorer victims were more greatly affected, and these findings are confirmed here. But one thing they state gracefully is that "although tower survivors may have shared a collective experience, individuals who were exposed to several of the most troubling and life-threatening events during the disaster were at the greatest risk of PTSD," that is, the experience may have been collective but the responses were individualistic. Another thing I would not have thought of but makes immediate sense is that "Working for an employer that sustained fatalities also increased risk." As I said, this is an incredible study of an unthinkable event.

J. A. Talbott, MD

Posttraumatic Stress Without Trauma in Children
Copeland WE, Keeler G, Angold A, et al (Duke Univ Med Ctr, Durham, NC)
Am J Psychiatry 167:1059-1065, 2010

Objective.—It remains unclear to what degree children show signs of posttraumatic stress disorder (PTSD) after experiencing low-magnitude stressors, or stressors milder than those required for the DSM-IV extreme stressor criterion.

Method.—A representative community sample of 1,420 children, ages 9, 11, and 13 at intake, was followed annually through age 16. Low-magnitude and extreme stressors as well as subsequent posttraumatic stress symptoms were assessed with the Child and Adolescent Psychiatric Assessment. Two measures of posttraumatic stress symptoms were used: having painful recall, hyperarousal, and avoidance symptoms (subclinical PTSD) and having painful recall only.

Results.—During any 3-month period, low-magnitude stressors occurred four times as often as extreme stressors (24.0% compared with 5.9%). Extreme stressors elicited painful recall in 8.7% of participants and subclinical PTSD in 3.1%, compared with 4.2% and 0.7%, respectively, for low-magnitude stressors. Because of their higher prevalence, however, low-magnitude stressors accounted for two-thirds of cases of painful recall and half of cases of subclinical PTSD. Moreover, exposure to low-magnitude stressors predicted symptoms even among youths with no prior lifetime exposure to an extreme stressor.

Conclusions.—Relative to low-magnitude stressors, extreme stressors place children at greater risk for posttraumatic stress symptoms. Nevertheless, a sizable proportion of children manifesting posttraumatic stress symptoms experienced only a low-magnitude stressor.

▶ I've been around long enough to have seen the waxing and waning of the emphasis on severity of trauma and subsequent symptoms and/or diagnoses. My medical school education and residency training occurred when *Diagnostic and Statistical Manual of Mental Disorders* (First Edition) (published in 1952) was still the diagnostic manual of the day. Here the term gross stress reaction ruled, and my most influential mentor, Lawrence C. Kolb, wrote articles and chapters using that term. But gross could mean an industrial explosion or car crash not necessarily a combat experience. *Diagnostic and Statistical Manual of Mental Disorders* (Second Edition) (1968) veered away from the gross descriptor toward calling such conditions adjustment disorders. Sometime after the Vietnam War, many of us who had served there and saw patients afterward were impressed by the lack of concordance between the severity of stressors and the severity of symptoms; that is, people who had been exposed to extremely horrible combat conditions sometimes had few consequences, while others who had seemingly mild stressors, even some who had desk jobs, had crippling aftereffects. *Diagnostic and Statistical Manual of Mental Disorders* (Third Edition) then (1980) reflected this by decoupling severity from symptoms but naming them posttraumatic stress disorders while placing them among anxiety disorders, which is a long way of getting to the point of this study that revealed that even though there tends to be a correlation between severity of stress and symptoms, it is not a one-to-one correlation. The authors' take-home message for clinicians is to not overlook the diagnosis just because children were exposed to low-magnitude stressors.

J. A. Talbott, MD

Mental Health Outcomes and Predictors of Chronic Disorders After the North Sea Oil Rig Disaster: 27-Year Longitudinal Follow-Up Study
Boe HJ, Holgersen KH, Holen A (Norwegian Univ of Science and Technology, Trondheim, Norway)
J Nerv Ment Dis 199:49-54, 2011

The present study examined long-term mental health outcomes following a major disaster, including the relative risks (RR) of developing psychiatric disorders. Trauma exposure and predisaster vulnerability factors were examined as predictors of chronic psychopathology. Standardized questionnaires measuring psychological distress were completed 5(½) months, 14 months, 5 years, and 27 years after the disaster. Twenty seven years after the disaster, 48 (79%) survivors and a matched comparison group of 62 (78%) nondisaster-exposed controls were assessed using the

TABLE 3.—Diagnoses in Survivors and Nonexposed Controls 27 Years After Disaster

Diagnoses	Survivors $n = 48$		Controls $n = 62$		RR (95% CI)
	%	n	%	n	
PTSD	6.1	3	1.6	1	3.88 (0.49–30.71)
Subsyndromal PTSD	14.6	7	—	0	—
Depressive disorders	14.6	7	6.5	4	2.26 (0.72–7.06)
Anxiety disorders	14.6	7	3.2	2	4.52* (1.14–17.94)
Somatoform disorders	10.4	5	—	0	—
Substance misuse disorders	4.2	2	1.6	1	2.60 (0.26–25.54)
Any psychopathological disorder[a]	33.3	16	9.7	6	3.44* (1.56–7.60)

PTSD indicates posttraumatic stress disorder; RR, relative risk; CI, confidence interval.
[a]Excluding subsyndromal PTSD.
*Fisher exact test $p < 0.05$, 2-tailed.

Structured Clinical Interview for DSM-IV, axis I Disorders. The prevalence of posttraumatic stress disorder among the survivors was 6.1%, and the risk of having a psychiatric disorder was more than 3 times higher than in the comparison group (RR = 3.44, 95% confidence interval = 1.6–7.6). Disaster exposure and general neurotic personality predicted chronic psychopathology, which was reported by 20.9% of the participants. Findings from this study suggest that increased risk of psychopathology persists 27 years after disaster. Both disaster exposure and vulnerable personality are important predictors of chronic psychopathology (Table 3).

▶ As tragic as the North Sea oil rig disaster in 1980 was (and I remember it well), where over half of the workers on it were killed, this long-term study provides an unusual window into a number of key issues regarding civilian disasters and, indeed, all stressful situations. First, as shown in Fig 2 in the original article, some persons get better over time. But second, the group never attains the degree of mental health as a comparison group of unstricken oil workers does, and third, as shown in Table 3, it is naive to think that stress only results in fully diagnosable posttraumatic stress disorder. Indeed, subsyndromal posttraumatic stress disorder, depressive, anxiety, and somatoform disorders are more common sequelae. The major clinical lessons then are that we can instill some hope in survivors of civilian accidents/disasters but we must be alert to questioning survivors not just about the classic symptoms of posttraumatic stress disorder, such as startle reactions, flashbacks, nightmares, avoidance, and hyperarousal, but also look for depression, anxiety, and somatic symptoms.

J. A. Talbott, MD

A Randomized Controlled Trial of the Safety and Promise of Cognitive-Behavioral Therapy Using Imaginal Exposure in Patients With Posttraumatic Stress Disorder Resulting From Cardiovascular Illness
Shemesh E, Annunziato RA, Weatherley BD, et al (Mount Sinai Med Ctr, NY; Momentum Res, Inc, Durham, NC; et al)
J Clin Psychiatry 72:168-174, 2011

Objective.—We investigated the physical safety of cognitive-behavioral therapy (CBT) utilizing imaginal exposure in patients who suffered from posttraumatic stress disorder (PTSD) following a life-threatening cardiovascular event.

Method.—In this phase I, prospective, single-blind trial conducted from April 2006 through April 2008, we randomly assigned 60 patients to receive either 3 to 5 sessions of imaginal exposure therapy (experimental group) or 1 to 3 educational sessions only (control group). Criteria for PTSD and other mental health disorders were evaluated according to *DSM-IV* using the full Structured Clinical Interview for *DSM-IV* (SCID). Safety assessments included patients' blood pressure and pulse before and after each study session and the occurrence of deaths, hospitalizations, repeat myocardial infarctions, or invasive procedures. We also investigated the effects of the treatment on PTSD symptoms (Impact of Event Scale and Posttraumatic Stress Disorder Scale), depression (Beck Depression Inventory-II), and the Clinical Global Impressions-Severity of Illness (CGI-S) scale.

Results.—There were no significant differences between the experimental and control groups and between exposure and nonexposure sessions in any of the safety measures. In addition, confidence intervals were such that the nonsignificant effects of exposure therapy were not of clinical concern. For example, the mean difference in systolic pressure between control and exposure sessions was 0.5 mm Hg (95% CI, −6.1 to 7.1 mm Hg). Nonsignificant improvements were found on all psychiatric measures in the experimental group, with a significant improvement in CGI-S in the entire cohort (mean score difference, −0.6; 95% CI, −1.1 to −0.1; $P = .02$) and a significant improvement in PTSD symptoms in a subgroup of patients with acute unscheduled cardiovascular events and high baseline PTSD symptoms (mean score difference, −1.2; 95% CI, −2.0 to −0.3; $P = .01$).

Conclusions.—Cognitive-behavioral therapy that includes imaginal exposure is safe and promising for the treatment of posttraumatic stress in patients with cardiovascular illnesses who are traumatized by their illness.

Trial Registration.—clinicaltrials.gov Identifier: NCT00364910.

▶ I semijokingly often say that I have never seen a study of the use of cognitive behavioral treatment (CBT) in any mental condition where it doesn't work better than what it's being compared with (in this case, an educational effort, not waiting list). As my readers may have noted, I'm a great fan of this treatment and found that it has drastically changed the way I view patients' illnesses and assess and treat them. As one who writes on posttraumatic stress disorders (PTSD), I am also amazed at the ever-expanding types of stresses that lead to PTSD. Years ago, our predecessors wrote about PTSD as a sequelae of war or combat, only later expanding it to grave civil disasters, such as industrial explosions. Now, however, we look for it in everyone from a burn victim to (as here) a cardiovascular patient. I'm pleased, but not surprised, that CBT (with imaginal exposure) is not only safe but effective. With so many of our nation's veterans, especially in Veterans Affairs facilities, suffering from chronic PTSD from WWII forward, CBT may well become a first-line treatment.

J. A. Talbott, MD

Prolonged Exposure Versus Dynamic Therapy for Adolescent PTSD: A Pilot Randomized Controlled Trial
Gilboa-Schechtman E, Foa EB, Shafran N, et al (Bar-Ilan Univ, Ramat-Gan, Israel; Univ of Pennsylvania, Philadelphia; et al)
J Am Acad Child Adolesc Psychiatry 49:1034-1042, 2010

Objective.—To examine the efficacy and maintenance of developmentally adapted prolonged exposure therapy for adolescents (PE-A) compared with active control time-limited dynamic therapy (TLDP-A) for decreasing posttraumatic and depressive symptoms in adolescent victims of single-event traumas.

Method.—Thirty-eight adolescents (12 to 18 years old) were randomly assigned to receive PE-A or TLDP-A.

Results.—Both treatments resulted in decreased posttraumatic stress disorder and depression and increased functioning. PE-A exhibited a greater decrease of posttraumatic stress disorder and depression symptom severity and a greater increase in global functioning than did TDLP-A. After treatment, 68.4% of adolescents beginning treatment with PE-A and 36.8% of those beginning treatment with TLDP-A no longer met diagnostic criteria for posttraumatic stress disorder. Treatment gains were maintained at 6- and 17-month follow-ups.

Conclusions.—Brief individual therapy is effective in decreasing posttraumatic distress and behavioral trauma-focused components enhance efficacy.

Clinical Trial Registry Information.—Prolonged Exposure Therapy Versus Active Psychotherapy in Treating Post-Traumatic Stress Disorder in Adolescents, URL: http://clinicaltrials.gov, unique identifier: NCT00183690.

▶ I chose this article for several reasons that I think deserve widespread notice. First, psychodynamic therapy has taken a backseat to cognitive behavioral therapy (CBT) in so many conditions and studies that it is reassuring to learn that here, at least, the old standard still has a role and as powerful an effect as CBT. I am among those amazed at how many studies have shown the effect of CBT on so many conditions in so many studies (the week this was written, a JAMA article demonstrated the effectiveness of not CBT but behavioral therapy on postprostatectomy incontinence[1]). Second, despite some people's preconceptions, dropout rates for psychodynamic therapy are not necessarily high; here they're identical (21%) to the CBT-type treatment. And third, as the authors state better than I could, "These (relatively) low drop-out rates and significant clinical gains were obtained by clinicians with modest experience in treatment of trauma...[which]...suggests that PE-A can be effectively disseminated to real-world settings."

J. A. Talbott, MD

Reference

1. Goode PS, Burgio KL, Johnson TM 2nd, et al. Behavioral therapy with or without biofeedback and pelvic floor electrical stimulation for persistent postprostatectomy incontinence: a randomized controlled trial. *JAMA*. 2011;305:151-159.

Violence

Barriers and facilitators of disclosures of domestic violence by mental health service users: qualitative study
Rose D, Trevillion K, Woodall A, et al (King's College London, UK; et al)
Br J Psychiatry 198:189-194, 2011

Background.—Mental health service users are at high risk of domestic violence but this is often not detected by mental health services.

Aims.—To explore the facilitators and barriers to disclosure of domestic violence from a service user and professional perspective.

Method.—A qualitative study in a socioeconomically deprived south London borough, UK, with 18 mental health service users and 20 mental health professionals. Purposive sampling of community mental health service users and mental healthcare professionals was used to recruit participants for individual interviews. Thematic analysis was used to determine dominant and subthemes. These were transformed into conceptual maps with accompanying illustrative quotations.

Results.—Service users described barriers to disclosure of domestic violence to professionals including: fear of the consequences, including fear of Social Services involvement and consequent child protection proceedings, fear that disclosure would not be believed, and fear that disclosure would lead to further violence; the hidden nature of the violence; actions of the perpetrator; and feelings of shame. The main themes for professionals concerned role boundaries, competency and confidence. Service users and professionals reported that the medical diagnostic and treatment model with its emphasis on symptoms could act as a barrier to enquiry and disclosure. Both groups reported that enquiry and disclosure were facilitated by a supportive and trusting relationship between the individual and professional.

Conclusions.—Mental health services are not currently conducive to the disclosure of domestic violence. Training of professionals in how to address domestic violence to increase their confidence and expertise is recommended.

▶ Domestic violence is a terrible problem (20% of women in England and Wales) made worse,[1] we have learned, by economic depression/recessions and alcohol and drug abuse. But I never thought much about the crossover between domestic violence and mental illness. Now that the authors have studied its relationship, it makes sense to be more alert. The authors found the barriers to reporting included: "fear of the consequences ... consequent child protection proceedings ... not be believed ... and fear that disclosure would lead to further violence" and shame.

It is interesting that the authors state that service providers and users felt that "a supportive and therapeutic relationship was necessary for enquiry and disclosure so that the issue could be explored further..." yet they go on to say that others have concluded that "the experience of being asked about domestic violence may be sufficient to facilitate disclosure, despite not having an established relationship with the interviewer."

J. A. Talbott, MD

Reference

1. Howard LM, Trevillion K, Khalifeh H, Woodall A, Agnew-Davies R, Feder G. Domestic violence and severe psychiatric disorders: prevalence and interventions. *Psychol Med*. 2010;40:881-893.

The Influence of Clinicians' Previous Trauma Exposure on Their Assessment of Child Abuse Risk

Regehr C, LeBlanc V, Shlonsky A, et al (Univ of Toronto, Ontario, Canada)
J Nerv Ment Dis 198:614-618, 2010

Research has identified high levels of trauma exposure and PTSD in professionals responsible for assessing children at risk for abuse. An important question arising is the influence of stress and trauma on professional judgment. This study examined the association between critical incident exposure, PTSD and workers' judgments of child risk. Ninety-six child protection workers participated in 2 simulated clinical interviews and subsequently completed standardized risk assessment measures. Workers reported high levels of exposure to critical events in the workplace and high levels of traumatic stress symptoms. Number of prior critical events encountered was negatively associated with assessment of risk. Level of traumatic stress symptoms was negatively associated with risk on one, but not other measures of risk. It is concluded that standardized measures for assessing a child's risk of abuse may be influenced by previous exposure to critical workplace events and levels of traumatic stress in workers.

▶ A number of years ago, I served for the first and last time as an expert witness at trial on a civil case involving 2 longshoremen whose legs had been crushed when a container on a container ship fell on them while unloading the cargo hold. I was serving because someone on the defendants' legal team knew of my involvement and interest in posttraumatic stress disorder post-Vietnam. At the time, I was on the mend from an accident where a taxi ran into me on a sidewalk, crushing my leg, which was in a huge plaster cast. I said to the legal team, "The moment the opposing lawyers see me crutching in, hardly able to walk to the stand, they'll throw me out. I'd have such a conflict of interest for the two longshoremen." "No way," they predicted. "No one will object." And no one did. But I knew my prior experience had to shape my current opinion of these men's situation. And so it does not surprise me that the opinions of people evaluating cases of child abuse are influenced by their own "previous exposure to critical workplace events and levels of traumatic stress ..." Two other issues are raised by this study though. The first is why are so many evaluators of child abuse carrying this risk factor (which leads to various hypotheses), and the second is, is there any harm done by overdiagnosing and overtreating child abuse victims, given its devastating impact? But those issues are for another study, another day.

J. A. Talbott, MD

Bipolar Disorder and Violent Crime: New Evidence From Population-Based Longitudinal Studies and Systematic Review
Fazel S, Lichtenstein P, Grann M, et al (Univ of Oxford, England; Karolinska Institutet, Stockholm, Sweden)
Arch Gen Psychiatry 67:931-938, 2010

Context.—Although bipolar disorder is associated with various adverse health outcomes, the relationship with violent crime is uncertain.

Objectives.—To determine the risk of violent crime in bipolar disorder and to contextualize the findings with a systematic review.

Design.—Longitudinal investigations using general population and unaffected sibling control individuals.

Setting.—Population-based registers of hospital discharge diagnoses, sociodemographic information, and violent crime in Sweden from January 1, 1973, through December 31, 2004.

Participants.—Individuals with 2 or more discharge diagnoses of bipolar disorder (n = 3743), general population controls (n = 37 429), and unaffected full siblings of individuals with bipolar disorder (n = 4059).

Main Outcome Measure.—Violent crime (actions resulting in convictions for homicide, assault, robbery, arson, any sexual offense, illegal threats, or intimidation).

Results.—During follow-up, 314 individuals with bipolar disorder (8.4%) committed violent crime compared with 1312 general population controls (3.5%) (adjusted odds ratio, 2.3; 95% confidence interval, 2.0-2.6). The risk was mostly confined to patients with substance abuse comorbidity (adjusted odds ratio, 6.4; 95% confidence interval, 5.1-8.1).

The risk increase was minimal in patients without substance abuse comorbidity (adjusted odds ratio, 1.3; 95% confidence interval, 1.0-1.5), which was further attenuated when unaffected full siblings of individuals with bipolar disorder were used as controls (1.1; 0.7-1.6). We found no differences in rates of violent crime by clinical subgroups (manic vs depressive or psychotic vs nonpsychotic). The systematic review identified 8 previous studies (n = 6383), with high heterogeneity between studies. Odds ratio for violence risk ranged from 2 to 9.

Conclusion.—Although current guidelines for the management of individuals with bipolar disorder do not recommend routine risk assessment for violence, this assertion may need review in patients with comorbid substance abuse.

▶ When we think of violence and the brain/mind, I suspect most of us think of the victimization of people suffering from schizophrenia or developmental disorders/mental retardation, the episodic violence perpetuated by people abusing drugs or alcohol, sociopathy, or plain old criminal behavior—we don't think of bipolar disorder. Because Sweden has such magnificent records, conclusions drawn from large-scale studies there carry extra weight. Interesting (to me anyway) was the fact that patients in manic states were not involved in violence more than those in depressive states. Not surprisingly, men are involved with violent incidents more than women. However, both interestingly and not surprisingly, most excess crimes in people with bipolar disorder occur with comorbid substance abuse. The implications are clear: do better assessments and better treatment of substance abuse in individuals with bipolar illness. One always wonders how transferable conclusions are from country to country, but in this case the shoe fits since assault rates are similar in both nations as are alcohol sales.

J. A. Talbott, MD

Effects of a Brief Intervention for Reducing Violence and Alcohol Misuse Among Adolescents: A Randomized Controlled Trial

Walton MA, Chermack ST, Shope JT, et al (Univ of Michigan, Ann Arbor)
JAMA 304:527-535, 2010

Context.—Emergency department (ED) visits present an opportunity to deliver brief interventions to reduce violence and alcohol misuse among urban adolescents at risk of future injury.

Objective.—To determine the efficacy of brief interventions addressing violence and alcohol use among adolescents presenting to an urban ED.

Design, Setting, and Participants.—Between September 2006 and September 2009, 3338 patients aged 14 to 18 years presenting to a level I ED in Flint, Michigan, between 12 PM and 11 PM 7 days a week completed a computerized survey (43.5% male; 55.9% African American). Adolescents reporting past-year alcohol use and aggression were enrolled in a randomized controlled trial (SafERteens).

Intervention.—All patients underwent a computerized baseline assessment and were randomized to a control group that received a brochure (n = 235) or a 35-minute brief intervention delivered by either a computer (n = 237) or therapist (n = 254) in the ED, with follow-up assessments at 3 and 6 months. Combining motivational interviewing with skills training, the brief intervention for violence and alcohol included review of goals, tailored feedback, decisional balance exercise, role plays, and referrals.

Main Outcome Measures.—Self-report measures included peer aggression and violence, violence consequences, alcohol use, binge drinking, and alcohol consequences.

Results.—About 25% (n = 829) of screened patients had positive results for both alcohol and violence; 726 were randomized. Compared with controls, participants in the therapist intervention showed self-reported reductions in the occurrence of peer aggression (therapist, −34.3%; control, −16.4%; relative risk [RR], 0.74; 95% confidence interval [CI], 0.61-0.90), experience of peer violence (therapist, −10.4%; control, +4.7%; RR, 0.70; 95% CI, 0.52-0.95), and violence consequences (therapist, −30.4%; control, −13.0%; RR, 0.76; 95% CI, 0.64-0.90) at 3 months. At 6 months, participants in the therapist intervention showed self-reported reductions in alcohol consequences (therapist, −32.2%; control, −17.7%; odds ratio, 0.56; 95% CI, 0.34-0.91) compared with controls; participants in the computer intervention also showed self-reported reductions in alcohol consequences (computer, −29.1%; control, −17.7%; odds ratio, 0.57; 95% CI, 0.34-0.95).

Conclusion.—Among adolescents identified in the ED with self-reported alcohol use and aggression, a brief intervention resulted in a decrease in the prevalence of self-reported aggression and alcohol consequences.

Trial Registration.—clinicaltrials.gov Identifier: NCT00251212.

▶ There are several things that caught my eye here:

1. The investment of 35 minutes in an intervention that reduces subsequent violence and alcohol abuse seems a wise investment in an increasingly violent and addictive world.

2. The fact that the intervention can be done via computer is quite frankly amazing and an index of how digitized our society has become.

3. Adolescents are extremely malleable and if we can have this sort of impact after 35 minutes, what else can be done to improve their lives and society?

The emergency room/department has become an interesting place. Once used for emergencies, it now functions as a walk-in clinic, Doc-in-the-box, treatment of last resort, and caring place for the uninsured and underinsured. In the late 1960s and 1970s, especially with the impact of deinstitutionalization and never-institutionalization, those who worked in or administered psychiatric emergency room/departments considered nonemergency cases as clutter, noise, or inappropriate. I wonder if our mindset isn't changing as we sense the opportunities for interventions rather than the burden of work?

J. A. Talbott, MD

Effect of an Advocacy Intervention on Mental Health in Chinese Women Survivors of Intimate Partner Violence: A Randomized Controlled Trial

Tiwari A, Fong DYT, Yuen KH, et al (The Univ of Hong Kong; et al)
JAMA 304:536-543, 2010

Context.—Intimate partner violence (IPV) against women can have negative mental health consequences for survivors; however, the effect of interventions designed to improve survivors' depressive symptoms is unclear.

Objective.—To determine whether an advocacy intervention would improve the depressive symptoms of Chinese women survivors of IPV.

Design, Setting, and Participants.—Assessor-blinded randomized controlled trial of 200 Chinese women 18 years or older with a history of IPV, conducted from February 2007 to June 2009 in a community center in Hong Kong, China.

Intervention.—The intervention group (n = 100) received a 12-week advocacy intervention comprising empowerment and telephone social support. The control group (n = 100) received usual community services including child care, health care and promotion, and recreational programs.

Main Outcome Measures.—Primary outcome was change in depressive symptoms (Chinese version of the Beck Depression Inventory II) between baseline and 9 months. Secondary outcomes were changes in IPV (Chinese Revised Conflict Tactics Scales), health-related quality of life (12-Item Short Form Health Survey), and perceived social support (Interpersonal Support Evaluation List) between baseline and 9 months. Usefulness of the intervention and usual community services was evaluated at 9 months.

Results.—At 3 months, the mean change in depressive symptom score was 11.6 (95% CI, 9.5 to 13.7) in the control group and 14.9 (95% CI, 12.4 to 17.5) in the intervention group; respective changes at 9 months were 19.6 (95% CI, 16.6 to 22.7) and 23.2 (95% CI, 20.4 to 26.0). Intervention effects at 3 and 9 months were not significantly different ($P=.86$). The intervention significantly reduced depressive symptoms by 2.66 (95% CI, 0.26 to 5.06; $P=.03$) vs the control, less than the 5-unit minimal clinically important difference. Statistically significant improvement was found in partner psychological aggression (-1.87 [95% CI, -3.34 to -0.40]; mean change at 3 months, 1.5 [95% CI, -1.0 to 3.9] in the control group and 0.3 [95% CI, -0.7 to 1.4] in the intervention group; mean change at 9 months, -6.4 [95% CI, -7.8 to -5.0] and -8.9 [95% CI, -10.6 to -7.2]) and perceived social support (2.18 [95% CI, 0.48 to 3.89]; meanchange at 3 months, 6.4 [95% CI, 4.9 to 7.8] and 9.2 [95% CI, 7.7 to 10.8]; mean change at 9 months, 12.4 [95% CI, 10.5 to 14.3] and 14.4 [95% CI, 12.7 to 16.1]) but not in physical assault, sexual coercion, or health-related quality of life. By end of study, more women in the intervention group found the advocacy intervention useful or extremely useful in improving intimate relationships vs those in the control group receiving usual community services (93.8% vs 81.7%; difference, 12.1% [95% CI, 2.1% to 22.0%]; $P=.02$) and in helping them to resolve conflicts with their intimate partners (97.5% vs 84.1%; difference, 13.4% [95% CI, 4.7% to 22.0%]; *P*=.001).

Conclusion.—Among community-dwelling abused Chinese women, an advocacy intervention did not result in a clinically meaningful improvement in depressive symptoms.

Trial Registration.—clinicaltrials.gov Identifier: NCT01054898.

▶ I have not chosen to discuss many articles on domestic or partner violence over the years, but given the incredible incidence of such in the United States, I feel compelled to comment. The American Bar Association gives the incidence in the United States using "… a 1995-1996 study conducted in the 50 States and the District of Columbia, [that found that] nearly 25% of women and 7.6% of men were raped and/or physically assaulted by a current or former spouse, cohabiting partner, or dating partner/acquaintance at some time in their lifetime (based on survey of 16,000 participants, equally male and female)."[1] In addition, as the authors of the study at hand (Tiwari et al) note, "Depression is one of the most common mental health sequelae of IPV. A meta-analysis of 18 studies has found a weighted mean prevalence of depression of 47.6% among abused women, 4 which is much higher than the lifetime rates of between 10.2% and 21.3% found in the general US female population." So the mental health impact on top of the incidence makes addressing the problem a public health and mental health issue. So it is discouraging to look over the literature over the past 25 years (during which my spouse has been interested in the area) and see how ineffective we have been at halting domestic violence through a host of residential, psychological and social programs, judicial means, and social pressures. The rate has apparently gone down, but no one knows to what to attribute it and since this intervention didn't seem to do much, there's much more to be done.

J. A. Talbott, MD

Reference

1. Tjaden P, Thoennes N; US Department of Justice. Extent, Nature, and Consequences of Intimate Partner Violence: Findings From the National Violence Against Women Survey. NCJ 181867. 2000. http://www.ojp.usdoj.gov/nij/pubssum/181867.htm. Accessed June 2, 2011.

Suicide

Treatment Engagement: A Neglected Aspect in the Psychiatric Care of Suicidal Patients
Lizardi D, Stanley B (Columbia Univ, NY; New York State Psychiatric Inst)
Psychiatr Serv 61:1183-1191, 2010

Objective.—Suicide remains a serious health problem in the United States and worldwide. Despite changing distributions in sex, race-ethnicity, and age and considerable efforts to reduce the incidence rate, the number of suicides has remained relatively stable. The transition from emergency services to outpatient services is a crucial but often neglected step in treating suicidal individuals. Up to 50% of attempters refuse recommended treatment, and up to 60% drop out after only one session. This point of intervention is crucial for patients at elevated risk of suicide to reduce imminent danger and to increase the chances that patients will follow up on recommended treatment.

Methods.—PubMed, MEDLINE, and PsycINFO databases were searched for empirical investigations of treatment engagement of suicide attempters. Keywords searched included treatment, intervention, engagement, adherence, compliance, utilization, participation, and suicide attempt. Mapped terms were also included. Thirteen articles were selected.

Results.—Studies that have examined the effectiveness of postdischarge contact with suicide attempters (phone, letter, and in-person visits) to increase treatment adherence have found some immediate effects after substantial contact that were not sustained. Simple referrals to outpatient care were not effective. Family group interventions for adolescents have improved adherence, as have brief interventions in the emergency department.

Conclusions.—Despite greater public awareness of suicide, heightened prevention effort, and increased efficacy of treatment interventions, success in reducing suicidal behavior has been limited. Developing brief interventions for use in emergency settings that can reduce suicide risk and enhance treatment follow-up has been a neglected aspect of suicide prevention and may help to reduce suicidal behavior.

▶ In the 1970s, in the heyday of naïveté about the goals of community psychiatry, tenets of reaching every patient in need, providing continuity of care, and making sure people were not lost "between the cracks," we were concerned about patients continuing in contact or treatment. (This was all lost, of course, with the advent of managed care in which one could make more money by keeping patients away). However, back then, one study (the author and title of which I've forgotten) looked at the frequency that patients showed up for appointments using 2 methods: handing them an appointment card versus introducing them to the provider who would see them and the setting in which they would be seen.

Guess what? That little bit of extra time and effort paid off in a drastically better stick-to-it-ness on transfer. Suicide is the leading cause of death in psychiatric illnesses, and many suicides can be prevented by treating the disease (or diseases) that leads to suicidal thoughts. Taking a public health rather than a cost-cutting approach, then, should induce us to work harder to make sure patients make the transition from emergency departments to outpatient settings. But will we, and will we ever learn?

J. A. Talbott, MD

Research

Attitudes of College Students Toward Mental Illness Stigma and the Misuse of Psychiatric Medications
Stone AM, Merlo LJ (Univ of Florida, Gainesville)
J Clin Psychiatry 72:134-139, 2011

Objective.—Mental illness stigma remains a significant barrier to treatment. However, the recent increase in the medical and nonmedical use of prescription psychiatric medications among college students seems to contradict this phenomenon. This study explored students' attitudes and experiences related to psychiatric medications, as well as correlates of psychiatric medication misuse (ie, attitudes toward mental illness and beliefs about the efficacy of psychiatric medications).

Method.—Data were collected anonymously via self-report questionnaires from April 2008 to February 2009. Measures included the Michigan Alcoholism Screening Test, the Drug Abuse Screening Test, Day's Mental Illness Stigma Scale, the Attitudes Toward Psychiatric Medication scale, and the Psychiatric Medication Attitudes Scale. Participants included 383 university students (59.2% female), recruited on the campus of a large state university or through online classes offered through the same university.

Results.—High rates of psychiatric medication misuse were shown (13.8%) when compared to rates of medical use (6.8%), and students with prescriptions for psychiatric drugs were also more likely to be misusers ($\chi^2 = 20.60$, $P < .001$). Psychiatric medication misusers reported less stigmatized beliefs toward mental illness, including lower anxiety around the mentally ill ($t = 3.26$, $P < .001$) as well as more favorable attitudes toward psychiatric medications ($t = 2.78$, $P < .01$) and stronger beliefs in the potential for recovery from mental illness ($t = -2.11$, $P < .05$). Students with more stigmatized beliefs had greater concerns about psychiatric medications and less favorable beliefs regarding their effectiveness. Reasons for misuse varied by medication class, with 57.1% of stimulant misusers noting help with studying as their primary reason for use and 33.3% of benzodiazepine misusers noting attempts to get high or "party" as their primary reason for misuse.

Conclusions.—Results suggest the need for improved education regarding the nature of mental illness, the appropriate use of psychiatric medications, and the potential consequences associated with abuse of these potent drugs.

▶ We have to be careful regarding how we see this research. No one wants to glorify or promote the misuse of psychiatric medications, even if reduced stigmatization is associated with such misuse. I suspect there are 2 groups of students here: (1) those that view mental illness, its treatment, and some if not all psychopharmacologic interventions as less stigmatizing and are more prone to misuse such medications, be they stimulants or anxiolytics (the 2 types of drugs singled out here); (2) those who have a more stigmatized view of the mentally ill, mental illness, its treatment, and psychopharmacologic interventions. The authors recommend "the need for improved education regarding the nature of mental illness [and I would add toward the more stigmatizing group], the appropriate use of psychiatric medications [for all students], and the potential consequences associated with abuse of these potent drugs [to the misusing group]."

J. A. Talbott, MD

Miscellaneous

Stigma in America: Has Anything Changed? Impact of Perceptions of Mental Illness and Dangerousness on the Desire for Social Distance: 1996 and 2006
Silton NR, Flannelly KJ, Milstein G, et al (Marymount Manhattan College, NY; Healthcare Chaplaincy, NY; City Univ of New York; et al)
J Nerv Ment Dis 199:361-366, 2011

Data from the 1996 and 2006 General Social Survey were analyzed to examine the relationship between the desire for social distance from individuals with mental illness and a number of factors that were thought to contribute to it, including perceptions of mental illness and dangerousness. Random samples of participants were assigned to one of four experimental conditions, in which they were read a vignette describing a character who presented with alcoholism, depression, schizophrenia, or minor problems. The desire for social distance from characters whose presenting problems were alcoholism or depression was significantly lower in 2006 than in 1996. The participants' perceptions that the character was mentally ill and/or dangerous to others partially mediated the association between presenting problem and social distance. Participants who were younger, white, better educated, and attended religious services more often required less social distance from the vignette characters than did their counterparts.

▶ Stigma regarding the mentally ill has been a concern of organizations, such as the American Psychiatric Association, for as long as I can remember. It is accepted wisdom that gradually over the past century, stigma has been reduced, and this is often attributed to deinstitutionalization (leading more nonafflicted citizens to be in close proximity to severely and chronically mentally ill persons), educational efforts and the rising acceptance of severe and chronic mental illnesses as brain disorders rather than the results of poor mothering, evil spirits, or moral weakness. This study is illustrative in showing that headway is being made into the reduction of such stigma, albeit slowly, and singles out 3 methods of improving the situation: protest (by which they really mean advocacy, if you go back to the source of their wording)[1] education, and contact. They conclude, however, that such efforts do not have the same impact regarding people suffering from schizophrenia as those with depression and alcoholism because such people are presumed to be more dangerous. I would add that this is probably the case because it is more difficult to understand, empathize, and "walk in the shoes" of actively psychotic patients than those suffering from other illnesses. More work is called for.

J. A. Talbott, MD

Reference

1. Corrigan PW, Penn DL. Lessons from social psychology on discrediting psychiatric stigma. *Am Psychol.* 1999;54:765-776.

Associations between Physical Activity and Physical and Mental Health—A HUNT 3 Study

Bertheussen GF, Romundstad PR, Landmark T, et al (Norwegian Univ of Science and Technology, Trondheim, Norway; Univ of Science and Technology, Trondheim, Norway)
Med Sci Sports Exerc 43:1220-1228, 2011

Purpose.—Health-related quality of life (HRQoL) has been characterized as the ultimate goal for health interventions such as physical activity (PA). We assessed how frequency, duration, and intensity of PA were related to HRQoL in younger (<65 yr) and older (≥65 yr) females and males.

Methods.—This population-based cross-sectional study explored associations between frequency, duration, and intensity of PA and physical and mental health. HRQoL was measured by SF-8 Health Survey. Frequency and duration were assessed by items validated in a previous HUNT study, and intensity was assessed by Borg RPE scale. Associations between PA and physical and mental health were estimated using general linear modeling.

Results.—A total of 4500 participants (56% females), age 19—91 yr, with mean age of 53 ± 15 yr, were included. Of these, 40% were less active than recommended by international guidelines. In general, mean physical health (PCS-8) in females and males was 47.4 ± 9.7 and 48.8 ± 8.9, and mental health (MCS-8) was 50.5 ± 8.0 and 51.9 ± 7.3, respectively. Age-adjusted association between PA and HRQoL was stronger for physical than mental health in both genders and age groups. The largest differences were between no exercise and exercise groups at any level for frequency, duration, and intensity of PA. We found no substantial gender differences in association between PA and HRQoL, but association was stronger in older (≥65 yr) than younger (<65 yr) females and males. Adjusting for socioeconomic factors and factors such as presence of diseases, body mass index, smoking habits, cohabitation, and disablement did not change the results.

Conclusions.—The study suggests that exercising at any level is associated with better physical and mental health in both genders compared with no exercise, particularly among the older individuals.

▶ Is this worth abstracting and commenting on? I think so, because despite the fact that one would expect the results, they need to be pounded home to everyone. We've mandated seat belts, we've cut smoking drastically, and in countries like France, with its strict, relatively new anti—drinking while driving laws (the Law Evin), alcohol consumption by drivers took a nosedive. Obesity, however, defies this trend, as sugar consumption, junk food eating, "couch-potatoing," and lack of exercise seem to be spreading. Depressed patients I've encouraged to exercise more often blame their inactivity on their disease and mood, and I can see their point. One day in Central Park in New York, I literally ran into a friend-colleague running pal of mine out for a jog with a patient; I was impressed but never offered to do it myself. Yet maybe that's what it would take. One additional point: the authors found the correlation was curvilinear and "The largest age-adjusted differences in physical and mental health scores were between those reporting 'no exercise' and 'any degree of exercise.'" Thus, anything is better than nothing.

J. A. Talbott, MD

"A Disease Like Any Other"? A Decade of Change in Public Reactions to Schizophrenia, Depression, and Alcohol Dependence
Pescosolido BA, Martin JK, Long JS, et al (Indiana Univ, Bloomington; Columbia Univ, NY)
Am J Psychiatry 167:1321-1330, 2010

Objective.—Clinicians, advocates, and policy makers have presented mental illnesses as medical diseases in efforts to overcome low service use, poor adherence rates, and stigma. The authors examined the impact of this approach with a 10-year comparison of public endorsement of treatment and prejudice.

Method.—The authors analyzed responses to vignettes in the mental health modules of the 1996 and 2006 General Social Survey describing individuals meeting DSM-IV criteria for schizophrenia, major depression, and alcohol dependence to explore whether more of the public 1) embraces neurobiological understandings of mental illness; 2) endorses treatment from providers, including psychiatrists; and 3) reports community acceptance or rejection of people with these disorders. Multivariate analyses examined whether acceptance of neurobiological causes increased treatment support and lessened stigma.

Results.—In 2006, 67% of the public attributed major depression to neurobiological causes, compared with 54% in 1996. High proportions of respondents endorsed treatment, with general increases in the proportion endorsing treatment from doctors and specific increases in the proportions endorsing psychiatrists for treatment of alcohol dependence (from 61% in 1996 to 79% in 2006) and major depression (from 75% in 1996 to 85% in 2006). Social distance and perceived danger associated with people with these disorders did not decrease significantly. Holding a neurobiological conception of these disorders increased the likelihood of support for treatment but was generally unrelated to stigma. Where associated, the effect was to increase, not decrease, community rejection.

Conclusions.—More of the public embraces a neurobiological understanding of mental illness. This view translates into support for services but not into a decrease in stigma. Reconfiguring stigma reduction strategies may require providers and advocates to shift to an emphasis on competence and inclusion.

▶ I realize as an editor/commenter I'm not supposed to merely repeat a study's findings and conclusions, but in this case, some things bear repeating. The authors looked at the 10 years between the Surgeon General's Report of 1996 and 2006. Their jumping off point was the statement that "the stigma attached to mental illness constituted the 'primary barrier' to treatment and recovery (1, p. viii)...[and]...could be reduced,...if people could be convinced that mental illnesses were 'real' brain disorders and not volitional behaviors." So they tested this supposition and found that from 1996 to 2006, people did attribute mental illnesses more to neurobiological causes, but measures of stigma (social distance and perceived danger) were not reduced much. So now the authors suggest we switch from this neurobiological cause effort to "a focus on the abilities, competencies, and community integration of persons with mental illness and substance use disorders." How exactly this new effort would be implemented is spelled out in another contribution that deserves a comment of its own.[1] It'll be interesting to see if in another decade this approach changes the situation.

J. A. Talbott, MD

Reference

1. Ware NC, Hopper K, Tugenberg T, Dickey B, Fisher D. Connectedness and citizenship: redefining social integration. *Psychiatr Serv.* 2007;58:469-474.

Measuring Quality of Mental Health Care: A Review of Initiatives and Programs in Selected Countries
Spaeth-Rublee B, IIMHL Clinical Leaders Group, Mental Health Quality Indicator Project (Columbia Univ, NY)
Can J Psychiatry 55:539-548, 2010

This review article presents a systematic review of grey literature describing current initiatives that assess the quality of mental health care in 12 countries, as collected by the International Initiative for Mental Health Leadership. There have been increased efforts in many countries to develop and implement mental health indicator schemes to measure and monitor the quality of mental health care at the national and subnational level. Most mental health indicator sets are part of larger health policy initiatives at the national and (or) provincial or state level, with indicators and domains regularly reviewed and revised. The indicator sets described in health care quality initiatives vary widely in their scope, intended use, and degree of development, and they often cut across a broad range of domains, reflecting not only a country's specific health system and how it is organized and structured but also the implementation of such schemes (that is, collection and analysis of data) and the sociopolitical realities that determine mental health priorities.

▶ This is an intriguing article, as much for what it doesn't say or conclude as for what it does. If you read only the abstract as reprinted above, you (or at least I) are left thinking: "what the deuce are they talking about?" I mean, what can one do with such disparate data that show that "quality initiatives vary widely in their scope, intended use, and degree of development, and they often cut across a broad range of domains, reflecting not only a country's specific health system and how it is organized and structured but also the implementation of such schemes." It is only when you read the results from each country—and they included Australia, Canada, England, Germany, Ireland, Japan, the Netherlands, New Zealand, Norway, Scotland, Taiwan, and the United States—that you begin to see how each country tries to measure quality of care. And then, in their Summary of Measures, you see that different countries measure different things, including access, efficiency, effectiveness, safety, and appropriateness of care, but using proxies such as waiting time and waiting lists for access and Global Assessment of Functioning scales for effectiveness, which may be a little like the drunk searching for his lost key where the light is good rather than where he dropped it. Granted different states/provinces and countries designed these measuring systems with different goals in mind and might be loath to have uniform reporting, but unless and until that happens, few comparisons can be made.

J. A. Talbott, MD

Transforming the Nation's Health: Next Steps in Mental Health Promotion
Power AK (US Dept of Health and Human Services, Rockville, MD)
Am J Public Health 100:2343-2346, 2010

The National Research Council and the Institute of Medicine have called for making the healthy mental, emotional and behavioral development of young people a national priority. The Substance Abuse and Mental Health Services Administration (SAMHSA) in the US Department of Health and Human Services is uniquely positioned to help develop national mental health policies that promote mental health and prevent mental illnesses.

In this article I describe the role of mental health in overall health, I make the case for a public health approach tomental health promotion and mental illness prevention, and I outline a strategy to promote individual, family, and community resilience. I also describe how SAMHSA works to achieve these goals.

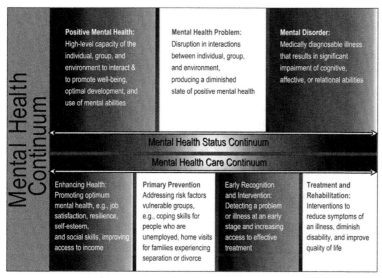

FIGURE 1.—Mental health viewed as a continuum. (Reprinted from Power AK. Transforming the nation's health: next steps in mental health promotion. *Am J Public Health*. 2010;100:2343-2346. Reprinted with permission from the American Public Health Association ©.)

Ultimately, true health reform will not succeed without a comprehensive, committed focus on the mental health needs of all Americans.

▶ This is an area that is in need of a serious relook. Ever since I can remember, people have been advocating mental health, not just treating mental illness. But in that time, little has happened. Oh, I suppose we had Head Start and lead paint elimination programs, and everyone understands the importance of secondary prevention (early recognition and intervention) and tertiary prevention (treatment and rehabilitation), but where is preprimary and primary prevention? It's like Stalin's comment, "How many divisions does the Pope have?" Preprimary efforts, that is, Enhancing Health, is specified here (Fig 1) as "Promoting optimum mental health, eg, job satisfaction, resilience, self-esteem, and social skills, improving access to income" and primary prevention as "addressing risk factors, vulnerable groups, eg, coping skills for people who are employed, home visits for families experiencing separation or divorce." Noble, worthy, and not new, but how? The author, who is at the Substance Abuse and Mental Health Services Administration, urges "Professionals in mental health and public health...[to]... band together to cultivate strong, enlightened leaders who acknowledge that the mental health implications of public policies are as important as—if not more important than—their political or economic impact." Terrific, but I see no plan, no specifics, and no sequences of actions—just a cri de coeur.

J. A. Talbott, MD

Impact of Patient Language Proficiency and Interpreter Service Use on the Quality of Psychiatric Care: A Systematic Review
Bauer AM, Alegría M (Cambridge Health Alliance, MA)
Psychiatr Serv 61:765-773, 2010

Objective.—This literature review examined the effects of patients' limited English proficiency and use of professional and ad hoc interpreters on the quality of psychiatric care.

Methods.—PubMed, PsycINFO, and CINAHL (Cumulative Index to Nursing and Allied Health Literature) were systematically searched for English-language publications from inception of each database to April 2009. Reference lists were reviewed, and expert sources were consulted. Among the 321 articles identified, 26 met inclusion criteria: peer-reviewed articles reporting primary data on clinical care for psychiatric disorders among patients with limited proficiency in English or in the provider's language.

Results.—Evaluation in a patient's nonprimary language can lead to incomplete or distorted mental status assessment. Although both untrained and trained interpreters may make errors, untrained interpreters' errors may have greater clinical impact, compromising diagnostic accuracy and clinicians' detection of disordered thought or delusional content. Use of professional interpreters may improve disclosure in patient-provider communications, referral to specialty care, and patient satisfaction.

Conclusions.—Little systematic research has addressed the impact of language proficiency or interpreter use on the quality of psychiatric care in contemporary U.S. settings. Findings are insufficient to inform evidence-based guidelines for improving quality of care among patients with limited English proficiency. Clinicians should be aware of the ways in which quality of care can be compromised when they evaluate patients in a nonprimary language or use an interpreter. Given U.S. demographic trends, future research should help guide practice and policy by addressing deficits in the evidence base.

▶ When I was in college years ago, I learned about translations and their quirks from a humorous episode. A misbehaving student from abroad was about to be sacked for neglect of his studies in favor of social activities and his family was summoned to talk to the dean. Since the dean didn't speak the student's tongue, when the mother appeared, the student offered to translate; for an hour the dean regaled her with her son's misdeeds ending with a summary in which he said that "if the student spent more time in the library and less in the local liquor store (which carried the name X College Provision Company) he'd have done well." The student duly translated to the mother how well he was doing and when asked about the Provision Company said it was where he bought his books. There's a moral here: use professional interpreters who know the situation. As MacKinnon and Michels pointed out some 40 years ago (1971) in their classic book "The Psychiatric Interview in Clinical Practice," to use patient's relatives or friends invites them to insert themselves and their opinions into the interview.[1] In my hospital, while we see largely Spanish-speaking foreigners, the hospital maintains an active roster of people speaking languages from all over and I think most of us agree with the authors that using professional translators or, when they are not available, professionals who can translate accurately, is a necessity to present errors in assessment, treatment, and understanding of treatment plans.

J. A. Talbott, MD

Reference

1. MacKinnon RA, Michels R. *The Psychiatric Interview in Clinical Practice.* Philadelphia, PA: W.B. Saunders; 1971.

A Feasibility Study of the Use of Asynchronous Telepsychiatry for Psychiatric Consultations

Yellowlees PM, Odor A, Parish MB, et al (Univ of California, Davis, Sacramento)
Psychiatr Serv 61:838-840, 2010

Objective.—This study examined the feasibility of conducting psychiatric consultations using asynchronous, or store-and-forward, video-based telepsychiatry.

Methods.—Video-recorded 20- to 30-minute assessments of 60 nonemergency, English-speaking adult patients in a medically underserved county in California were uploaded along with other patient data to a Web-based record. Two psychiatrists then used the record to provide psychiatric consultations to the referring primary care providers.

Results.—Eighty-five percent of patients received diagnoses of mood disorders, 32% diagnoses of substance use disorders, 53% diagnoses of anxiety disorders, and 5% other axis I diagnoses. Psychiatrists recommended short-term medication changes for 95% of the patients and provided guidelines for possible future changes.

Conclusions.—This study—the first study of asynchronous telepsychiatry to be published—demonstrated the feasibility of this approach. This type of assessment should not replace the face-to-face psychiatric interview, but it may be a very helpful additional process that improves access to care and expertise.

▶ I thought this was a most interesting study for several reasons.

As we become more technologically dependent and sophisticated, the ease and familiarity of using electronic communication becomes more obvious.

While our parents may not have been comfortable with computers, our children and grandchildren are madly texting by the time they enter high school. The one I'm most familiar with makes her own films, edits and distributes them, all with the nonchalance of our parents making a phone call.

We enter doctors' offices and are unfazed by being asked to fill out histories and reviews on systems electronically, our pictures are taken as we enter and leave the country, and if we want information, whether it be on films or diseases, we turn more quickly to Wikipedia than the library.

And as the authors point out, other specialties have pioneered in synchronous telemedicine and asynchronous consultations long before us. At my medical school, trauma experts showed the Army that it was cheaper and better to walk and talk medical corpsmen through emergency procedures in the field, than train everyone in all the complex interventions they might face.

So it is logical and quite reassuring to learn that psychiatric consultations cannot be done face to face and in real time. Certainly I still like to meet patients and size them up in person, but for rural populations, this could much more efficiently replace circuit riders, bush pilot documents, and satellite clinics.

J. A. Talbott, MD

6 Clinical Psychiatry

Introduction

Once again this year, I had a rich amount of literature to choose from. This makes me even more convinced of the wisdom of this type of format, where an interested reader can sample the best articles from large areas of psychiatry.

As usual, I began with our largest clinical and research area, ie, depression. There are multiple advances in the treatment arena with a new antidepressant vilazodone, research about combining medications, atypicals in depression, and attempts to match depression treatments to patients. In the non-medication arena, there are continuing studies of repetitive transcranial magnetic stimulation (rTMS), deep brain stimulation for resistant depression, and acupuncture as augmenting therapy. There are articles about psychotherapy versus antidepressants, as well as mindfulness and cognitive behavioral therapy (CBT). These are complemented with studies of risk for depression, including the genetic variance of the serotonin transporter promoter gene. In the bipolar area, I included studies about atypicals, about antidepressants in bipolar depression, and an article about rTMS in bipolar depression. There is a good guide for clinicians about monitoring kidney function for lithium-treated patients, as well as basic science studies of brain abnormalities in this disorder.

I have included good studies in the suicide area with risk in adolescents, men in the postpartum period, and in lesbian, gay, and bisexual youth. There is also a follow-up article about the use of antiepileptic drugs and suicide risk.

In the anxiety area, I included articles on CBT, psychodynamic psychotherapy, computer-assisted CBT, and a parent-based group intervention in children. There are articles detailing deep brain stimulation in obsessive-compulsive disorder (OCD) and dealing with the use of atypicals in anxiety disorders. There are studies in hippocampal volume differences in posttraumatic stress disorder (PTSD) among veterans and evidence of a deletion in the tropomyosin-related kinase B in anxiety.

In the schizophrenia section this year, there are articles I included on advances in treatment with comparison of atypicals in neuroleptic-induced tardive dyskinesia, a new medicine asenapine, high-dose quetiapine in resistant schizophrenia, comparison of sertindole and risperidone in treatment resistant patients versus standard care, and positive effects of early treatment of psychosis. I also included an article about a genetic variant predisposing patients to diabetes in schizophrenia and 2 interesting articles investigating whether there are progressive brain changes in schizophrenia.

In the substance abuse area, I continued to follow the relationship of the use of cannabis and anxiety and depression and other psychiatric disorders. There is also a fascinating treatment-oriented article documenting the value of gabapentin added to naltrexone to treat alcohol dependence.

In the general psychiatry section this year, we have articles about the abnormal brain circuitry in Tourette syndrome, migraine and antidepressants, body dysmorphic disorder, pharmacotherapy of paraphilias, a review of electroconvulsive therapy (ECT), as well as a novel syndrome in which antibiotics appear to induce the serotonin syndrome.

In the miscellaneous section, there are articles about traumatic brain injury and psychiatric disorders in children, atypicals in Alzheimer disease, counter-transference in eating disorders, placental abruption and anxiety and depression, sleep medicine in college students, the long-term effect of insomnia on headaches, as well as sleep disturbances and death rates. There is an interesting follow-up to a theme we have followed for years with a survey documenting the change in public opinion about psychiatric disorders over the last decade.

In the psychiatry in general medicine section, there is a very interesting neuropsychiatric syndrome induced by the commonly utilized Z-pack antibiotics.

All in all, it was again an excellent year for articles that affect the daily practice of clinical psychiatry.

James C. Ballenger, MD

Depression

A pilot study of acupuncture augmentation therapy in antidepressant partial and non-responders with major depressive disorder

Yeung AS, Ameral VE, Chuzi SE, et al (Massachusetts General Hosp, Boston)
J Affect Disord 130:285-289, 2011

Background.—Acupuncture is widely used for treating major depressive disorder (MDD). There is evidence supporting acupuncture as an antidepressant monotherapy, but its efficacy as augmentation in antidepressant partial and non-responders has not been well-investigated.

Methods.—Thirty subjects (47% female, mean age 48 ± 11 years) with a history of SCID-diagnosed MDD and partial or non-response after ≥8 weeks of antidepressant therapy were assigned 8 weeks of standardized 30-min open acupuncture augmentation sessions on a weekly (n = 24) or twice-weekly (n = 6) basis. Change in the Hamilton-D-17 score was the primary outcome measure, and response rates (based on HAM-D-17 score improvement of ≥50%) the secondary outcome.

Results.—Twenty subjects (40% female; 18 in weekly and 2 in twice-weekly treatment) completed the study. In the intent-to-treat (ITT) sample

(N = 30), HAM-D-17 scores decreased from 18.5 ± 3.8 to 11.2 ± 5.3 in the weekly group (p < 0.001), and from 18.5 ± 3.3 to 11.8 ± 4.8 in the twice-weekly group (p = 0.03). Improvement did not differ significantly between treatment arms (p = 0.76). Response rates were 47% for all ITT subjects, 50% for the weekly group and 33% for the twice-weekly group (p = 0.66). The most common side effects included soreness/pain (n = 7), bruising (n = 4), and mild bleeding (n = 1) at the needle site. One subject discontinued because of side effects (pain).

Limitations.—Open design, small sample, polypharmacy with anti-depressants.

Conclusions.—Once or twice-weekly acupuncture augmentation was safe, well-tolerated and effective in antidepressant partial and non-responders, suggesting good feasibility in outpatient settings. Replication in controlled trials is warranted.

▶ These authors began with a claim that acupuncture is now widely used to treat major depressive disorder (MDD). They actually studied whether its use to augment antidepressant partial and nonresponders was effective. They compared 30 subjects with MDD who had not responded optimally to at least 8 weeks of antidepressant therapy, and these patients were assigned 8 weeks of 30-minute open acupuncture augmentation sessions either once or twice weekly. In fact, they saw significant drops in the Hamilton Depression scores dropping 18.5 to approximately 11.2 for the weekly group, and 11.8 in the twice weekly group. It would appear that treatment did work, but twice a week was not more efficacious than once a week. This is interesting, and I would like to know how commonly acupuncture is actually used to treat depressed people either in psychiatric or nonpsychiatric settings.

J. C. Ballenger, MD

A Randomized, Double-Blind, Placebo-Controlled 8-Week Study of Vilazodone, a Serotonergic Agent for the Treatment of Major Depressive Disorder

Khan A, Cutler AJ, Kajdasz DK, et al (Northwest Clinical Res Ctr, Bellevue, WA; Univ of Florida, Gainesville; a division of Clinical Data, Inc, New Haven, CT; et al)
J Clin Psychiatry 72:441-447, 2011

Objective.—To evaluate the efficacy, and further establish the safety profile, of oral once-daily vilazodone, a potent and selective serotonin 1A receptor partial agonist and reuptake inhibitor, in the treatment of major depressive disorder (MDD).

Method.—This phase 3, randomized, double-blind, placebo-controlled, 8-week study (conducted March 2008—February 2009) enrolled 481 adults with *DSM-IV-TR*-defined MDD. Patients received vilazodone (titrated to 40 mg/d) or placebo. The primary efficacy endpoint was change in

Montgomery-Asberg Depression Rating Scale (MADRS) total score from baseline to end of treatment. Secondary efficacy measures included MADRS and 17-item Hamilton Depression Rating Scale (HDRS-17) response and change in HDRS-17, HDRS-21, Hamilton Anxiety Rating Scale (HARS), Clinical Global Impressions-Severity of Illness (CGI-S), and Clinical Global Impressions-Improvement (CGI-I) scores. The Changes in Sexual Functioning Questionnaire (CSFQ) was administered at baseline and week 8.

Results.—Vilazodone-treated patients had significantly greater improvement ($P = .009$) according to the MADRS than placebo patients (intent-to-treat; least-squares mean changes: -13.3, -10.8). MADRS response rates were significantly higher with vilazodone than placebo (44% vs 30%, $P = .002$). Remission rates for vilazodone were not significantly different based on the MADRS (vilazodone, 27.3% vs placebo, 20.3%; $P = .066$) or HDRS-17 (vilazodone, 24.2% vs placebo, 17.7%; $P = .088$). Vilazodone-treated patients had significantly greater improvements from baseline in HDRS-17 ($P = .026$), HDRS-21 ($P = .029$), HARS ($P = .037$), CGI-S ($P = .004$), and CGI-I ($P = .004$) scores than placebo patients. Rates of discontinuation due to adverse events were 5.1% (vilazodone) and 1.7% (placebo). The most common adverse events (vilazodone vs placebo) were diarrhea (31% vs 11%), nausea (26% vs 6%), and headache (13% vs 10%). Treatment-related effects on sexual function as measured by the CSFQ were small and similar to placebo. Effects on weight were no different from placebo.

Conclusions.—Vilazodone 40 mg/d was well tolerated and effective in adult patients with MDD.

Trial Registration.—clinicaltrials.gov Identifier: NCT00683592.

▶ Although I have not been involved in the studies, I have heard about vilazodone for several years, and it has just recently been released after receiving approval by the Food and Drug Administration (FDA) to treat depression. This agent is interesting because it is a potent and selective serotonin reuptake inhibitor, as well as a 1A receptor partial agonist. It is clearly effective in depression, and the FDA approval was based on 2 effective studies. Results are comparable with most antidepressants in terms of efficacy and side effects, with 2 very important exceptions. What actually makes this drug exciting is that treatment-related side effects on sexual function and weight gain were actually comparable with placebo. If this continues to be the case with more chronic therapy, then this drug will become a very popular one to add to our treatment armamentarium.

J. C. Ballenger, MD

Antidepressant Drug Compliance: Reduced Risk of MI and Mortality in Depressed Patients
Scherrer JF, Garfield LD, Lustman PJ, et al (St Louis Veterans Affairs Med Ctr, MO; et al)
Am J Med 124:318-324, 2011

Background.—The long-term risk of myocardial infarction (MI) associated with use of antidepressants is uncertain, especially for nontricyclic antidepressants. The present study uses a national Veterans Affairs cohort to test whether antidepressants increase or decrease risk of MI and all-cause mortality.

Methods.—US Department of Veterans Affairs patient records were analyzed to identify a cohort free of cardiovascular disease in fiscal years 1999 and 2000, aged 25-80 years, who had an International Classification of Diseases, Ninth Revision, Clinical Modification code indicating an episode of depression (n = 93,653). Incident MI and all-cause mortality were modeled in patients who received 12 weeks or more of antidepressant pharmacotherapy as compared with 0-11 weeks during follow-up. Age-adjusted Cox proportional hazard models were computed before and after adjusting for baseline sociodemographics and time-dependent covariates.

Results.—Receipt of 12 or more weeks of continuous antidepressant therapy was associated with significantly reduced rates of incident MI across classes of antidepressants: selective serotonin reuptake inhibitor (SSRIs) (hazard ratio [HR] 0.48; 95% confidence interval [CI], 0.44-0.52), serotonin-norepinephrine reuptake inhibitors (SNRIs) (HR 0.35; 95% CI, 0.32-0.40), tricyclic antidepressants (TCAs) (HR 0.39; 95% CI, 0.34-0.44), and "Other" (HR 0.41; 95% CI, 0.37-0.45). Risk of all-cause mortality also was decreased with receipt of 12 weeks of pharmacotherapy with all classes of antidepressants (SSRI, SNRI, TCA, Other), with HRs ranging from 0.50 to 0.66.

Conclusions.—Across classes of antidepressants, 12 weeks of pharmacotherapy appears to be safe in terms of MI risk. Although the mechanism for this association remains uncertain, it is possible that compliance with pharmacotherapy for depression reflects compliance with cardiovascular medications. It also is possible that a direct drug effect or improved depressed mood may attenuate the risk of MI in depressed patients.

▶ Unlike other studies, this study using patient records from the US Department of Veterans Affairs found that receiving 12 weeks or more of continuous antidepressants was associated with actually significantly reduced rates of myocardial infarction (MI) across all types of antidepressants. All-cause mortality was also decreased with all classes. It is actually uncertain whether patients willing to take medicines for depression may also be more compliant with their cardiovascular medications, which may explain these results. This is an important study contributing to this debate.

J. C. Ballenger, MD

Childhood Predictors of Use and Costs of Antidepressant Medication by Age 24 Years: Findings from the Finnish Nationwide 1981 Birth Cohort Study

Gyllenberg D, Sourander A, Niemelä S, et al (Univ of Helsinki and Helsinki Univ Hosp, Finland; the Univ of Turku and Turku Univ Hosp, Finland; et al)
J Am Acad Child Adolesc Psychiatry 50:406-415, 2011

Objective.—Prior studies on antidepressant use in late adolescence and young adulthood have been cross-sectional, and prospective associations with childhood psychiatric problems have not been examined. The objective was to study the association between childhood problems and lifetime prevalence and costs of antidepressant medication by age 24 years.

Method.—A total of 5,547 subjects from a nation-wide birth cohort were linked to the National Prescription Register. Information about parent- and teacher-reported conduct, hyperkinetic and emotional symptoms, and self-reported depressive symptoms was gathered at age 8 years. The main outcome measure was national register-based lifetime information about purchases of antidepressants between ages 8 and 24 years. In addition, antidepressant costs were analyzed using a Heckman maximum likelihood model.

Results.—In all, 8.8% of males and 13.8% of females had used antidepressants between age 13 and 24 years. Among males, conduct problems independently predicted later antidepressant use. In both genders, self-reported depressive symptoms and living in other than a family with two biological parent at age 8 years independently predicted later antidepressant use. Significant gender interactions were found for conduct and hyperkinetic problems, indicating that more males who had these problems at age 8 have used antidepressants compared with females with the same problems.

Conclusions.—Childhood psychopathology predicts use of antidepressants, but the type of childhood psychopathology predicting antidepressant use is different among males and females.

▶ Previous studies of antidepressant use in adolescence and young adulthood have all been cross-sectional, but this study was able to look at the link of childhood problems and lifetime use of antidepressants by age 24. The authors included 5547 individuals from a nationwide birth cohort linked to the national prescription registry. They were able to use information from parents and teachers about conduct, hyperkinetic and emotional symptoms, and depressive symptoms to predict future antidepressant use between the ages of 8 and 24 years. Interestingly, 8.8% of males and 13.8% of females used antidepressants between the ages of 13 and 24 years. In males, it was conduct problems that predict a later antidepressant use. In both genders, depressive symptoms and being in a family other than one with 2 biological parents at the age of 8 years both predicted later antidepressant uses. It was an interesting but albeit not a surprising result; however, the level of antidepressant use in adolescents and young adults is notable. I would have to guess that Finland is not that different from the rest of the developed world in availability and use of antidepressants, making this an interesting study.

J. C. Ballenger, MD

Combining Medications to Enhance Depression Outcomes (CO-MED): Acute and Long-Term Outcomes of a Single-Blind Randomized Study
Rush AJ, Trivedi MH, Stewart JW, et al (Duke–Natl Univ of Singapore Graduate Med School; Univ of Texas Southwestern Med Ctr at Dallas; Univ of Pittsburgh, PA; et al)
Am J Psychiatry 168:689-701, 2011

Objective.—Two antidepressant medication combinations were compared with selective serotonin reuptake inhibitor monotherapy to determine whether either combination produced a higher remission rate in first-step acute-phase (12 weeks) and long-term (7 months) treatment.

Method.—The single-blind, prospective, randomized trial enrolled 665 outpatients at six primary and nine psychiatric care sites. Participants had at least moderately severe nonpsychotic chronic and/or recurrent major depressive disorder. Escitalopram (up to 20 mg/day) plus placebo, sustained-release bupropion (up to 400 mg/day) plus escitalopram (up to 20 mg/day), or extended-release venlafaxine (up to 300 mg/day) plus mirtazapine (up to 45 mg/day) was delivered (1:1:1 ratio) by using measurement-based care. The primary outcome was remission, defined as ratings of less than 8 and less than 6 on the last two consecutive applications of the 16-item Quick Inventory of Depressive Symptomatology—Self-Report. Secondary outcomes included side effect burden, adverse events, quality of life, functioning, and attrition.

Results.—Remission and response rates and most secondary outcomes were not different among treatment groups at 12 weeks. The remission rates were 38.8% for escitalopram-placebo, 38.9% for bupropion-escitalopram, and 37.7% for venlafaxine-mirtazapine, and the response rates were 51.6%−52.4%. The mean number of worsening adverse events was higher for venlafaxine-mirtazapine (5.7) than for escitalopram-placebo (4.7). At 7 months, remission rates (41.8%−46.6%), response rates (57.4%−59.4%), and most secondary outcomes were not significantly different.

Conclusions.—Neither medication combination outperformed monotherapy. The combination of extended-release venlafaxine plus mirtazapine may have a greater risk of adverse events.

▶ These authors at the University of Texas Southwestern followed up on some promising work, that is, that beginning treatment for depression with 2 antidepressants appeared to be better than either one alone. These promising results led to this trial called Combining Medications to Enhance Depression Outcomes (CO-MED) trial, which was a 7-month, single-blind, randomized, placebo-controlled trial to follow up on this idea (N = 660 outpatients). Patients were randomly assigned to escitalopram plus placebo, bupropion plus escitalopram, or venlafaxine plus mirtazapine. The primary outcome was symptom remission at 12 weeks. Unfortunately, they failed to find that remission rates or even response rates were different at either 12 weeks or 7 months later. Not only were the combination treatments not more effective, they had significantly more side effects. This is a very disappointing result of a very promising simple intervention and one that I had already incorporated into my practice.

J. C. Ballenger, MD

Daily Left Prefrontal Repetitive Transcranial Magnetic Stimulation for Acute Treatment of Medication-Resistant Depression
George MS, Post RM (Med Univ of South Carolina, Charleston; Ralph H. Johnson VA Med Ctr, Charleston; George Washington Univ School of Medicine, DC; et al)
Am J Psychiatry 168:356-364, 2011

After much controversy over the past 15 years, the data now demonstrate that daily left prefrontal rTMS for at least several weeks treats acute depression in a subset of moderately but not extremely treatment-resistant patients with unipolar illness. The effects are about as large as those of medication in this group, but not as large as ECT. The debate and research thus now shift from determining whether rTMS works in the acute setting to trying to improve the technology and maximizing its clinical effectiveness, utility, and durability. Research is also now focusing on whether rTMS can be used as a maintenance treatment and whether it is effective in depression subgroups, such as adolescents, patients with bipolar depression, and depressed patients with anxiety disorders and other comorbidities.

It is not yet clear which subgroups of depressed patients are most likely to benefit from rTMS. The trials to date have largely been performed in mildly to moderately treatment-resistant adult unipolar patients in an acute episode. Thus, for a newly depressed patient, prescribing an antidepressant medication would be more expeditious and less expensive than delivering rTMS as it is currently performed. The place of rTMS in the treatment algorithm is likely to continue to evolve as new data become available. Currently, one might use rTMS to treat depression in patients who have tried at least one antidepressant medication and did not respond adequately (or were unable to tolerate the treatment) and some form of targeted psychotherapy. In patients who respond to rTMS, one should attempt to maintain the remission with prophylactic oral medications. If the patient relapses or does not tolerate the medication side effects, one can reapply rTMS, as in the patient described in the vignette, and perhaps even attempt maintenance TMS despite the meager supporting evidence.

▶ In this article in the *American Journal of Psychiatry*, the authors, 2 of my oldest colleagues, provide an excellent case history and review of the current evidence base for repetitive transcranial stimulation (rTMS). The bottom line is that the data now demonstrate that daily left prefrontal rTMS for at least several weeks does treat acute depression in moderately, but not extremely, treatment-resistant patients with unipolar illness. The point now is to try to determine the various parameters and patient groups in which it will be effective. Data at this point support the conclusion that with newly depressed patients, an antidepressant might be easier and less expensive; however, in patients who have not responded to at least 1 antidepressant and psychotherapy or don't tolerate anti-depressant therapy, it might be reasonable to proceed to rTMS. It is unclear what we should do to maintain remission, but we probably should use oral medications and reapply rTMS if medication does not work, despite the limited evidence that this will be effective.

J. C. Ballenger, MD

Deep Brain Stimulation for Treatment-Resistant Depression: Follow-Up After 3 to 6 Years
Kennedy SH, Giacobbe P, Rizvi SJ, et al (Univ Health Network, Toronto, Ontario, Canada; Univ of Toronto, Ontario, Canada; Emory Univ School of Medicine, Atlanta, GA)
Am J Psychiatry 168:502-510, 2011

Objective.—A prevalence of at least 30% for treatment-resistant depression has prompted the investigation of alternative treatment strategies. Deep brain stimulation (DBS) is a promising targeted approach involving the bilateral placement of electrodes at specific neuroanatomical sites. Given the invasive and experimental nature of DBS for treatment-resistant depression, it is important to obtain both short-term and long-term effectiveness and safety data. This report represents an extended follow-up of 20 patients with treatment-resistant depression who received DBS to the subcallosal cingulate gyrus (Brodmann's area 25).

Method.—After an initial 12-month study of DBS, patients were seen annually and at a last follow-up visit to assess depression severity, functional outcomes, and adverse events.

Results.—The average response rates 1, 2, and 3 years after DBS implantation were 62.5%, 46.2%, and 75%, respectively. At the last follow-up visit (range=3−6 years), the average response rate was 64.3%. Functional impairment in the areas of physical health and social functioning progressively improved up to the last follow-up visit. No significant adverse events were reported during this follow-up, although two patients died by suicide during depressive relapses.

Conclusions.—These data suggest that in the long term, DBS remains a safe and effective treatment for treatment-resistant depression. Additional trials with larger samples are needed to confirm these findings.

▶ A treatment option that is under development for the 30% of depressed patients who are treatment resistant is deep brain stimulation (DBS). These authors report on the follow-up of 20 patients who received DBS bilaterally in the subcallosal cingulate gyrus (Brodmann area 25). The average response rates 1, 2, and 3 years after DBS were 62.5%, 46.2%, and 75.0%, respectively. At the end of 3 to 6 years, the average response rate was 64.3%. There were significant improvements in physical health and social functioning and no significant adverse events, although 2 patients died by suicide during depressive episodes. Despite its invasive nature, these results clearly establish DBS as one of the promising treatments in this difficult area.

J. C. Ballenger, MD

Mindfulness-based cognitive therapy vs cognitive behaviour therapy as a treatment for non-melancholic depression
Manicavasgar V, Parker G, Perich T (Black Dog Inst, New South Wales, Australia; Univ of NSW, Randwick, Australia)
J Affect Disord 130:138-144, 2011

Aim.—To examine the comparative effectiveness of Mindfulness-Based Cognitive Therapy (MBCT) and Cognitive Behaviour Therapy (CBT) as treatments for non-melancholic depression.

Method.—Participants who met criteria for a current episode of major depressive disorder were randomly assigned to either an 8-week MBCT (n = 19) or CBT (n = 26) group therapy condition. They were assessed at pre-treatment, 8-week post-group, and 6- and 12-month follow-ups.

Results.—There were significant improvements in pre- to post-group depression and anxiety scores in both treatment conditions and no significant differences between the two treatment conditions. However, significant differences were found when participants in the two treatment conditions were dichotomized into those with a history of four or more episodes of depression vs those with less than four. In the CBT condition, participants with four or more previous episodes of depression demonstrated greater improvements in depression than those with less than four previous episodes. No such differences were found in the MBCT treatment condition. No significant differences in depression or anxiety were found between the two treatment conditions at 6- and 12-month follow-ups.

Limitations.—Small sample sizes in each treatment condition, especially at follow-up.

Conclusions.—MBCT appears to be as effective as CBT in the treatment of current depression. However, CBT participants with four or more previous episodes of depression derived greater benefits at 8-week post-treatment than those with less than four episodes.

▶ These authors compared mindfulness-based cognitive therapy (MBCT) with cognitive behavior therapy (CBT) for nonmelancholic depression and randomly assigned 19 patients to MBCT and 26 to CBT. They were followed up after 8 weeks of treatment and at 6 and 12 months. There were significant improvements in both groups but no significant difference between. Interestingly, the MBCT patients who had 4 or more previous episodes of depression did better than the patients with less than 4 previous episodes. This is obviously a surprising finding that the patients with the more severe condition actually responded better to CBT. These findings will have to be followed up and confirmed in a large patient sample.

J. C. Ballenger, MD

Psychotherapy Versus Second-Generation Antidepressants in the Treatment of Depression: A Meta-Analysis
Spielmans GI, Berman MI, Usitalo AN (Metropolitan State Univ, St Paul, MN; Dartmouth Med School, Lebanon, NH)
J Nerv Ment Dis 199:142-149, 2011

Most meta-analyses have concluded that psychotherapy and pharmacotherapy yield roughly similar efficacy in the short-term treatment of depression, with psychotherapy showing some advantage at long-term follow-up. However, a recent meta-analysis found that selective serotonin reuptake inhibitors medications were superior to psychotherapy in the short-term treatment of depression. To incorporate results of several recent trials into the meta-analytic literature, we conducted a meta-analysis of trials which directly compared psychotherapy to second-generation antidepressants (SGAs). Variables potentially moderating the quality of psychotherapy or medication delivery were also examined, to allow the highest quality comparison of both types of intervention. Bona fide psychotherapies showed equivalent efficacy in the short-term and slightly better efficacy on depression rating scales at follow-up relative to SGA. Non-bona fide therapies had significantly worse short-term outcomes than medication $(d = 0.58)$. No significant differences emerged between treatments in terms of response or remission rates, but non-bona fide therapies had significantly lower rates of study completion than medication (odds ratio $= 0.55$). Bona fide psychotherapy appears as effective as SGAs in the short-term treatment of depression, and likely somewhat more effective than SGAs in the longer-term management of depressive symptoms.

▶ These authors performed an interesting meta-analysis of the comparative efficacy of psychotherapy versus pharmacotherapy in the short-term treatment of depression. Several recent reports suggested that perhaps selective serotonin reuptake inhibitor medications were superior to psychotherapy. However, incorporating those trials and the previous ones led to the same original finding of no significant difference between psychotherapy and second-generation antidepressants. It is also interesting that some articles show that medication treatment can actually be ultimately more expensive than psychotherapy, a finding that most third-party payers and patients find hard to believe. In this day and age, it is even hard for patients to believe that psychotherapy works as well as antidepressants, but that evidence seems very clear. Despite the drift of opinion expressed in the media, medications have not supplanted in efficacy or, in my experience, even popularity, with most patients. It is hard for many patients to understand why a pill would help fix their problems, or it seems to be a less elegant approach to them than psychotherapy. Obviously, one of the major issues is financial support for this very valuable treatment.

J. C. Ballenger, MD

Residual Symptoms in Depressed Outpatients Who Respond by 50% But Do Not Remit to Antidepressant Medication

McClintock SM, Husain MM, Wisniewski SR, et al (Univ of Texas Southwestern Med Ctr at Dallas; Univ of Pittsburgh, PA; et al)
J Clin Psychopharmacol 31:180-186, 2011

Little is known about the quantity or quality of residual depressive symptoms in patients with major depressive disorder (MDD) who have responded but not remitted with antidepressant treatment. This report describes the residual symptom domains and individual depressive symptoms in a large representative sample of outpatients with nonpsychotic MDD who responded without remitting after up to 12 weeks of citalopram treatment in the Sequenced Treatment Alternatives to Relieve Depression (STAR*D) study. Response was defined as 50% or greater reduction in baseline 16-item Quick Inventory of Depressive Symptomatology—Self-Report (QIDS-SR$_{16}$) by treatment exit, and remission as a final QIDS-SR$_{16}$ of less than 6. Residual symptom domains and individual symptoms were based on the QIDS-SR$_{16}$ and classified as either persisting from baseline or emerging during treatment. Most responders who did not remit endorsed approximately 5 residual symptom domains and 6 to 7 residual depressive symptoms. The most common domains were insomnia (94.6%), sad mood (70.8%), and decreased concentration (69.6%). The most common individual symptoms were midnocturnal insomnia (79.0%), sad mood (70.8%), and decreased concentration/decision making (69.6%). The most common treatment-emergent symptoms were midnocturnal insomnia (51.4%) and decreased general interest (40.0%). The most common persistent symptoms were midnocturnal insomnia (81.6%), sad mood (70.8%), and decreased concentration/decision making (70.6%). Suicidal ideation was the least common treatment-emergent symptom (0.7%) and the least common persistent residual symptom (17.1%). These findings suggest that depressed outpatients who respond by 50% without remitting to citalopram treatment have a broad range of residual symptoms. Individualized treatments are warranted to specifically address each patient's residual depressive symptoms.

▶ That a large percentage of depressed patients do not completely respond to antidepressant therapy has become widely recognized and even forms a U.S. Food and Drug Administration indication for treatment. These authors studied these residual symptoms in a large representative sample of outpatients with nonpsychotic major depressive disorder. These are patients who failed to remit with 12 weeks of citalopram treatment in the STAR*D study. Responders who did not remit had approximately 5 residual symptoms. The most common symptom domains were insomnia (94.6%), sad mood (70.8%), and decreased concentration (69.6%). The most common individual symptoms were middle-of-the-night awakening (79%), sad mood (70.8%), and decreased concentration/decision making (69.6%). This is obviously a fairly broad set of symptoms that we do not yet know how to deal with. Obviously, many of us now have added atypical antipsychotics to treatment of partially remitted patients based on good data, but this remains a huge unsettled issue.

J. C. Ballenger, MD

Risk factors for chronic depression — A systematic review
Hölzel L, Härter M, Reese C, et al (Univ Med Ctr Freiburg, Germany; et al)
J Affect Disord 129:1-13, 2011

Background.—One of five patients with an acute depressive episode develops chronic depression. Risk factors for a current depressive episode to become chronic are insufficiently known. This review was conducted to examine which factors represent a risk factor for the development of chronic depression for patients diagnosed with a depressive episode.

Method.—Medline, Psycinfo, ISI Web of Science, CINHAL and BIOSIS Previews were searched up until September 2007, complemented by hand-searching in the December 1987 to December 2007 issues of *Journal of Affective Disorders* and investigating reference lists of included articles and existing reviews. On the basis of a formal checklist, two investigators independently decided which studies to include or exclude.

Results.—25 relevant primary studies with a total of 5192 participants were included in the systematic review. Overall the methodological quality of the included studies was found to be sufficient. Data synthesis was performed via vote counting. The following risk factors were identified: *younger age at onset, longer duration of depressive episode,* and *family history of mood disorders.* Psychological comorbidity i.e. *anxiety disorders, personality disorders* and *substance abuse, low level of social integration, negative social interaction* and *lower severity of depressive symptoms* repeatedly appeared concurrently with chronic depression.

Limitations.—Most included studies were cross-sectional thus drawing causal conclusions with regard to risk factors proved to be difficult.

Conclusion.—Risk factors for a current depressive episode to become chronic were identified. To date only few significant longitudinal studies on this topic are available.

▶ Although almost 20% of depressive episodes develop into chronic depression, we do not know yet what the predictors are of this adverse condition. These authors picked the 25 most relevant studies for a total of 5192 participants to identify risk factors. These were shown to include younger age of onset, longer duration of depressive episode, and a family history of mood disorders. Comorbidity with anxiety disorders, personality disorders, substance abuse, poor social integration, as well as the severity of depressive symptoms repeatedly occurred with the chronic depression. Studies of this type are highly important.

J. C. Ballenger, MD

Stigma and Depression During Pregnancy: Does Race Matter?
O'Mahen HA, Henshaw E, Jones JM, et al (Univ of Exeter, UK; Denison Univ, Granville, OH; et al)
J Nerv Ment Dis 199:257-262, 2011

Rates of depression treatment are low in pregnant women, particularly Black women. Stigma is an important barrier to treatment, but little research has examined how depression stigma differs in Blacks and Whites; a key purpose of this study. Participants were 532 pregnant women recruited in obstetrics settings, who responded to measures of stigma and mood. Black women reported more depression stigma than White women, regardless of their depression status, and were more likely to endorse the view that depression should be kept secret, than White women. In White women, stigma increased as a function of depression status (current, past, never). White women's perceptions of depression stigma were positively correlated with their beliefs about keeping depression secret. Secrecy and depression stigma were uncorrelated in Black women. There are important racial differences in the way depression stigma functions in pregnant women. Implications for engaging women in mental health treatment are discussed.

▶ We have been following the issues of depression and pregnancy. This study involved 532 pregnant women in obstetrical settings. Interestingly, black women reported more depression stigma than white women and were much more likely to feel that their depression should be kept a secret than white women. This is yet another issue to be considered in this clinically vulnerable group.

J. C. Ballenger, MD

The effects of continuous antidepressant treatment during the first 6 months on relapse or recurrence of depression
Kim K-H, Lee S-M, Paik J-W, et al (Health Insurance Review and Assessment Service, Seoul, Republic of Korea; Kyung Hee Univ, Seoul, Republic of Korea; et al)
J Affect Disord 132:121-129, 2011

Background.—To examine whether continuous antidepressant treatment during the first 6 month reduces the risk of relapse/recurrence of depression in South Korea.

Methods.—We used National Health Insurance Data covering the period from 2001 through 2004. The study population consisted of 117,087 adult patients who received antidepressants after being diagnosed with depression. The continuous antidepressant was defined as evidence of antidepressant prescriptions for 75% of the first 6 months of treatment. Relapse or recurrence during the next 18-month period was defined by evidence of a new episode requiring antidepressant treatment, psychiatric hospitalization, electroconvulsive therapy, emergency department visit or attempted suicide. We compared the relapse/recurrence rate during the 18-month follow-up period in patients receiving continuous treatment and those who discontinued early using a Cox's proportional hazard model.

Results.—Patients receiving continuous antidepressant treatment experienced a lower risk of relapse/recurrence (Hazard ratio: 0.42, 95% CI: 0.40−0.44). Three or more follow-up visits in the first 3 months also reduced the risk of relapse/recurrence. Factors associated with a significant increase of relapse/recurrence were comorbid medical illness, anxiety disorder, and alcohol abuse. The small benefit of SSRIs was appeared only in the early discontinued treatment subgroup, not in the continuous treatment subgroup.

Limitations.—We were not able to consider the antidepressant utilization pattern.

Conclusions.—Continuous antidepressant treatment and frequent follow-up visits during the acute phase were associated with a significant reduction in the likelihood of relapse or recurrence of depression. Our results provide important evidence on the effectiveness of antidepressant treatment in South Korea.

▶ I found this article interesting because it examined a question of whether what we have learned in the United States about depression relapse is also true in South Korea. The authors were able to use a database of 117 087 adult patients who received antidepressants for depression. Similar to what we have learned in the United States, continuous antidepressant treatment resulted in a lower risk of relapse and recurrence over the following 18 months. The authors observed that 3 or more follow-up visits to the clinician reduced risk of relapse. Factors influencing relapse were comorbid medical illness, anxiety disorder, and alcohol abuse. This finding in an Asian population was of particular interest to me, because I had once chaired a very interesting consensus conference in which we compared symptom pictures and treatments of depression in Japan compared with the West. It was somewhat surprising to our Japanese colleagues and some of our social anthropologists that with few exceptions, psychiatric disorders in Japan, particularly depression and anxiety, are very similar to those in the West; however, treatment advances, like the ones in this article, are generally 15 to 20 years behind the West.

J. C. Ballenger, MD

The Serotonin Transporter Promoter Variant (5-HTTLPR), Stress, and Depression Meta-analysis Revisited: Evidence of Genetic Moderation

Karg K, Burmeister M, Shedden K, et al (Univ of Wuerzburg, Germany; Univ of Michigan, Ann Arbor)
Arch Gen Psychiatry 68:444-454, 2011

Context.—Two recent meta-analyses assessed the set of studies exploring the interaction between a serotonin transporter promoter polymorphism (5-HTTLPR) and stress in the development of depression and concluded that the evidence did not support the presence of the interaction. However, even the larger of the meta-analyses included only 14 of the 56 studies that have assessed the relationship between 5-HTTLPR, stress, and depression.

Objective.—To perform a meta-analysis including all relevant studies exploring the interaction.

Data Sources.—We identified studies published through November 2009 in PubMed.

Study Selection.—We excluded 2 studies presenting data that were included in other larger studies.

Data Extraction.—To perform a more inclusive meta-analysis, we used the Liptak-Stouffer z score method to combine findings of primary studies at the level of significance tests rather than the level of raw data.

Data Synthesis.—We included 54 studies and found strong evidence that 5-HTTLPR moderates the relationship between stress and depression, with the 5-HTTLPR s allele associated with an increased risk of developing depression under stress ($P = .00002$). When stratifying our analysis by the type of stressor studied, we found strong evidence for an association between the s allele and increased stress sensitivity in the childhood maltreatment ($P = .00007$) and the specific medical condition ($P = .0004$) groups of studies but only marginal evidence for an association in the stressful life events group ($P = .03$). When restricting our analysis to the studies included in the previous meta-analyses, we found no evidence of association (Munafò et al studies, $P = .16$; Risch et al studies, $P = .11$). This suggests that the difference in results between meta-analyses was due to the different set of included studies rather than the meta-analytic technique.

Conclusion.—Contrary to the results of the smaller earlier meta-analyses, we find strong evidence that the studies published to date support the hypothesis that 5-HTTLPR moderates the relationship between stress and depression.

▶ One of the most intriguing findings in psychiatry in recent history has been the seemingly explanatory relationship reported between the serotonin transporter promoter polymorphism (5-HTTLPR) and stress in the development of depression. Two recent meta-analyses failed to support the presence of this interaction; however, these authors performed a larger meta-analysis including all relevant studies exploring the interaction. Very interestingly, they found strong evidence that the 5-HTTLPR allele polymorphism does moderate the relationship between depression and stress with the 5-HTTLPR s allele being associated with increased risk of depression under stress ($P = .00002$). They were also able to look at the type of stress and found strong evidence for the association of the s allele and increased stress sensitivity from childhood maltreatment ($P = .00007$) and specific medical conditions ($P = .0004$) but more marginal evidence in the stressful life events group ($P = .03$). When they put their analytic method to the studies that had been included in the previous meta-analyses, they too found no evidence of association, suggesting that the difference in the results is related to the difference in included studies rather than technique.

J. C. Ballenger, MD

Trajectories of Depressive Episodes and Hypertension Over 24 Years: The Whitehall II Prospective Cohort Study
Nabi H, Chastang J-F, Lefèvre T, et al (Institut National de la Santé et de la Recherche Médicale, Villejuif, France; Laboratory of Medical Information Processing/Institut National de la Santé et de la Recherche Médicale U650/ IFR 148, Brest, France; et al)
Hypertension 57:710-716, 2011

Prospective data on depressive symptoms and blood pressure are scarce, and the impact of age on this association is poorly understood. The present study examines longitudinal trajectories of depressive episodes and the probability of hypertension associated with these trajectories over time. Participants were 6889 men and 3413 women, London-based civil servants aged 35 to 55 years at baseline, followed for 24 years between 1985 and 2009. Depressive episode (defined as scoring ≥4 on the General Health Questionnaire-Depression subscale or using prescribed antidepressant medication) and hypertension (systolic/diastolic blood pressure ≥140/ 90 mm Hg or use of antihypertensive medication) were assessed concurrently at 5 medical examinations. In the fully adjusted longitudinal logistic regression analyses based on generalized estimating equations using age as the time scale, participants in the "increasing depression" group had a 24% ($P<0.05$) lower risk of hypertension at ages 35 to 39 years compared with those in the "low/transient depression" group. However, there was a faster age-related increase in hypertension in the increasing depression group, corresponding with a 7% ($P<0.01$) greater increase in the odds of hypertension for each 5-year increase in age. A higher risk of hypertension in the first group of participants was not evident before 55 years of age. A similar pattern of association was observed in men and women, although it was stronger in men. This study suggests that the risk of hypertension increases with repeated experience of depressive episodes over time and becomes evident in later adulthood.

▶ This is a remarkable study of 6889 men and 3413 women who were civil servants in Great Britain who were followed for 24 years in terms of depressive episodes and hypertension. The participants who had "increasing depression" had a 24% lower risk of hypertension compared with those who had "low/transient depression" in the ages from 35 to 39. In contrast, there was a faster age-related increase in hypertension in the group that had increasing depression, corresponding to a 7% greater increase in the odds of having hypertension for each 5-year increase in age. This higher risk in the first group of participants was not evident until they were 55 years of age. This pattern was observed in men and women but was stronger in men. This again suggests that paying attention to psychiatric issues is important in that depression over time appears to lead to an increased risk of hypertension.

J. C. Ballenger, MD

A pooled analysis of two randomised, placebo-controlled studies of extended release quetiapine fumarate adjunctive to antidepressant therapy in patients with major depressive disorder
Bauer M, El-Khalili N, Datto C, et al (Technische Universität Dresden, Germany; Alpine Clinic, Lafayette, IN; AstraZeneca Pharmaceuticals, Wilmington, DE; et al)
J Affect Disord 127:19-30, 2010

Background.—Two positive studies evaluated adjunctive extended release quetiapine fumarate (quetiapine XR) in patients with major depressive disorder (MDD) showing inadequate response to antidepressant treatment. This preplanned, pooled analysis provides an opportunity for subgroup analyses investigating the influence of demographic and disease-related factors on observed responses. Additional post hoc analyses examined the efficacy of quetiapine XR against specific depressive symptoms including sleep.

Methods.—Data were analysed from two 6-week, multicentre, double-blind, randomised, placebo-controlled studies, prospectively designed to be pooled. Patients received once-daily quetiapine XR 150 mg/day ($n = 309$), 300 mg/day ($n = 307$) or placebo ($n = 303$) adjunctive to ongoing antidepressant therapy. The primary endpoint was change from randomisation to Week 6 in MADRS total score. Other assessments included MADRS response ($\geq 50\%$ decrease in total score) and remission (total score ≤ 8), change from randomisation in HAM-D, HAM-A, PSQI global and CGI-S scores.

Results.—Quetiapine XR (150 and 300 mg/day) reduced MADRS total scores vs placebo at every assessment including Week 6 (-14.5, -14.8, -12.0; $p < 0.001$ each dose) and Week 1 (-7.8, -7.3, -5.1; $p < 0.001$ each dose). For quetiapine XR 150 and 300 mg/day and placebo, respectively at Week 6: MADRS response 53.7% ($p = 0.063$), 58.3% ($p < 0.01$) and 46.2%; MADRS remission 35.6% ($p < 0.01$), 36.5% ($p < 0.001$) and 24.1%. Quetiapine XR 150 and 300 mg/day significantly improved HAM-D, HAM-A, PSQI and CGI-S scores at Week 6 vs placebo. Quetiapine XR demonstrated broad efficacy, independent of factors including concomitant antidepressant.

Limitations.—Fixed dosing; lack of active comparator.

Conclusions.—Adjunctive quetiapine XR is effective in patients with MDD and an inadequate response to antidepressant therapy, with improvement in depressive symptoms seen as early as Week 1.

▶ We continue to try to find the role for the new second-generation antipsychotics, including quetiapine (Seroquel). This article presented results from two 6-week, multicenter, double-blind, placebo-controlled trials adding quetiapine XR 150 and 300 mg compared with placebo added to antidepressant therapy. Not surprisingly, both doses of quetiapine reduced depression scores greater than placebo at every assessment from week 1. Both doses appeared relatively similar, and both led to significantly greater remission rates (approximately 35% vs 24% placebo). This is one of a series of studies showing that quetiapine, either by itself or adjunctively with antidepressants, is effective in the treatment of unipolar depression and, in other trials, for bipolar depression. It is increasingly clear that the second-generation antipsychotics are useful in the treatment of depression and their original indications in schizophrenia and bipolar mania.

J. C. Ballenger, MD

Antidepressant Exposure as a Predictor of Clinical Outcomes in the Treatment of Resistant Depression in Adolescents (TORDIA) Study
Sakolsky DJ, Perel JM, Emslie GJ, et al (Western Psychiatric Inst and Clinic, Pittsburgh, PA; Univ of Texas Southwestern Med Ctr at Dallas; et al)
J Clin Psychopharmacol 31:92-97, 2011

This paper examines the relationship between plasma concentration of antidepressant and both clinical response and adverse effects in treatment-resistant depressed adolescents. Adolescents (n = 334) with major depression who had not responded to a selective serotonin reuptake inhibitor (SSRI) were randomized to 1 of 4 treatments: switch to another SSRI (fluoxetine, citalopram, or paroxetine), switch to venlafaxine, switch to SSRI plus cognitive behavior therapy, or switch to venlafaxine plus cognitive behavior therapy. Adolescents who did not improve by 6 weeks had their dose increased. Plasma concentrations of medication and metabolites were measured at 6 weeks in 244 participants and at 12 weeks in 204 participants. Adolescents treated with citalopram whose plasma concentration was equal to or greater than the geometric mean (GM) showed a higher response rate compared to those with less than the GM, with parallel but nonsignificant findings for fluoxetine. A dose increase of citalopram or fluoxetine at week 6 was most likely to result in response when it led to a change in concentration from less than the GM at 6 weeks to the GM or greater at week 12. Plasma levels of paroxetine, venlafaxine, or O-desmethylvenlafaxine were not related to clinical response. Exposure was associated with more cardiovascular and dermatologic side effects in those receiving venlafaxine.

Antidepressant concentration may be useful in optimizing treatment for depressed adolescents receiving fluoxetine or citalopram.

▶ We have struggled with the appropriate antidepressant treatment in adolescents, because many, if not most, trials have failed to show efficacy. This study examines the issue of whether blood levels would be useful to maximize response. In a complex study of 244 patients, they compared fluoxetine, citalopram, paroxetine, venlafaxine, and various combinations and switches. Adolescents who did not improve after 6 weeks had their doses increased, and plasma levels were measured at 6 and 12 weeks. They were able to show that those adolescents treated with citalopram whose plasma concentration was greater than or equal to the geometric mean (GM) did show a higher response rate than those whose plasma concentration was lower than the GM, with similar but nonsignificant findings for fluoxetine. The dose increase in citalopram or fluoxetine at 6 weeks led to a change in concentration from less than the GM to greater than the GM at week 12. These results suggest that with citalopram, and maybe fluoxetine, measuring serum levels of antidepressants might be an important addition to the way we treat depressed adolescents.

J. C. Ballenger, MD

Behavioural activation delivered by the non-specialist: phase II randomised controlled trial
Ekers D, Richards D, McMillan D, et al (Durham Univ, UK; Univ of Exeter, UK; Univ of York, UK)
Br J Psychiatry 198:66-72, 2011

Background.—Behavioural activation appears as effective as cognitive-behaviour therapy (CBT) in the treatment of depression. If equally effective, then behavioural activation may be the preferred treatment option because it may be suitable for delivery by therapists with less training. This is the first randomised controlled trial to look at this possibility.

Aims.—To examine whether generic mental health workers can deliver effective behavioural activation as a step-three high-intensity intervention.

Method.—A randomised controlled trial (ISRCTN27045243) comparing behavioural activation ($n = 24$) with treatment as usual ($n = 23$) in primary care.

Results.—Intention-to-treat analyses indicated a difference in favour of behavioural activation of -15.79 (95% CI -24.55 to -7.02) on the Beck Depression Inventory-II and Work and Social Adjustment Scale (mean difference -11.12, 95% CI -17.53 to -4.70).

Conclusions.—Effective behavioural activation appears suitable for delivery by generic mental health professionals without previous experience as therapists. Large-scale trial comparisons with an active comparator (CBT) are needed.

▶ This randomized controlled trial compared behavioral activation in 24 depressed patients with primary care usual treatment (n = 23). Behavioral activation was, in fact, more effective. This is a potentially important lead in the issue of dissemination of effective treatment to large numbers of depressed patients in primary care. Behavioral activation appears to be as effective as cognitive behavioral therapy, and because it can be delivered by therapists with relatively little training, it could be an effective dissemination strategy. It obviously deserves further exploration.

J. C. Ballenger, MD

Cognitive-emotional reactivation during deep transcranial magnetic stimulation over the prefrontal cortex of depressive patients affects antidepressant outcome
Isserles M, Rosenberg O, Dannon P, et al (Hadassah-Hebrew Univ Med Ctr, Jerusalem, Israel; Tel-Aviv Univ, Israel; et al)
J Affect Disord 128:235-242, 2011

Background.—Transcranial magnetic stimulation (TMS) enables non-surgical activation of specific brain areas. TMS over the prefrontal cortex (PFC) is emerging as a significant tool that can augment or replace non/partially effective antidepressant medications. Deep TMS (DTMS) utilizes newly developed coils that enable effective stimulation of deeper cortical layers involved in the pathophysiology of depression.

Objectives.—We aimed to assess the H1-DTMS coil as an add-on to antidepressants in treating patients with major depression. We also intended to evaluate whether the antidepressant outcome of DTMS treatment is affected by a cognitive-emotional procedure performed during stimulation.

Methods.—57 patients were enrolled in the study that included 4 weeks of daily 20 Hz stimulation sessions and additional 4 weekly sessions as a short maintenance phase. Two subgroups of patients received either positive or negative cognitive-emotional reactivation along with the stimulation sessions.

Results.—21 of 46 patients (46%) who received at least 10 stimulation sessions achieved response (improvement of ≥50% in the Hamilton Depression Rating Scale (HDRS)) and 13 of them (28%) achieved remission (HDRS-24 ≤ 10) by the end of the daily treatment phase. Improvements were smaller in the negatively reactivated group and Beck Depression Inventory scores were not significantly improved in this group.

Conclusions.—DTMS over the PFC proved to be safe and effective in augmenting antidepressant medications. Negative cognitive-emotional reactivation can disrupt the therapeutic effect of DTMS. A large sham controlled study is required to further establish the effectiveness of DTMS as an augmentation treatment and the role of cognitive reactivation during stimulation.

▶ The efficacy of traditional transcranial magnetic stimulation (TMS) is presumably limited by its inability to stimulate deep in the cortex. Recently developed deep TMS coils do allow more effective stimulation in deeper levels. These authors evaluated 57 patients who were stimulated for 4 weeks with daily 20-Hz stimulation sessions and an additional 4 weekly sessions as a short maintenance phase. They did observe that 46% of their 46 patients receiving 10 sessions responded with greater than or equal to a 50% drop in their Hamilton Depression Rating Scale and 13 of them (28%) achieved remission. This is certainly a promising result and bears further study to define the range of efficacy for repetitive TMS.

J. C. Ballenger, MD

Personalized Medicine for Depression: Can We Match Patients With Treatments?
Simon GE, Perlis RH (Group Health Res Inst, Seattle, WA; Massachusetts General Hosp, Boston)
Am J Psychiatry 167:1445-1455, 2010

Objective.—Response to specific depression treatments varies widely among individuals. Understanding and predicting that variation could have great benefits for people living with depression.

Method.—The authors describe a conceptual model for identifying and evaluating evidence relevant to personalizing treatment for depression. They review evidence related to three specific treatment decisions: choice between antidepressant medication and psychotherapy, selection of a specific antidepressant medication, and selection of a specific psychotherapy. They then discuss potential explanations for negative findings as well as implications for research and clinical practice.

Results.—Many previous studies have examined general predictors of outcome, but few have examined true moderators (predictors of differential response to alternative treatments). The limited evidence indicates that some specific clinical characteristics may inform the choice between antidepressant medication and psychotherapy and the choice of specific antidepressant medication. Research to date does not identify any biologic or genetic predictors of sufficient clinical utility to inform the choice between medication and psychotherapy, the selection of specific medication, or the selection of a specific psychotherapy.

Conclusions.—While individuals vary widely in response to specific depression treatments, the variability remains largely unpredictable. Future research should focus on identifying true moderator effects and should consider how response to treatments varies across episodes. At this time, our inability to match patients with treatments implies that systematic follow-up assessment and adjustment of treatment are more important than initial treatment selection.

▶ This recent *American Journal of Psychiatry* article by Drs Simon and Perlis provides a significant review of the clinical choices we must make in treating depressed patients. The authors attempted to use available evidence in the literature to develop algorithms for which patients should receive antidepressants versus psychotherapy, as well as which specific antidepressant and which specific psychotherapy. Perhaps not surprisingly, they concluded that the literature is inadequate at this point to answer these questions. They suggested that this is where the research in the near future must go. The authors leave us with the clinical understanding that at present, following up and changing treatments that do not work is more important than which treatment is chosen initially. Although we would have hoped for more, this is actually a valuable conclusion to guide us clinically and, interestingly, in our arguments with insurance companies or others about what the empirically supported treatments of depression are.

J. C. Ballenger, MD

Bipolar Disorder

Abnormal frontal cortex white matter connections in bipolar disorder: A DTI tractography study

Lin F, Weng S, Xie B, et al (Wuhan Inst of Physics and Mathematics, People's Republic of China; Renmin Hosp of Wuhan Univ, People's Republic of China; et al)
J Affect Disord 131:299-306, 2011

Objective.—In bipolar disorder, white matter abnormalities have been reported with region-of-interest and voxel-based methods; however, deficits in specific white matter tracts cannot be localized by these methods. Therefore, in this study, we aimed to investigate the white matter tracts that mediate connectivity of the frontal cortex using diffusion tensor imaging (DTI) tractography.

Methods.—Eighteen patients with bipolar disorder and sixteen age- and gender-matched healthy subjects underwent DTI examinations. Frontal cortex white matter tracts, including the anterior thalamic radiation (ATR), uncinate fasciculus (UF), superior longitudinal fasciculus (SLF), cingulum, and inferior fronto-occipital fasciculus (IFO) were reconstructed by DTI tractography, and we calculated the mean fractional anisotropy (FA) for each fiber tract. The values were compared between groups by repeated measures analysis of variance with age and gender as covariates, which allowed us to investigate significant differences between the tracts.

Results.—When compared with healthy controls, the patients with bipolar disorder showed significantly decreased FA in the ATR and UF, and a trend towards lower FA in the SLF and cingulum. However, there were no FA differences between groups in the IFO.

Conclusions.—Our study indicates that bipolar patients show abnormalities within white matter tracts connecting the frontal cortex with the temporal and parietal cortices and the fronto-subcortical circuits. These findings suggest that alterations in the connectivity of white matter tracts in the frontal cortex might contribute to the neuropathology of bipolar disorder.

▶ These authors followed previous research that suggested that there are deficits in specific white matter tracts in the brain in bipolar patients, but previous methods have not allowed direct exploration of that issue. They used diffusion sensor imaging tractography in 18 patients with bipolar disorder matched with 16 well-matched healthy controls. They found that the patients with bipolar disorder showed significantly decreased fractional anisotropy in the anterior thalamic radiation and uncinate fasciculus. These results allowed them to conclude that there were abnormalities in the white matter tracts connecting the frontal lobe with the temporal parietal cortices and the fronto-subcortical circuits, and they postulate that this might be part of the underlying neuropathology of bipolar disorder. This is yet another very interesting article about how the advances of neuroimaging have allowed us to better conceptualize the pathology of the disorders we treat.

J. C. Ballenger, MD

Aggression, ADHD symptoms, and dysphoria in children and adolescents diagnosed with bipolar disorder and ADHD
Doerfler LA, Connor DF, Toscano PF Jr (Univ of Massachusettes Med School, Worcester; Univ of Connecticut Health Ctr, Farmington)
J Affect Disord 131:312-319, 2011

Background.—This study had two objectives: (1) examine characteristics of aggression in children and adolescents diagnosed with bipolar disorder and (2) determine whether the CBCL pediatric bipolar disorder profile differentiated youngsters with bipolar disorder from youngsters with ADHD.

Method.—Children and adolescents referred to a pediatric psychopharmacology clinic were systematically evaluated for psychopathology using a psychiatrist-administered diagnostic interview, parent- and teacher-report rating scales assessing the child's behavior, and child-completed self-report scales. In this sample, 27 children and adolescents were diagnosed with bipolar disorder and 249 youngsters were diagnosed with ADHD without co-occurring bipolar disorder. These two groups were compared to determine whether there were significant differences on various measures of psychopathology.

Results.—Youngsters diagnosed with bipolar disorder were more verbally aggressive and exhibited higher levels of reactive aggression than youngsters with ADHD without co-occurring bipolar disorder. Youngsters with bipolar disorder also reported higher levels of depressive symptoms than youngsters with ADHD without bipolar disorder. The CBCL pediatric bipolar disorder profile did not accurately identify youngsters diagnosed with bipolar disorder.

Conclusions.—The present findings present a picture of manic youngsters as verbally aggressive and argumentative, who respond with anger when frustrated. Youngsters diagnosed with bipolar disorder and ADHD exhibited significant levels of impulsive behavior and attention problems, but youngsters with bipolar disorder also exhibited significant levels of aggressive behavior and dysphoric mood. Finally, the CBCL pediatric bipolar disorder profile did not accurately identify youngsters who were diagnosed with bipolar disorder.

▶ Almost from the the time we began diagnosing children with bipolar disorder, there has been a debate about the difficulties differentiating children with bipolar disorder from those with attention deficit hyperactivity disorder (ADHD). These workers compared 27 children and adolescents diagnosed with bipolar disorder with 249 with ADHD without co-occurring bipolar disorder. They were in fact able to discern clear differences in their psychopathology. Children with bipolar disorder were more verbally aggressive with higher levels of reactive aggression than children with ADHD without bipolar disorder. They also had higher dysphoric depressive symptoms and responded with anger when frustrated.

J. C. Ballenger, MD

An estimate of the minimum economic burden of bipolar I and II disorders in the United States: 2009
Dilsaver SC (Comprehensive Doctors Med Group, Inc, Arcadia, CA)
J Affect Disord 129:79-83, 2011

Objective.—To conduct an analysis yielding estimates of the direct and indirect costs accruing from bipolar I and II disorders in 2009. The last analysis of these costs pertained to 1991.

Methods.—The analysis presented is based on recent epidemiological data, a measure of the increase in the cost of health care services and commodities between 1991 and December 31, 2009, a measure of the increase in the cost of living after partialing out of the costs of health care between 1991 and December 31, 2009 and adjustment for growth in the population of the United States between 1991 and 2009 to calculate the direct and indirect costs of bipolar I and II disorders.

Results.—The estimated direct and indirect costs of bipolar I and II disorders in 2009 were 30.7 and 120.3 billion dollars, respectively. The estimated total economic burden imposed by these disorders was 151.0 billion dollars. The increase in costs between 1991 and 2009 was not entirely due to inflation. Bipolar I and II disorders are now estimated to have a combined prevalence exceeding that used in the calculation of costs for 1991 by 1.6154-fold. Direct costs escalated out of proportion (2.2393-fold) to indirect costs (1.6148-fold).

Limitations.—The analysis required the acceptance assumptions that likely resulted in a net-underestimation of costs and did not take the entirety of the bipolar spectrum into account.

Conclusions.—The findings have implications for the formulation of public policy. The lifetime prevalences of not only bipolar I and II disorders but also the high prevalence of the entire body of bipolar spectrum disorders, the suffering that they create and the economic burden imposed by them render them worthy of having a high priority in the formulation of plans for the delivery of health care services, planning educational programs for the public and informing policymakers.

▶ These authors were able to generate estimates of direct and indirect costs of bipolar I and II disorders in the United States in 2009. Direct costs were $30.7 billion and indirect were $120.3 billion. A combined $151 billion is bad enough, but the authors also point out that these estimates do not include the rest of the bipolar spectrum; therefore, actual estimates would be higher. They make a much-needed pitch that this is an area that needs greater attention in terms of education and public policy thinking.

J. C. Ballenger, MD

Association Between Prior Authorization for Medications and Health Service Use by Medicaid Patients with Bipolar Disorder
Lu CY, Adams AS, Ross-Degnan D, et al (Harvard Med School, Boston, MA)
Psychiatr Serv 62:186-193, 2011

Objective.—This study examined the association between a Medicaid prior-authorization policy for second-generation antipsychotic and anticonvulsant agents and medication discontinuation and health service use by patients with bipolar disorder.

Methods.—A pre-post design with a historical comparison group was used to analyze Maine Medicaid and Medicare claims data. A total of 946 newly treated patients were identified during the eight-month policy (July 2003—February 2004), and a comparison group of 1,014 was identified from the prepolicy period (July 2002—February 2003). Patients were stratified by number of visits to community mental health centers (CMHCs) before medication initiation (proxy for illness severity): CMHC attenders, at least two visits; nonattenders, fewer than two. Changes in rates of medication discontinuation and outpatient, emergency room, and hospital visits were estimated.

Results.—Compared with nonattenders, at baseline CMHC attenders had substantially higher rates of comorbid mental disorders and use of medications and health services. The policy was associated with increased medication discontinuation among attenders and nonattenders, reductions in mental health visits after discontinuation among attenders (−.64 per patient per month; p<.05), and increases in emergency room visits after discontinuation among nonattenders (−.16 per patient per month; p<.05). During the eight-month policy period, the policy had no detectable impact on hospitalization risk.

Conclusions.—The prior-authorization policy was associated with increased medication discontinuation and subsequent changes in health service use. Although small, these unintended effects raise concerns about quality of care for a group of vulnerable patients. Long-term consequences of prior-authorization policies on patient outcomes warrant further investigation.

▶ These authors used an opportunity when the Maine Medicaid and Medicare group established a prior authorization for second-generation antipsychotics and anticonvulsant agents. They followed 946 newly treated patients with bipolar illness and compared them with 1014 patients who were treated prior to the institution of this policy. Interestingly, the policy was associated with increased discontinuation of medication, reduction in mental health visits, and increases in emergency room visits in some patients, but it had no effect on hospitalization risks. These are surprising negative results from a seemingly innocuous policy change, but not actually surprising if the administrator who did it gave it any thought.

J. C. Ballenger, MD

Differences between bipolar I and bipolar II disorders in clinical features, comorbidity, and family history

Baek JH, Park DY, Choi J, et al (Samsung Med Ctr, Seoul, Republic of Korea; et al)
J Affect Disord 131:59-67, 2011

Background.—The present study was designed to investigate whether bipolar II disorder (BP-II) has different characteristics from bipolar I disorder (BP-I), not only in manic severity but also in clinical features, prior course, comorbidity, and family history, sufficiently enough to provide its nosological separation from BP-I.

Methods.—Comprehensive clinical evaluation was performed based on information available from ordinary clinical settings. Seventy-one BP-I and 34 BP-II patients were assessed using the Diagnostic Interview for Genetic Studies, Korean version. Psychiatric assessment for first-degree relatives ($n = 374$) of the probands was performed using the modified version of the Family History-Research Diagnostic Criteria.

Results.—The frequency of depressive episodes was higher in BP-II ($p = 0.009$) compared to BP-I. Further, seasonality ($p = 0.035$) and rapid-cycling course ($p = 0.062$) were more common in BP-II. Regarding manic expression, 'elated mood' was predominant in BP-II whereas 'elated mood' and 'irritable mood' were equally prevalent in BP-I. With regard to depressive symptoms, psychomotor agitation, guilty feeling, and suicidal ideation were more frequently observed in BP-II. BP-II patients exhibited a higher trend of lifetime co-occurrence of an axis I diagnosis ($p = 0.09$), and a significantly higher incidence of phobia and eating disorder. The overall occurrence rate of psychiatric illness in first-degree relatives was 15.4% in BP-I and 26.5% in BP-II ($p = 0.01$). Major depression ($p = 0.005$) and substance-related disorder ($p = 0.051$) were more prevalent in relatives of BP-II probands.

Conclusion.—Distinctive characteristics of BP-II were identified in the current study and could be adopted to facilitate the differential diagnosis of BP-I and BP-II in ordinary clinical settings.

▶ The authors studied 71 patients with bipolar I disorder (BP-I) and 34 patients with bipolar II disorder (BP-II) and 374 of their first-degree relatives. They did in fact find differences between BP-I and BP-II symptomatology. The frequency of depressive episodes was significantly ($P = .009$) higher in BP-II patients as well as seasonality ($P = .035$), and rapid cycling ($P = .062$). "Elated mood" was more predominant in BP-II, whereas "elated mood" and "irritable mood" were approximately equal in frequency in BP-I. These more severe symptom pictures in BP-II were certainly surprising for this supposedly "simpler and milder" form of bipolar disorder.

J. C. Ballenger, MD

The seasonality of bipolar affective disorder: Comparison with a primary care sample using the Seasonal Pattern Assessment Questionnaire
Shand AJ, Scott NW, Anderson SM, et al (Royal Cornhill Hosp, Aberdeen, UK; Univ of Aberdeen, UK)
J Affect Disord 132:289-292, 2011

Background.—In contrast with recurrent unipolar depression, relatively little is known about the seasonality of depressive episodes in bipolar affective disorder (BAD).

Method.—We compared responses on the Seasonal Pattern Assessment Questionnaire (SPAQ) between a cohort of 183 patients with BAD and a large sample of patients in primary care (N = 4746). Comparisons were adjusted for age and gender.

Results.—27% of the BAD patients fulfilled SPAQ criteria for Seasonal Affective Disorder (SAD. This gave an adjusted odds ratio of 3.73 (95% confidence intervals 2.64 to 5.27) in comparison with the rate among the primary care samples. Global seasonality scores were significantly higher among BAD patients (adjusted mean difference 1.73, 95% CI 0.97 to 2.49, p < 0.001).

Limitations.—The SPAQ was originally designed as a screening instrument rather than as a case-finding instrument.

Conclusions.—Vigilance for seasonal symptom recurrence in BAD may be important with regard to management and relapse prevention.

▶ In this large sample of 183 patients with bipolar affective disorder (BAD), 7% actually fulfilled criteria for seasonal affective disorder, 4 times that seen in a large comparison primary care group. The authors make a plea that given how frequently this seems to occur, it may be important in the management and prevention of BAD patients.

J. C. Ballenger, MD

A clinical review of aripiprazole in bipolar depression and maintenance therapy of bipolar disorder
Yatham LN (Univ of British Columbia, Vancouver, Canada)
J Affect Disord 128:S21-S28, 2011

Background.—Bipolar disorder is a chronic, recurrent disorder with a significant negative impact on quality of life. Effective treatments are available for acute mania. In contrast, there is a lack of consensus on the treatment of acute bipolar depression and long treatment options for bipolar disorder require more study. Aripiprazole is FDA approved for the treatment of acute mania. This paper reviews current data on the efficacy of aripiprazole in the treatment of acute bipolar depression and in maintenance therapy of bipolar disorder.

Methods.—PubMed and abstracts of recent conferences were searched for randomized, double-blind studies that investigated the efficacy of aripiprazole in acute bipolar depression or maintenance therapy of bipolar disorder.

Results.—Two studies assessed the efficacy of aripiprazole monotherapy in the treatment of acute bipolar depression. These showed that although aripiprazole significantly reduced depressive symptoms early in treatment, the results were not significantly different from placebo at the primary end point of week 8. As to long-term treatment, aripiprazole was superior to placebo in delaying time to relapse for manic episodes, but not for depressive episodes after 26 and 100 weeks of maintenance therapy. Aripiprazole was as effective as lithium, and adjunctive aripiprazole with lithium or valproate was more effective than placebo plus lithium or valproate, in preventing a manic relapse. Reductions in manic and mixed relapse rates compared to placebo were achieved in a study combining aripiprazole with lamotrigine; however, the results were not statistically significant. Similar to other maintenance studies, depressive relapse rates were not significantly reduced compared to placebo.

Limitations.—Negative findings for aripiprazole in the treatment of acute bipolar depression have been attributed to high study doses, rapid titration, and high placebo rates. A recent post-hoc analysis demonstrated that aripiprazole was more effective in patients with severe depressive symptoms, particularly for patients on a lower dose. Further research is needed to confirm this finding. The inability of aripiprazole to reduce the time to depressive relapse during maintenance therapy may be due to the recruitment of patients with an index manic episode and a consequent lower incidence of depressive relapses. Therefore, studies using a depression index episode are needed to appropriately evaluate relapse prevention.

Conclusions.—Although aripiprazole has proven efficacy for acute mania and the prevention of mania, the evidence available thus far does not support the efficacy of aripiprazole for the treatment of acute bipolar depression and prevention of depressive relapse. Further studies with appropriate doses and a depressive index episode are needed to clarify the role of aripiprazole in bipolar disorder.

▶ In the field, we are still searching for appropriate treatments for bipolar depression and the maintenance therapy of bipolar disorder. There are 2 recent studies of aripiprazole monotherapy in acute bipolar depression that demonstrated reduced depressive symptoms early in treatment, although they were not significantly different from placebo at week 8. In long-term studies, aripiprazole has been shown to be superior to placebo in delaying time to relapse from manic episodes, but not depressive episodes, after 26 and 100 weeks of maintenance therapy. It was as effective as lithium, and adjunctive aripiprazole with lithium or valproate was more effective than placebo plus lithium or valproate in preventing a manic relapse. Given the entire literature, the authors conclude that although aripiprazole has sufficient demonstrated efficacy in acute mania and the prevention of mania, the available evidence does not support efficacy for aripiprazole in acute bipolar depression or in the prevention of depressive relapses. They caution that the studies have not used the appropriate index episode (ie, depression) and that may be the cause of failure to see a placebo aripiprazole difference. However, as we struggle to find appropriate maintenance therapy, it appears that aripiprazole does not yet seem to fill the bill entirely.

J. C. Ballenger, MD

A Clinician's Guide to Monitoring Kidney Function in Lithium-Treated Patients

Jefferson JW (Healthcare Technology Systems, Madison, WI)
J Clin Psychiatry 71:1153-1157, 2010

Objective.—Bipolar disorder treatment guidelines recommend kidney-function monitoring at regular intervals for patients taking lithium, but they tend not to provide specifics with regard to what to measure and how to ensure that the results most accurately reflect true kidney function. This overview clarifies those practical aspects of monitoring that are often overlooked or misunderstood.

Data Sources.—Utilized English language materials were obtained by PubMed searches (1970–2009), from the Lithium Information Center database, and from books. Search terms included *lithium, kidney function, creatinine, creatinine clearance, GFR, GFR prediction equations, albuminuria,* and *urine concentration.*

Data Synthesis.—Urine osmolality most accurately reflects urine concentrating ability, although specific gravity is usually adequate for clinical purposes. Serum creatinine concentration can be influenced by extrarenal factors, but even when these are controlled, it remains a less than ideal measure of glomerular filtration rate (GFR). Prediction equations are used commonly to estimate GFR and are an advance over serum creatinine alone, but even they are not as useful when GFR is only mildly impaired. Urine albumin measurement is important, but it requires greater standardization and sensitivity to maximize its potential.

Conclusions.—The safe and effective use of lithium requires regular monitoring of kidney function. Doing so effectively requires knowledge of what to measure, how to ensure accurate results, and how to properly interpret them.

▶ Jeff Jefferson from Madison, Wisconsin, has for some time been our field's monitor about the appropriate use of lithium. In this article, he recommends what he thinks are the appropriate monitoring intervals of kidney function for patients taking lithium. From the data he has collected for his Lithium Information Center database, he discusses this entire area and suggests changes in the way that we have been generally operating. He thinks that the data justify using glomerular filtration rates (GFR) rather than serum creatinine alone since creatinine is more frequently influenced by extra renal factors. However, even the GFR is limited when it is in the mildly impaired range. I recommend this article for practicing clinicians who are using lithium, which I hope includes any and all clinicians treating bipolar patients.

J. C. Ballenger, MD

Adjunctive Armodafinil for Major Depressive Episodes Associated With Bipolar I Disorder: A Randomized, Multicenter, Double-Blind, Placebo-Controlled, Proof-of-Concept Study

Calabrese JR, Ketter TA, Youakim JM, et al (Case Western Reserve Univ, Cleveland, OH; Stanford Univ School of Medicine, CA; Cephalon, Inc, Frazer, PA; et al)
J Clin Psychiatry 71:1363-1370, 2010

Objective.—To evaluate the efficacy and safety of armodafinil, the longer-lasting isomer of modafinil, when used adjunctively in patients with bipolar depression.

Method.—In this 8-week, multicenter, randomized, double-blind, placebo-controlled study conducted between June 2007 and December

2008, patients who were experiencing a major depressive episode associated with bipolar I disorder (according to *DSM-IV-TR* criteria) despite treatment with lithium, olanzapine, or valproic acid were randomly assigned to adjunctive armodafinil 150 mg/d (n = 128) or placebo (n = 129) administered once daily in the morning. The primary outcome measure was change from baseline in the total 30-item Inventory of Depressive Symptomatology, Clinician-Rated (IDS-C$_{30}$) score. Secondary outcomes included changes from baseline in scores on the Montgomery-Åsberg Depression Rating Scale, among other psychological symptom scales. Statistical analyses were performed using analysis of covariance (ANCOVA), with study drug and concurrent mood stabilizer treatment for bipolar disorder as factors and the corresponding baseline value as a covariate. A pre-specified sensitivity analysis was done using analysis of variance (ANOVA) if a statistically significant treatment-by-baseline interaction was found. Tolerability was also assessed.

Results.—A significant baseline-by-treatment interaction in the total IDS-C$_{30}$ score ($P = .08$) was found. Patients administered adjunctive armodafinil showed greater improvement in depressive symptoms as seen in the greater mean ± SD change on the total IDS-C$_{30}$ score (-15.8 ± 11.57) compared with the placebo group (-12.8 ± 12.54) (ANOVA: $P = .044$; ANCOVA: $P = .074$). No differences between treatment groups were observed in secondary outcomes. Adverse events reported more frequently in patients receiving adjunctive armodafinil were headache, diarrhea, and insomnia. Armodafinil was not associated with an increased incidence and/ or severity of suicidality, depression, or mania or with changes in metabolic profile measurements.

Conclusions.—In this proof-of-concept study, adjunctive armodafinil 150 mg/d appeared to improve depressive symptoms according to some, but not all, measures and was generally well tolerated in patients with bipolar depression.

Trial Registration.—clinicaltrials.gov Identifier: NCT00481195.

▶ One of the new medications and medication classes that we now have available is the wakefulness-promoting agent, modafinil, and its longer-lasting isomer, armodafinil. I personally have found modafinil to be useful in depression, and this has been backed up by the literature. This 8-week, multicenter, randomized, double-blind, placebo-controlled trial studied this issue in a large sample of bipolar depressed individuals who had failed to respond despite treatment with lithium, olanzapine, or valproaic acid. They were administered armodafinil (150 mg/d, n = 128) or placebo (n = 129) each morning. Patients on armodafinil did show greater improvement in their depressive symptoms compared with the placebo group on many, but not all, of the outcome measures used. Side effects on armodafinil included headache, diarrhea, and insomnia. Although this was a proof-of-concept study, its size and design do allow us preliminary understanding that this, like modafinil, is potentially quite useful in the treatment of bipolar depression.

J. C. Ballenger, MD

Antidepressants for the Acute Treatment of Bipolar Depression: A Systematic Review and Meta-Analysis

Sidor MM, MacQueen GM (Univ of Texas, Dallas; Univ of Calgary, Alberta, Canada)
J Clin Psychiatry 72:156-167, 2011

Objective.—The role of antidepressants in the acute treatment of bipolar depression remains a contentious issue. A previous meta-analysis of randomized controlled trials (RCTs) concluded that antidepressants were effective and safe for bipolar depression. Several trials published since then suggest that antidepressants may not be as beneficial as previously concluded. The current systematic review and meta-analyses reexamine the efficacy and safety of antidepressant use for the acute treatment of bipolar depression.

Data Sources.—EMBASE, MEDLINE, CINAHL, PsycINFO, and the Cochrane Central Register of Controlled Trials databases were searched for double- blind RCTs published from 2003 to 2009 using the following diagnostic medical subject heading (MESH) terms: *bipolar disorder, bipolar depression, bipolar I disorder, bipolar II disorder, bipolar III disorder, bipolar mania, cyclothymia, manic depressive psychosis, mixed mania and depression, and rapid cycling and bipolar disorder.* Databases of trial registries were also searched for unpublished RCTs. These searches were supplemented by hand searches of relevant articles and review articles.

Study Selection.—Trials that compared acute (<16 wk) antidepressant treatment with either an active drug or a placebo comparator in adult bipolar patients, depressive phase were eligible for inclusion. Main outcome measures were clinical response, remission, and affective switch.

Data Synthesis.—Six RCTs (N = 1,034) were identified since publication in 2004 of the first meta-analysis that assessed antidepressant use in the acute treatment of bipolar depression. These studies were combined with earlier studies for a total of 15 studies containing 2,373 patients. Antidepressants were not statistically superior to placebo or other current standard treatment for bipolar depression. Antidepressants were not associated with an increased risk of switch. Studies that employed more sensitive criteria to define switch did report elevated switch rates for antidepressants.

Conclusions.—Although antidepressants were found to be safe for the acute treatment of bipolar depression, their lack of efficacy may limit their clinical utility. Further high-quality studies are required to address the existing limitations in the literature.

▶ This is an issue that I have followed in past years because of the evidence that antidepressants are not effective in bipolar depression, yet almost all bipolar patients are on antidepressants. The authors searched the published and some of the unpublished trials in the bipolar spectrum. They used 6 randomized controlled trials published since 2004 and combined those with earlier studies giving them a total of 15 studies with 2373 patients. In this cumulative litera- ture, the antidepressants were not statistically superior to placebo, but they did find that they were not associated with an increased risk of switching mood states, except in trials where they used more sensitive criteria for switches. This remains an interesting and important study for clinicians to think about because most clinicians and most patients clamor for antidepres- sants when they become depressed, but they may not be effective in this condition.

J. C. Ballenger, MD

Clinical Predictors Associated With Duration of Repetitive Transcranial Magnetic Stimulation Treatment for Remission in Bipolar Depression: A Naturalistic Study
Cohen RB, Brunoni AR, Boggio PS, et al (Centro Brasileiro de Estimulacao Magnetica Transcraniana, Sao Paulo, Brazil; Univ of Sao Paulo, Brazil; Mackenzie Presbyterian Univ, Sao Paulo, Brazil)
J Nerv Ment Dis 198:679-681, 2010

Repetitive transcranial magnetic stimulation (rTMS) has been widely tested and shown to be effective for unipolar depression. Although it has also been investigated for bipolar depression (BD), there are only few rTMS studies with BD. Here, we investigated 56 patients with BD who received rTMS treatment until remission (defined as Hamilton Depression Rating Scores ≤ 7). We used simple and multiple logistic regressions to identify clinical and demographic predictors associated with duration of treatment (defined as <15 vs. >15 rTMS sessions). Age, refractoriness, number of prior depressive episodes, and severe depression at baseline were associated with a longer rTMS treatment. In the multivar- iate analysis, refractoriness (likelihood ratio $(LR) = 4.33$; $p < 0.01$) and baseline severity $(LR = 0.18$, $p < 0.01)$ remained significant predictors. Our preliminary study showed that, in remitted patients, refractoriness and severity of index episode are associated with the need of a longer rTMS treatment; providing preliminary evidence of important factors associated with rTMS parameters adjustment.

▶ This study fills a gap in our understanding of repetitive transcranial magnetic stimulation (rTMS) in that they studied 56 patients with bipolar depression. Although we have growing knowledge of the effectiveness of rTMS in unipolar depression, we have few studies in bipolar depression. They studied the number of treatments used to develop a remission and used the cutoff of less than 15 and more than 15 rTMS sessions. They were able to demonstrate in this prelim- inary study that the severity of the index episode and their measure of refracto- riness to previous treatments predicted the need for longer rTMS treatments. I was impressed when I visited clinicians in Brazil and other South American and some European countries how well accepted rTMS is in those areas, prob- ably because of its ease of administration. There were many clinicians who were strong advocates based on experience with huge numbers of patients they had treated clinically. It is my sense that rTMS is on the verge of being much more widely used in the United States, which, in my opinion, is a very appropriate step forward in our field.

J. C. Ballenger, MD

Complexity of Pharmacologic Treatment Required for Sustained Improvement in Outpatients With Bipolar Disorder
Post RM, Altshuler LL, Frye MA, et al (George Washington Univ, DC; Univ of California, Los Angeles; Mayo Clinic, Rochester, MN; et al)
J Clin Psychiatry 71:1176-1186, 2010

Objective.—To evaluate the clinical correlates of and types of naturalistic treatments associated with sustained improvement/remission for at least 6 months in outpatients with bipolar disorder.

Method.—Five hundred twenty-five outpatients with bipolar disorder (77.7% bipolar I) gave informed consent, had their mood rated daily on the National Institute of Mental Health Life Chart Method for a minimum of at least 1 year, and recorded all medications. Demographics and clinical characteristics of patients with a "sustained response" (ratings of "improved" or "very much improved" on the Clinical Global Impressions-Bipolar Version for a period of at least 6 months) versus nonresponders were compared. The study was conducted from 1996 to 2002.

Results.—Of the 429 patients who were ill at study entry, 195 (45.5%) showed a sustained response; 54.5% showed no or insufficient response. A mean of 2.98 medications was given at time of improvement, which occurred after a mean of 18 months of participation in the study. Lithium and valproate were the medications most frequently prescribed at the time of improvement and had among the highest overall success rates. Equally complex regimens were employed in the nonresponders who, however, had a more adverse clinical course prior to network entry. Nonresponders were ultimately exposed to more antidepressants and antipsychotics than the sustained responders.

Conclusions.—A mean of 1.5 years and at times highly complex medication regimens were required to achieve a sustained response for 6 months during naturalistic outpatient treatment of bipolar disorder. Delineating the clinical and biologic correlates of individual response to combination treatment is a very high clinical research priority, as is developing new treatment strategies for the large proportion of patients who fail to respond in a sustained fashion.

▶ This is another valuable contribution from my old colleague Bob Post and the Stanley Network of bipolar researchers that he developed across the country. In this publication, they followed 525 outpatients with bipolar disorder (77.7% bipolar I) who had daily ratings of their mood for at least a year. They rated the patients who reached a sustained response of "improved" or "very much improved" for at least 6 months versus nonresponders. Interestingly, 45.5% showed a sustained response, but 54.5% showed no response or an insufficient response, although they were on a mean of 2.9 medications. Lithium and valproate were the 2 medications with the highest overall success, although these medicines and complex regimens were also used in the nonresponders who were ultimately exposed to even more antipsychotics and antidepressants than the responders. They were able to state that even with very complex medication regimens used by these very experienced bipolar researcher clinicians, it took a minimum of 18 months for less than half of the patients to obtain a sustained response. This study documents well that even in the most experienced hands, bipolar I outpatients in most cases are not doing well despite aggressive and sometimes heroic medication regimens. This is no surprise to those of us who try to treat these patients. Despite the progress of new and old medications in this condition, it remains a very difficult-to-treat condition.

J. C. Ballenger, MD

Suicide

Availability of Mental Health Service Providers and Suicide Rates in Austria: A Nationwide Study
Kapusta ND, Posch M, Niederkrotenthaler T, et al (Med Univ of Vienna, Austria)
Psychiatr Serv 61:1198-1203, 2010

Objective.—Evidence shows that access to mental health services may have an impact on mental health outcomes such as suicide rates. This small-area analysis examined whether the availability of professionals providing mental health treatment in Austria had an effect on regional suicide rates.

Methods.—A hierarchical Bayesian model accounting for spatially correlated random effects using an intrinsic conditional autoregressive prior that incorporated the neighborhood structure of districts and that assumed a Poisson distribution for the observed number of suicides was used to estimate the effects of access to mental health care (population density of general practitioners, psychiatrists, and psychotherapists) in Austria.

Results.—Regional socioeconomic factors were correlated with the density of psychiatrists and psychotherapists. Only the number of psychotherapists per 10,000 population had a significant effect on suicide rates (relative risk [RR]=.97, 95% confidence interval [CI]=.94 −.997, and absolute risk reduction [ARR]=−.62, CI=−1.20 to −.11); however, after adjustment for socioeconomic factors (in particular urbanicity as indicated by population density, average income, and proportion of non-Catholics), the observed effects were no longer significant. In the final model, only the socioeconomic component remained significant (RR=.94, CI=.88 −.99), and ARR=−1.17, CI=−2.34 to −.05).

Conclusions.—The availability of specialized mental health service providers was associated with regional socioeconomic factors, and these factors appeared to be stronger predictors of suicide rates than the availability of providers. Therefore, suicide prevention efforts need to acknowledge that availability of services is only one aspect of access to care; a more influential factor is whether availability satisfies local demand.

▶ These authors studied the availability of psychotherapists per 10 000 of the population in Austria and found a significant effect on suicide rates; however, adjusting for socioeconomic factors changed the findings and conclusions. Ultimately, they concluded that availability of specialized mental health providers was associated with regional socioeconomic factors and those factors appeared to be stronger predictors of suicide rates than the availability of providers. They concluded that suicide prevention efforts need to deal with the fact that availability of services is only one aspect of access to care, and a more influential issue was whether availability actually meets local demand. This is a common sense conclusion, and it is refreshing to see that they realized that availability is most powerful when it actually meets the demand for that service.

J. C. Ballenger, MD

Clinical and Psychosocial Predictors of Suicide Attempts and Nonsuicidal Self-Injury in the Adolescent Depression Antidepressants and Psychotherapy Trial (ADAPT)
Wilkinson P, Kelvin R, Roberts C, et al (Cambridge Univ, England, UK; Manchester Univ, England, UK; Royal Manchester Children's Hosp, Pendlebury, England, UK)
Am J Psychiatry 168:495-501, 2011

Objective.—The authors assessed whether clinical and psychosocial factors in depressed adolescents at baseline predict suicide attempts and nonsuicidal self-injury over 28 weeks of follow-up.

Method.—Participants were 164 adolescents with major depressive disorder taking part in the Adolescent Depression Antidepressants and Psychotherapy Trial (ADAPT). Clinical symptoms, family function, quality of current personal friendships, and suicidal and nonsuicidal self-harm were assessed at baseline. Suicidal and nonsuicidal self-harm thoughts and behaviors were assessed during 28 weeks of follow-up.

Results.—High suicidality, nonsuicidal self-injury, and poor family function at entry were significant independent predictors of suicide attempts over the 28 weeks of follow-up. Nonsuicidal self-injury over the follow-up period was independently predicted by nonsuicidal self-injury, hopelessness, anxiety disorder, and being younger and female at entry.

Conclusions.—Both suicidal and nonsuicidal self-harm persisted in depressed adolescents receiving treatment in the ADAPT study. A history of nonsuicidal self-injury prior to treatment is a clinical marker for subsequent suicide attempts and should be as carefully assessed in depressed youths as current suicidal intent and behavior.

▶ These authors used the data from the Adolescent Depression Antidepressants and Psychotherapy Trial (ADAPT). The participants were 164 depressed adolescents followed for 28 weeks. They found that in fact high suicidality and nonsuicidal self-injury and poor family function at entry were significant predictors of suicide attempts over the 28 weeks. Also, suicidal self-injury was predicted by hopelessness, anxiety disorder, being younger and female at entry, and a previous nonsuicidal self-injury. These appear to be clear markers for subsequent difficulty and obviously need to be assessed in any depressed adolescent.

J. C. Ballenger, MD

Risk of suicide and mixed episode in men in the postpartum period
Quevedo L, da Silva RA, Coelho F, et al (Catholic Univ of Pelotas, Brazil; et al)
J Affect Disord 132:243-246, 2011

Objectives.—To assess suicide risk in men with mood disorders at the postpartum period.

Methods.—We conduct a longitudinal study with 650 men whose child has born from April 2007 to May 2008 at maternity hospital. The first assessment was in the antenatal period and the second within 30 to 60 days postpartum. Suicide risk, anxiety disorders, hypomanic, manic and mixed episodes were assessed by the Mini International Neuropsychiatric Interview (MINI).

Results.—The prevalence of suicide risk in fathers in postpartum was of 4.8%. Fathers with postpartum depression were 20.97 (CI: 5.74; 76.53) more likely to present suicide risk and those with mixed episodes showed a chance of 46.50 (CI: 10.52; 205.53) times higher than those who did not suffer from any mood disorder.

Conclusion.—Mixed episodes are common in fathers at postpartum, posing a higher suicide risk than depressive and manic/hypomanic episodes. Therefore, in order to reduce the suicide risk, clinicians should address and treat adequately mixed affective states in this specific population.

▶ This article provides a look at the flip side of the risk of depression in pregnancy. These authors assessed the suicide risk in men with mood disorders in the postpartum period. What they found was that the suicidal risk in fathers in this period was 4.8%. Men with postpartum depression were almost 21 times more likely to present with suicide risk, and those with mixed episodes had a chance almost 47 times higher than those without a mood disorder. This is a fairly striking conclusion that depressed episodes are common in new fathers and pose a significant suicidal risk. It is clear that pregnancy and postpartum pose a higher risk for mothers and now for fathers as well, particularly mothers and fathers who have a history or risk of depression.

J. C. Ballenger, MD

Suicidal risk and suicide attempts in people treated with antiepileptic drugs for epilepsy

Machado RA, Espinosa AG, Melendrez D, et al (Natl Neurology Inst, Plaza, Havana City, Cuba; Psychiatry Hospital (Eduardo Berbabé Ordaz Dupungé), Boyero, Havana City, Cuba; Roosevelt Univ, Cuba)
Seizure 20:280-284, 2011

Objective.—To determine whether antiepileptic drugs constitute in themselves an independent risk factor for suicidality in patients with epilepsy.

Methods.—One hundred and thirty one patients with epilepsy were recruited and followed-up during 5 years. A detailed medical history, neurological examination, EEGs, Mini-International Neuropsychiatric Interview, executive function, and MRI were assessed. Systematically collected data were used to assess suicidality. Multiple regression analysis was carried out to examine predictive associations between clinical variables, psychiatric disorders, antiepileptic drugs and suicidality.

Results.—We identified two AEDs related with suicide attempts (PHB and LTG) and four with suicidal risk: PHB, PRM, PHT and LTG, but the increased of risk diminished or disappeared when psychiatric comorbidity and other well established risk factors for suicidality were analyzed. We found a significant proportion of patients with depressive episodes associated with Topiramate, Phenitoin, Phenobarbital and Lamotrigine.

Conclusion.—Antiepileptic drugs probably do not have an impact on suicidality.

▶ One of the disturbing questions recently has been whether anticonvulsant drugs increase suicidality. These authors examined this issue in 131 patients with epilepsy and followed them for 5 years. Although they found a significant number of patients on various antiepileptic drugs with increased suicidal risks, when all of the relevant issues of comorbidity and well-established risk factors were considered, they found no increase in suicidality among patients on antiepileptic drugs. This is a welcome report that these drugs are seemingly safe since we are using them to such a great extent in psychiatry and neurology.

J. C. Ballenger, MD

The Social Environment and Suicide Attempts in Lesbian, Gay, and Bisexual Youth

Hatzenbuehler ML (Columbia Univ, NY)
Pediatrics 127:896-903, 2011

Objective.—To determine whether the social environment surrounding lesbian, gay, and bisexual youth may contribute to their higher rates of suicide attempts, controlling for individual-level risk factors.

Methods.—A total of 31 852 11th grade students (1413 [4.4%] lesbian, gay, and bisexual individuals) in Oregon completed the Oregon Healthy Teens survey in 2006–2008. We created a composite index of the social environment in 34 counties, including (1) the proportion of same-sex couples, (2) the proportion of registered Democrats, (3) the presence of gay-straight alliances in schools, and (4) school policies (nondiscrimination and antibullying) that specifically protected lesbian, gay, and bisexual students.

Results.—Lesbian, gay, and bisexual youth were significantly more likely to attempt suicide in the previous 12 months, compared with heterosexuals (21.5% vs 4.2%). Among lesbian, gay, and bisexual youth, the risk of attempting suicide was 20% greater in unsupportive environments compared to supportive environments. A more supportive social environment was significantly associated with fewer suicide attempts, controlling for sociodemographic variables and multiple risk factors for suicide attempts, including depressive symptoms, binge drinking, peer victimization, and physical abuse by an adult (odds ratio: 0.97 [95% confidence interval: 0.96–0.99]).

Conclusions.—This study documents an association between an objective measure of the social environment and suicide attempts among lesbian, gay, and bisexual youth. The social environment appears to confer risk for suicide attempts over and above individual-level risk factors. These results have important implications for the development of policies and interventions to reduce sexual orientation-related disparities in suicide attempts.

▶ These authors studied 31 852 11th grade students in Oregon. They document that lesbian, gay, and bisexual youth were significantly more likely to attempt suicide in the previous 12 months, 21.5% compared with 4.2% of heterosexuals. The risk of attempting suicide was 20% greater in nonsupportive environments (school and home). This much greater risk is not surprising, but it is so high that it has clear policy implications in schools as well as at home.

J. C. Ballenger, MD

Anxiety

A Deletion in Tropomyosin-Related Kinase B and the Development of Human Anxiety

Ernst C, Wanner B, Brezo J, et al (McGill Univ, Montreal, Quebec, Canada; Univ of Montréal, Canada)
Biol Psychiatry 69:604-607, 2011

Background.—The tropomyosin-related kinase B (TrkB)/brain-derived neurotrophic factor system has been associated with psychiatric disorders, and animal models of defects in this system suggest that it might have a particular role in anxiety.

Methods.—DNA sequencing and cloning were used to identify a mutation in *TrkB*, and four different cell lines were used to assess functionality. Clinical samples were from a 22-year longitudinal cohort representative of the Quebec general population ($n = 640$ subjects), randomly selected when they were in kindergarten. Anxiety-related traits were measured with the Social Behaviour Questionnaire, the Diagnostic Assessment of Personality Pathology-Brief Questionnaire, and the Diagnostic Interview Schedule for DSM-IIIR.

Results.—An 11 base pair deletion in *TrkB* is significantly associated with increases in anxiety traits during childhood and the development of anxiety disorders in adulthood. We found that this deletion impaired transcription in some human cell lines.

Conclusions.—The identification of this deletion provides additional support for the role of TrkB in modulating anxiety-related traits in human.

▶ As some of you may know, I have been interested in the development and treatment of anxiety disorders for some time. These authors report a very interesting and potentially important study, although a somewhat complicated one. They did DNA sequencing and cloning and identified a mutation in the tropomyosin-related kinase B (TrkB)/brain-derived neurotrophic factor system. They followed 640 subjects in Quebec for a 22-year longitudinal study beginning when these kids were in kindergarten. They measured their anxiety-related traits throughout this period. Strikingly, they did find that the 11 base pair depletion in TrkB was significantly associated with an increase in anxiety traits during childhood and the development of anxiety disorders when these kids reached adulthood. This is consistent with previous research and a very interesting finding.

J. C. Ballenger, MD

A Randomized Controlled Trial of Cognitive-Behavioral Therapy for Generalized Anxiety Disorder With Integrated Techniques From Emotion-Focused and Interpersonal Therapies

Newman MG, Castonguay LG, Borkovec TD, et al (The Pennsylvania State Univ)
J Consult Clin Psychol 79:171-181, 2011

Objective.—Recent models suggest that generalized anxiety disorder (GAD) symptoms may be maintained by emotional processing avoidance and interpersonal problems.

Method.—This is the first randomized controlled trial to test directly whether cognitive-behavioral therapy (CBT) could be augmented with the addition of a module targeting interpersonal problems and emotional processing. Eighty-three primarily White participants (mean age = 37) with a principle diagnosis of GAD were recruited from the community. Participants were assigned randomly to CBT plus supportive listening

($n = 40$) or to CBT plus interpersonal and emotional processing therapy ($n = 43$) within a study using an additive design. Doctoral-level psychologists with full-time private practices treated participants in an outpatient clinic. Using blind assessors, participants were assessed at pretreatment, posttreatment, 6-month, 1-year, and 2-year follow-up with a composite of self-report and assessor-rated GAD symptom measures (the Penn State Worry Questionnaire; T. J. Meyer, M. L. Miller, R. L. Metzger, & T. D. Borkovec, 1990; Hamilton Anxiety Rating Scale; M. Hamilton, 1959; assessor severity rating; State—Trait Anxiety Inventory-Trait Version; C. D. Spielberger, R. L. Gorsuch, R. Lushene, P. R. Vagg, & G. A. Jacobs, 1983) as well as with indices of clinically significant change.

Results.—Mixed models analysis of all randomized participants showed very large within-treatment effect sizes for both treatments ($CI = [-.40, -.28]$, $d = 1.86$) with no significant differences at post ($CI = [-.09, .07]$, $d = .07$) or 2-year follow-up ($CI = [-.01, .01]$), $d = .12$). There was also no statistical difference between compared treatments on clinically significant change based on chi-square analysis.

Conclusions.—Interpersonal and emotional processing techniques may not augment CBT for all GAD participants.

Trial Registry Name.—ClinicalTrials.gov, Identifier: NCT00951652.

▶ These authors performed a large randomized trial of 83 participants with generalized anxiety disorder (GAD). They report that this is the first randomized controlled trial to test whether adding a module targeting interpersonal problems and emotional processing would add to the cognitive-behavioral therapy effects in this patient population. The study was well controlled and found no difference between the CBT with and without the other modules of interpersonal and emotional processing target therapy. It is striking that this is another study showing that CBT has large treatment effects in GAD into a 1-year follow-up. It seems clear that CBT should be a frequently offered treatment for GAD, but I do not think it is, at least for psychiatrists who are generally unfamiliar with CBT therapy for GAD.

J. C. Ballenger, MD

Deep Brain Stimulation of the Nucleus Accumbens for Treatment-Refractory Obsessive-Compulsive Disorder
Denys D, Mantione M, Figee M, et al (Univ of Amsterdam, the Netherlands; et al)
Arch Gen Psychiatry 67:1061-1068, 2010

Context.—Obsessive-compulsive disorder (OCD) is a chronic psychiatric disorder that affects 2% of the general population. Even when the best available treatments are applied, approximately 10% of patients remain severely afflicted and run a long-term deteriorating course of OCD.

Objective.—To determine whether bilateral deep brain stimulation of the nucleus accumbens is an effective and safe treatment for treatment-refractory OCD.

Design.—The study consisted of an open 8-month treatment phase, followed by a double-blind crossover phase with randomly assigned 2-week periods of active or sham stimulation, ending with an open 12-month maintenance phase.

Setting.—Academic research.

Patients.—Sixteen patients (age range, 18-65 years) with OCD according to DSM-IV criteria meeting stringent criteria for refractoriness to treatment were included in the study.

Interventions.—Treatment with bilateral deep brain stimulation of the nucleus accumbens.

Main Outcome Measures.—Primary efficacy was assessed by score change from baseline on the Yale-Brown Obsessive Compulsive Scale (Y-BOCS). Responders were defined by a score decrease of at least 35% on the Y-BOCS.

Results.—In the open phase, the mean (SD) Y-BOCS score decreased by 46%, from 33.7 (3.6) at baseline to 18.0 (11.4) after 8 months ($P<.001$). Nine of 16 patients were responders, with amean (SD) Y-BOCS score decrease of 23.7 (7.0), or 72%. In the double-blind, sham-controlled phase (n=14), the mean (SD) Y-BOCS score difference between active and sham stimulation was 8.3 (2.3), or 25% ($P=.004$). Depression and anxiety decreased significantly. Except for mild forgetfulness and word-finding problems, no permanent adverse events were reported.

Conclusion.—Bilateral deep brain stimulation of the nucleus accumbens may be an effective and safe treatment for treatment-refractory OCD.

Clinical Trial Registration.—isrctn.org Identifier: ISRCTN23255677.

▶ This Dutch group has been studying bilateral deep brain stimulation of the nucleus accumbens in patients with refractory obsessive-compulsive disorder (OCD). This article reports their open trial of an 8-month treatment using a double-blind crossover random assignment with 2 weeks of either active or sham stimulation and then following the patients for 12 months. They studied 16 patients using the Yale-Brown Obsessive Compulsive Scale (Y-BOCS) scores, which decreased by 46% from 33.7 at baseline to 18.8 after 8 months. Nine of the 16 patients had good responses with a mean Y-BOCS decrease of 23.7, which is a 72% drop. The difference between sham and active treatment was 8.3 or 25%. Interestingly, depression and anxiety also decreased significantly and there were few adverse events beyond mild forgetfulness and word-finding problems. They argue, and I would concur, that this treatment should be considered in severe, treatment-resistant OCD patients.

J. C. Ballenger, MD

Therapeutic Interventions Related to Outcome in Psychodynamic Psychotherapy for Anxiety Disorder Patients

Slavin-Mulford J, Hilsenroth M, Weinberger J, et al (Massachusetts General Hosp & Harvard Med School, Boston; Adelphi Univ, Garden City, NY)
J Nerv Ment Dis 199:214-221, 2011

This is the first study with acceptable inter-rater reliability to examine specific therapeutic techniques related to change in anxiety disorder patients during short-term psychodynamic psychotherapy. The study first examined the effectiveness of short-term psychodynamic psychotherapy and results showed significant and positive pre-/post-treatment changes on both patient and independent clinical ratings for anxiety, global symptomatology, relational, social, and occupational functioning. Likewise, the majority of patients (76%) reported anxiety symptoms within a normal distribution at termination. Importantly, psychodynamic interventions rated early in treatment (third/fourth session) were positively related to changes in anxiety symptoms. Further, results showed that several individual psychodynamic techniques were meaningfully related to outcome including (1) focusing on wishes, fantasies, dreams, and early memories; (2) linking current feelings or perceptions to the past; (3) highlighting patients' typical relational patterns; and (4) helping patients to understand their experiences in new ways. Clinical applications are discussed.

▶ The authors contend that this is the first study of specific therapeutic techniques that resulted in positive change in patients with anxiety disorder during short-term psychodynamic psychotherapy. They were able to show that 76% of the patients at the end of treatment no longer met the criteria for their anxiety disorder. They were also able to show that the specific psychodynamic techniques were significantly related to outcome, including (1) focusing on wishes, fantasies, dreams, and early memories; (2) linking current feelings to the past; (3) highlighting the particular patient's relationship patterns; and (4) helping patients to understand their experiences in new ways. This was an interesting documentation that short-term psychodynamic therapy is effective. This is good news for a lot of psychiatrists who practice this type of psychiatry, but who are often criticized for not having adequate empirical support for that practice.

J. C. Ballenger, MD

A New Parenting-Based Group Intervention for Young Anxious Children: Results of a Randomized Controlled Trial

Cartwright-Hatton S, McNally D, Field AP, et al (Univ of Manchester, UK; Central Manchester Foundation Trust, UK; Univ of Sussex, UK)
J Am Acad Child Adolesc Psychiatry 50:242-251, 2011

Objective.—Despite recent advances, there are still no interventions that have been developed for the specific treatment of young children who have anxiety disorders. This study examined the impact of a new, cognitive—behaviorally based parenting intervention on anxiety symptoms.

Method.—Families of 74 anxious children (aged 9 years or less) took part in a randomized controlled trial, which compared the new 10-session, group-format intervention with a wait-list control condition. Outcome measures included blinded diagnostic interview and self-reports from parents and children.

Results.—Intention-to-treat analyses indicated that children whose parent(s) received the intervention were significantly less anxious at the end of the study than those in the control condition. Specifically, 57% of those receiving the new intervention were free of their primary disorder, compared with 15% in the control condition. Moreover, 32% of treated children were free of any anxiety diagnosis at the end of the treatment period, compared with 6% of those in the control group. Treatment gains were maintained at 12-month follow-up.

Conclusions.—This new parenting-based intervention may represent an advance in the treatment of this previously neglected group. Clinical trial registration information: Anxiety in Young Children: A Randomized Controlled Trial of a New Cognitive-Behaviourally Based Parenting Intervention; http://www.isrctn.org/; ISRCTN12166762.

▶ I'm delighted to see the attention being paid in the recent literature to developing treatment for young children who have anxiety disorders for which we only have a few well-studied treatments. These authors studied 74 anxious children in a randomized, controlled trial comparing a new 10-session group format with a wait list condition. In fact, they did see that with the parents who received the intervention, their children had significantly less anxiety at the end of the study compared with those in the controlled condition. Of the children whose parents received the intervention, 57% of them had resolved their anxiety disorder compared with only 15% in the controlled condition. These gains were maintained at 12 months. This cognitively based group parent treatment seems effective and could be potentially disseminated given its relatively short duration and group delivery.

J. C. Ballenger, MD

Acute Stress Disorder as a Predictor of Posttraumatic Stress Disorder: A Systematic Review
Bryant RA (Univ of New South Wales, Sydney, Australia)
J Clin Psychiatry 72:233-239, 2011

Objective.—The utility of the acute stress disorder diagnosis to describe acute stress reactions and predict subsequent posttraumatic stress disorder (PTSD) was evaluated.

Data Sources.—A systematic search was conducted in the PsycINFO, MEDLINE, and PubMed databases for English-language articles published between 1994 and 2009 using keywords that combined *acute stress disorder and posttraumatic stress disorder.*

Study Selection.—Studies were selected that assessed for acute stress disorder within 1 month of trauma exposure and assessed at a later time for PTSD, using established measures of acute stress disorder and PTSD.

Data Extraction.—For each study, capacity of the acute stress disorder diagnosis to predict PTSD was calculated in terms of sensitivity, specificity, and positive and negative predictive power. For studies that reported subsyndromal acute stress disorder, the same analyses were calculated for cases that initially satisfied subsyndromal acute stress disorder criteria.

Data Synthesis.—Twenty-two studies were identified as suitable for analysis (19 with adults and 3 with children). Diagnosis of acute stress disorder resulted in half the rate of distressed people in the acute phase being identified relative to including cases with subsyndromal acute stress disorder. In terms of prediction, the acute stress disorder diagnosis had reasonable positive predictive power (proportion of people with acute stress disorder who later developed PTSD). In contrast, the sensitivity (proportion of people who developed PTSD who initially met criteria for acute stress disorder) was poor.

Conclusions.—The acute stress disorder diagnosis does not adequately identify the majority of people who will eventually develop PTSD. There is a need to formally describe acute stress reactions, but this goal may be achieved more usefully by describing the broad range of initial reactions rather than by attempting to predict subsequent PTSD.

▶ This has been an issue that we have debated for some time (ie, in what percentage of individuals does the acute stress disorder diagnosis predict the evolution of posttraumatic stress disorder [PTSD]). This has a practical significance in places where there are very frequent traumatic events, like Israel. Ari Shalev, a PTSD expert in Israel, has argued the extreme practical significance of this question. He and his colleagues in Israel need to know how many individuals obviously traumatized by a bombing or a similar trauma should be treated beyond their emergency room visit. The authors of this article found 22 studies suitable for their analysis. Of traumatized adults distressed with subsyndromal stress disorder, only about half met the diagnosis of acute stress disorder. The diagnosis of acute stress disorder had reasonably positive predictive power for PTSD development, although the sensitivity was low. Unfortunately, this analysis cannot help us identify well most people who will eventually develop PTSD. We will continue to struggle with this issue at this point.

J. C. Ballenger, MD

Aripiprazole: A clinical review of its use for the treatment of anxiety disorders and anxiety as a comorbidity in mental illness
Katzman MA (START Clinic for the Mood and Anxiety Disorders, Toronto, Ontario, Canada)
J Affect Disord 128:S11-S20, 2011

Background.—Although anxiety disorders are common, optimal treatment is elusive. More than half of anxiety patients treated with an adequate course of antidepressants fail to fully improve: treatment resistance, residual symptoms, and recurrence/relapse remain a challenge. Recently, atypical antipsychotics have been considered for treatment-resistant anxiety disorders. This review will explore the available data for the role of aripiprazole in the treatment of anxiety.

Methods.—PubMed and conference abstracts were searched for randomized, double-blind studies that investigated the efficacy of aripiprazole in anxiety; its efficacy in bipolar disorder and depression was also explored for comparison.

Results.—A number of studies have shown atypical antipsychotics to be effective in anxiety, and currently available data suggest that aripiprazole augmentation in patients with anxiety disorders is likely as effective as other atypical antipsychotic drugs. Although there have been no randomized, controlled trials, aripiprazole has been found to be effective in treating anxiety disorders in two open-label trials. This combined with the larger data base demonstrating its utility in bipolar disorder and depression, its safety profile and its unique mechanism of action, make aripiprazole for anxiety an intriguing avenue of exploration.

Limitations.—Data from large randomized, controlled trials on the use of atypical antipsychotics for anxiety in general, and aripiprazole in particular, are currently lacking.

Conclusion.—The results of open-label trials of aripiprazole in anxiety provide enough support to warrant its further study. This, combined with a larger data base demonstrating its utility in bipolar disorder and depression, its safety profile and its unique mechanism of action, make aripiprazole for anxiety an intriguing avenue of exploration.

▶ These authors explore the recent suggestion that atypical antipsychotics may be a valuable adjunctive treatment in anxiety. At this point, at least half of anxiety patients have a poor response to antidepressants or residual symptoms or high relapse. A number of studies suggest that atypical antipsychotics are effective in treating bipolar illness or depression. At this point, there are no controlled trials with aripiprazole in anxiety but 2 open-label trials suggesting efficacy in anxiety conditions. This lack of controlled trials plus its unique mechanism of action suggest aripiprazole should be studied further in the anxiety disorders.

J. C. Ballenger, MD

Computer-Assisted Cognitive Behavioral Therapy for Child Anxiety: Results of a Randomized Clinical Trial

Khanna MS, Kendall PC (Univ of Pennsylvania, Philadelphia; Temple Univ, Philadelphia, PA)
J Consult Clin Psychol 78:737-745, 2010

Objective.—This study examined the feasibility, acceptability, and effects of Camp Cope-A-Lot (CCAL), a computer-assisted cognitive behavioral therapy (CBT) for anxiety in youth.

Method.—Children (49; 33 males) ages 7–13 (M = 10.1 ± 1.6; 83.7% Caucasian, 14.2% African American, 2% Hispanic) with a principal anxiety disorder were randomly assigned to (a) CCAL, (b) individual CBT (ICBT), or (c) a computer-assisted education, support, and attention (CESA) condition. All therapists were from the community (school or counseling psychologists, clinical psychologist) or were PsyD or PhD trainees with no experience or training in CBT for child anxiety. Independent diagnostic interviews and self-report measures were completed at pre- and posttreatment and 3-month follow-up.

Results.—At posttreatment, ICBT or CCAL children showed significantly better gains than CESA children; 70%, 81%, and 19%, respectively, no longer met criteria for their principal anxiety diagnosis. Gains were maintained at follow-up, with no significant differences between ICBT and CCAL. Parents and children rated all treatments acceptable, with CCAL and ICBT children rating higher satisfaction than CESA children.

Conclusions.—Findings support the feasibility, acceptability and beneficial effects of CCAL for anxious youth. Discussion considers the potential of computer-assisted treatments in the dissemination of empirically supported treatments.

▶ This study from the University of Pennsylvania addresses an important area: anxiety in children. They compared a computer-assisted cognitive behavioral therapy (CBT) called Camp Cope-A-Lot (CCAL) with individual CBT (ICBT) or computer-assisted education, support, and attention (CESA). Both the active treatment of CCAL and ICBT led to significantly greater improvement (70%, 81%, and 19%, respectively) in the number of individuals who no longer met criteria for their principal anxiety diagnoses. Improvements were maintained at follow-up, with no significant differences between them. We have now reached the point where we have empirically supported treatments from research settings but are largely confounded by how to apply these in a public health oriented way. This study is quite interesting and promising in that it shows a very acceptable and effective computer-assisted program that the children and parents accepted.

J. C. Ballenger, MD

Effect of Acute Psychological Stress on Prefrontal GABA Concentration Determined by Proton Magnetic Resonance Spectroscopy

Hasler G, van der Veen JW, Grillon C, et al (Univ of Berne, Switzerland; Natl Inst of Mental Health, Bethesda, MD)
Am J Psychiatry 167:1226-1231, 2010

Objective.—Impaired function of the central gamma-aminobutyric acid (GABA) system, which provides the brain's major inhibitory pathways, is thought to play an important role in the pathophysiology of anxiety disorders. The effect of acute psychological stress on the human GABA-ergic system is still unknown, however. The purpose of this study was to determine the effect of acute stress on prefrontal GABA levels.

Method.—A recently developed noninvasive magnetic resonance spectroscopy method was used to measure changes in the GABA concentration of the prefrontal cortex in 10 healthy human subjects during a threat-of-shock condition and during a safe condition (two sessions on different days). The main outcome measure was the mean GABA concentration within a $3 \times 3 \times 2$-cm^3 voxel selected from the medial prefrontal cortex.

Results.—Prefrontal GABA decreased by approximately 18% in the threat-of-shock condition relative to the safe condition. This reduction was specific to GABA, since the concentrations of N-acetyl-aspartate, choline-containing compounds, and glutamate/glutamine levels obtained in the same spectra did not change significantly.

Conclusions.—This result appeared compatible with evidence from preclinical studies in rodents, which showed rapid presynaptic down-regulation of GABA-ergic neurotransmission in response to acute psychological stress. The molecular mechanism and functional significance of this reduced inhibitory effect of acute psychological stress in relation to impaired GABA-ergic function in anxiety disorders merit further investigation.

▶ One of the greatest biological leads we have in the brain pathology related to the anxiety disorders is the hypothesis that central gamma-aminobutyric acid (GABA) systems, which are the major inhibitory pathways of the brain, might be involved. These authors examined the effect of acute stress on prefrontal GABA levels by noninvasive magnetic resonance spectroscopy in 10 healthy subjects in threat-of-shock conditions versus safe conditions. They found that prefrontal GABA was decreased by 18% in the threat-of-shock condition compared with the safe condition and that this reduction was specific to GABA. Human evidence is consistent with evidence from rodents showing rapid presynaptic down regulation of GABA neurotransmission in the context of acute psychological stress. This is yet another example of the steady progress we are making in the neurobiology of the psychiatric disorders toward more basic and clear pathophysiologies of the conditions we try to treat.

J. C. Ballenger, MD

Hippocampal Volume Differences in Gulf War Veterans with Current Versus Lifetime Posttraumatic Stress Disorder Symptoms

Apfel BA, Ross J, Hlavin J, et al (Univ of California, San Francisco; Veterans Affairs Med Ctr, San Francisco, CA; et al)
Biol Psychiatry 69:541-548, 2011

Background.—Decreased hippocampal volume is described in posttraumatic stress disorder (PTSD) and depression. However, it is not known whether it is a risk factor for the development of PTSD or a consequence of PTSD. We sought to determine the effects of PTSD and depressive symptoms on hippocampal volume.

Methods.—Clinical and magnetic resonance imaging data were collected in a cross sectional study of 244 Gulf War veterans. Measures included lifetime and current Clinician Administered PTSD Scale, Hamilton Depression Scale, Life Stressor Checklist, and Lifetime Drinking History. Magnetic resonance imaging data were acquired with a 1.5-T scanner and analyzed with automated and semiautomated image processing techniques.

Results.—Eighty-two veterans had lifetime PTSD, 44 had current PTSD, and 38 had current depression. In the linear regression analysis, current PTSD symptoms (standardized coefficient $\beta = -.25$, $p = .03$) but neither lifetime PTSD symptoms nor current depression were associated with smaller hippocampal volume. Gender, age, history of early life trauma, education, lifetime and current alcohol use, current marijuana use, and treatment with antidepressants did not have independent effects. Participants with chronic PTSD had, on average, a smaller hippocampus compared with those with remitted PTSD.

Conclusions.—The finding that current but not lifetime PTSD symptom severity explains hippocampal size raises two possibilities: either a small hippocampus is a risk factor for lack of recovery from PTSD (trait) or PTSD effects on hippocampal volume are reversible once PTSD symptoms remit and the patient recovers (state).

▶ Although we have observed decreased hippocampal volume in posttraumatic stress disorder (PTSD) and in depression, we do not know whether this is a risk factor or consequence of the trauma in PTSD. These authors were able to use MRI data from 244 Gulf War veterans to approach this issue. They studied 82 who had lifetime PTSD, 44 with chronic PTSD, and 38 with chronic depression. They observed that having current PTSD symptoms was significantly associated with decreased hippocampal volume but neither lifetime PTSD nor current depression were. They were also able to rule out a host of other possibilities, including early trauma, education, alcohol and drug use, and treatment with antidepressants, which did not have any significant effects. That current, but not lifetime, PTSD was associated with small hippocampal size raises 2 major possibilities. One is that a small hippocampus may be a risk factor for failing to recover from PTSD; the other is that hippocampal shrinkage may be reversed when individuals with PTSD recover. Both of these are important possibilities with differing implications, and we will have to look forward to studies that will tease apart this question.

J. C. Ballenger, MD

Schizophrenia

A Randomized Controlled Trial of Risperidone and Olanzapine for Schizophrenic Patients With Neuroleptic-Induced Tardive Dyskinesia

Chan H-Y, Chiang S-C, Chang C-J, et al (Taoyuan Mental Hosp, Taiwan; Natl Yang-Ming Univ, Taipei, Taiwan; et al)

J Clin Psychiatry 71:1226-1233, 2010

Objective.—To compare the efficacy of risperidone and olanzapine in schizophrenic patients with tardive dyskinesia on treatment with first-generation antipsychotics.

Method.—We conducted a 24-week, rater-blinded, flexible-dose study. Sixty patients with *DSM-IV* schizophrenia (n = 58) or schizoaffective disorder (n = 2) met the *DSM-IV* research criteria for neuroleptic-induced tardive dyskinesia and were randomly assigned to a risperidone or olanzapine group. The primary outcome was a comparison of the change in the total scores on the Abnormal Involuntary Movement Scale (AIMS) from baseline to study end point between the groups. The study was conducted from July 2000 to June 2004.

Results.—The mean ± SD doses of risperidone and olanzapine from baseline to study end point were 1.9 ± 0.7 to 4.1 ± 1.4 mg/d and 8.1 ± 2.0 to 12.6 ± 5.4 mg/d, respectively. There were no statistically significant differences in demographic data, severity of tardive dyskinesia, or psychotic symptoms between risperidone and olanzapine groups at baseline assessment. Both groups showed significant improvement in mean ± SD AIMS total scores (risperidone: −7.4 ± 6.9, $P < .0001$; olanzapine: −6.2 ± 8.0, $P = .0002$). However, there was a more statistically significant change in the slope of AIMS total scores in the risperidone group than in the olanzapine group ($P = .0001$).

Conclusions.—Our findings demonstrated that olanzapine may not have better potential for tardive dyskinesia improvement than risperidone did. Double-blinded, fixed dose studies with a larger sample size on schizophrenic patients with tardive dyskinesia from different ethnic groups are needed to confirm the results of our study.

Trial Registration.—clinicaltrials.gov Identifier NCT00621998.

▶ Tardive dyskinesia (TD) continues to be a problem, but it is hoped that the number of new cases is decreasing with the use of second-generation antipsychotics. These Taiwanese authors conducted a 24-week blinded study in 60 patients who had neuroleptic-induced TD. Patients were randomly assigned to risperidone or olanzapine, and both groups showed significant improvement in Abnormal Involuntary Movement Scale scores, with significant superior response seen in the risperidone group. This is somewhat surprising because risperidone has been observed to have more acute extrapyramidal side effects and therefore might be thought to have less efficacy than olanzapine. However, this study would certainly argue the reverse, and larger studies clearly are necessary.

J. C. Ballenger, MD

A Randomized Placebo-Controlled Trial of Asenapine for the Prevention of Relapse of Schizophrenia After Long-Term Treatment

Kane JM, Mackle M, Snow-Adami L, et al (Zucker Hillside Hospital, Glen Oaks, NY; Merck, Rahway, NJ; et al)
J Clin Psychiatry 72:349-355, 2011

Objective.—Long-term efficacy of asenapine in preventing schizophrenia relapse was assessed in a 26-week double-blind, placebo-controlled trial that followed 26 weeks of open-label treatment.

Method.—Stable schizophrenia patients (*DSM-IV-TR* criteria) who were cross-titrated from previous medication to sublingual asenapine and remained stable during 26 weeks of open-label treatment were eligible for 26 weeks of double-blind treatment, with randomization to continued asenapine or switch to placebo. Time to relapse/impending relapse (primary endpoint, as usually determined by specific scores on the Positive and Negative Syndrome Scale and the Clinical Global Impressions-Severity of Illness Scale) and discontinuation for any reason (key secondary endpoint) were assessed by survival analyses for asenapine versus placebo. The study was conducted from May 2005 through June 2008.

Results.—Of 700 enrolled patients treated with open-label asenapine, 386 entered (asenapine, n = 194; placebo, n = 192) and 207 completed (n = 135; n = 72) the double-blind phase. Times to relapse/impending relapse and discontinuation for any reason were significantly longer with asenapine than with placebo (both $P < .0001$). Incidence of relapse/impending relapse was lower with asenapine than placebo (12.1% vs 47.4%, $P < .0001$). The modal dosage of asenapine was 10 mg twice daily in both phases. During the double-blind phase, the incidence of adverse events (AEs) considered serious with asenapine and placebo was 3.1% and 9.9%, respectively; incidence of extrapyramidal symptom-related AEs was 3.1% and 4.7%, respectively. The most frequently reported AEs with asenapine versus placebo were anxiety (8.2%; 10.9%), increased weight (6.7%; 3.6%), and insomnia (6.2%; 13.5%). The incidence of clinically significant weight gain ($\geq$ 7% increase from double-blind baseline) was 3.7% with asenapine and 0.5% with placebo.

Conclusions.—Long-term treatment with asenapine was more effective than placebo in preventing relapse of schizophrenia and appeared to be safe and well tolerated.

Trial Registration.—clinicaltrials.gov Identifier NCT00150176.

▶ These authors studied a large number of patients with schizophrenia who were treated initially in a double-blind placebo-controlled trial of asenapine. After stabilization, they were then randomized into a study comparing continued asenapine to placebo. Not surprisingly, the patients remaining on asenapine did much better and were well significantly longer (*P* < .0001) than those on placebo. Also, the incidence of relapse was significantly lower (12.1% vs 47.4% on placebo). The dose of asenapine was 10 mg twice a day in both phases of the study, and side effects, except for weight gain, were generally better with the medication than placebo. In particular, the extrapyramidal symptoms were 3.1% with asenapine and 4.7% in placebo. Weight gain of 7% or more was only 3.7% with asenapine versus 0.5% with placebo. This appears to be an effective and well-tolerated medication.

J. C. Ballenger, MD

A Randomized, Double-Blind, Parallel-Group, Fixed-Dose, Clinical Trial of Quetiapine at 600 Versus 1200 mg/d for Patients With Treatment-Resistant Schizophrenia or Schizoaffective Disorder

Lindenmayer J-P, Citrome L, Khan A, et al (Manhattan Psychiatric Ctr, NY; Nathan S. Kline Inst for Psychiatric Res, Orangeburg, NY; et al)
J Clin Psychopharmacol 31:160-168, 2011

Quetiapine is often prescribed at doses higher than those approved by regulatory authorities, with limited evidence from controlled trials. The objective of this study was to assess the safety, tolerability, and efficacy of high-dose quetiapine (1200 mg/d) compared with a standard dose of 600 mg/d among patients with *Diagnostic and Statistical Manual of Mental Disorders, Fourth Edition*, schizophrenia or schizoaffective disorder hospitalized at 2 state-operated psychiatric facilities. In order to be eligible for randomization, subjects were required to prospectively fail to demonstrate an initial therapeutic response during a 4-week run-in phase with quetiapine at 600 mg/d (immediate release and dosed twice a day). Lack of an adequate initial response was defined a 15% or lower decrease in the Positive and Negative Syndrome Scale total score. Patients were then randomized to either continue quetiapine at 600 mg/d for an additional 8 weeks or to receive 1200 mg/d quetiapine instead. No significant differences were observed between the high dose (n = 29) and standard dose (n = 31) groups in change from baseline to endpoint on extrapyramidal symptoms, electrocardiographic changes, or most laboratory measures between groups. There was a significant difference between groups for triglycerides (*P* = 0.035), and post hoc tests revealed a decrease in triglycerides from baseline (mean [SD], 162.7 [59.3] mg/dL) to endpoint (mean [SD], 134.8 [62.7] mg/dL) for the 600 mg/d group (*P* = 0.019). The mean change in the Positive and Negative Syndrome Scale total score did not differ between groups. In conclusion, quetiapine at 1200 mg/d, although reasonably tolerated, did not confer any advantages over quetiapine at 600 mg/d among patients who had failed to demonstrate an adequate response to a prospective 4-week trial of 600 mg/d.

▶ These authors performed a valuable study in patients with schizophrenia who did not respond to 4 weeks of treatment of a dose of 600 mg a day of quetiapine, the dose approved by regulatory agencies, to examine whether increased doses would be the proper next step to take. They randomly assigned patients who did not respond to therapy at 600 mg to an additional 8 weeks at 600 mg versus receiving 1200 mg a day. Interestingly, although it was well tolerated, the increase of quetiapine to 1200 mg did not make any significant difference in clinical response. This is a particularly valuable and clinically relevant study because clinicians are faced with this type of question all the time, and limited evidence had suggested higher doses might be helpful.

J. C. Ballenger, MD

ANXA7, PPP3CB, DNAJC9, and *ZMYND17* Genes at Chromosome 10q22 Associated with the Subgroup of Schizophrenia with Deficits in Attention and Executive Function
Liu C-M, Fann CS-J, Chen C-Y, et al (Natl Taiwan Univ Hosp, Yunlin; Inst of Biomed Science, Academia Sinica, Taipei, Taiwan; Natl Taiwan Univ, Taipei; et al)
Biol Psychiatry 70:51-58, 2011

Background.—A genome scan of Taiwanese schizophrenia families suggested linkage to chromosome 10q22.3. We aimed to find the candidate genes in this region.

Methods.—A total of 476 schizophrenia families were included. Hierarchical clustering method was used for clustering families to homogeneous subgroups according to their performances of sustained attention and executive function. Association analysis was performed using family-based association testing and TRANSMIT. Candidate associated regions were identified using the longest significance run method. The relative messenger RNA expression level was determined using real-time reverse transcriptase polymerase chain reaction.

Results.—First, we genotyped 18 microsatellite markers between D10S1432 and D10S1239. The maximum nonparametric linkage score was 2.79 on D10S195. Through family clustering, we found the maximum nonparametric linkage score was 3.70 on D10S195 in the family cluster with deficits in attention and executive function. Second, we genotyped 79 single nucleotide polymorphisms between D10S1432 and D10S580 in 90 attention deficit and execution deficit families. Association analysis indicated significant transmission distortion for nine single nucleotide polymorphisms. Using the longest significance run method, we identified a 427-kilobase region as a significant candidate region, which encompasses nine genes. Third, we studied messenger RNA expression of these nine genes in Epstein-Barr virus-transformed lymphoblastic cells. In schizophrenic patients, there was significantly lower expression of *ANXA7*, *PPP3CB*, and *DNAJC9* and significantly higher expression of *ZMYND17*.

Conclusions.—*ANXA7, PPP3CB, DNAJC9,* and *ZMYND17* genes are potential candidate genes for schizophrenia, especially in patients with deficits in sustained attention and executive function. The responsible functional variants remained to be clarified.

▶ These authors have taken us one step closer to understanding the genetic contribution to schizophrenia. They did a large study of schizophrenia in 476 families in Taiwan and discovered a suggested linkage to chromosome 10q22.3. They found sufficient data to identify that in schizophrenic patients there was significantly lower expression of *ANXA7*, *PPP3CB*, and *DNAJC9* and significantly higher expression of *ZMYND17*. This was particularly seen in patients with deficits in sustained attention and executive functioning. These cognitive difficulties are some of the most problematic abnormalities seen in schizophrenia. This is an exciting advance in this area.

J. C. Ballenger, MD

Are There Progressive Brain Changes in Schizophrenia? A Meta-Analysis of Structural Magnetic Resonance Imaging Studies
Olabi B, Ellison-Wright I, McIntosh AM, et al (Univ of Edinburgh, UK; Avon and Wiltshire Mental Health Partnership Natl Health Service Trust, Salisbury, UK; et al)
Biol Psychiatry 70:88-96, 2011

Background.—It is well established that schizophrenia is associated with structural brain abnormalities, but whether these are static or progress over time remains controversial.

Methods.—A systematic review of longitudinal volumetric studies using region-of-interest structural magnetic resonance imaging in patients with schizophrenia and healthy control subjects. The percentage change in volume between scans for each brain region of interest was obtained, and data were combined using random effects meta-analysis.

Results.—Twenty-seven studies were included in the meta-analysis, with 928 patients and 867 control subjects, and 32 different brain regions of interest. Subjects with schizophrenia showed significantly greater decreases over time in whole brain volume, whole brain gray matter, frontal gray and white matter, parietal white matter, and temporal white matter volume, as well as larger increases in lateral ventricular volume, than healthy control subjects. The time between baseline and follow-up magnetic resonance imaging scans ranged from 1 to 10 years. The differences between patients and control subjects in annualized percentage volume change were −.07% for whole brain volume, −.59% for whole brain gray matter, −.32% for frontal white matter, −.32% for parietal white matter, −.39% for temporal white matter, and +.36% for bilateral lateral ventricles.

Conclusions.—These findings suggest that schizophrenia is associated with progressive structural brain abnormalities, affecting both gray and white matter. We found no evidence to suggest progressive medial temporal lobe involvement but did find evidence that this may be partly explained by heterogeneity between studies in patient age and illness duration. The causes and clinical correlates of these progressive brain changes should now be the focus of investigation.

▶ This is another study using a meta-analytic technique of 27 studies consisting of 928 patients and 867 control subjects and studying 32 different brain regions with MRI volumetric techniques. The patients with schizophrenia did show significantly greater decreases over time in whole brain volume, whole brain gray matter, frontal gray and white matter, parietal white matter, and temporal white matter volume, as well as larger increases in lateral ventricular volume compared with controls in scans ranging from 1 to 10 years of follow-up. This is yet another study to find these progressive brain changes in schizophrenia with increasingly strong evidence.

J. C. Ballenger, MD

At-Risk Variant in *TCF7L2* for Type II Diabetes Increases Risk of Schizophrenia

Hansen T, Ingason A, Djurovic S, et al (Copenhagen Univ Hosp, Denmark; Oslo Univ Hosp—Ullevål, Norway; et al)
Biol Psychiatry 70:59-63, 2011

Background.—Schizophrenia is associated with increased risk of type II diabetes and metabolic disorders. However, it is unclear whether this comorbidity reflects shared genetic risk factors, at-risk lifestyle, or side effects of antipsychotic medication.

Methods.—Eleven known risk variants of type II diabetes were genotyped in patients with schizophrenia in a sample of 410 Danish patients, each matched with two healthy control subjects on sex, birth year, and month. Replication was carried out in a large multinational European sample of 4089 patients with schizophrenia and 17,597 controls (SGENE+) using Mantel–Haenszel test.

Results.—One type II diabetes at-risk allele located in *TCF7L2*, rs7903146 [T], was associated with schizophrenia in the discovery sample ($p = .0052$) and in the replication with an odds ratio of 1.07 (95% confidence interval 1.01−1.14, $p = .033$).

Conclusion.—The association reported here with a well-known diabetes variant suggests that the observed comorbidity is partially caused by genetic risk variants. This study also demonstrates how genetic studies can successfully examine an epidemiologically derived hypothesis of comorbidity.

▶ We have followed the issue of the relationship of diabetes and depression for several years. There appears to be a bidirectional increased risk in both disorders, but it is unclear whether this is related to the presence of the other condition, genetic issues, lifestyle differences, or side effects of the antipsychotics. In this very well-done study, 410 Danish patients were matched with healthy controls. A replication study was carried out across a European sample of 489 patients with schizophrenia and 17 597 controls. They, in fact, did find that a type-II diabetes at-risk allele located at TCF7L2, rs7903146[T] was associated with schizophrenia in the first sample and then again in the replication sample. This is a well-known diabetes variant and lends even more evidence that the comorbidity is caused by a genetic risk variance.

J. C. Ballenger, MD

Brain Volume Changes After Withdrawal of Atypical Antipsychotics in Patients With First-Episode Schizophrenia
Boonstra G, van Haren NEM, Schnack HG, et al (Univ Med Ctr Utrecht, The Netherlands; et al)
J Clin Psychopharmacol 31:146-153, 2011

The influence of antipsychotic medication on brain morphology in schizophrenia may confound interpretation of brain changes over time. We aimed to assess the effect of discontinuation of atypical antipsychotic medication on change in brain volume in patients. Sixteen remitted, stable patients with first-episode schizophrenia, schizoaffective or schizophreniform disorder and 20 healthy controls were included. Two magnetic resonance imaging brain scans were obtained from all subjects with a 1-year interval. The patients either discontinued (n = 8) their atypical antipsychotic medication (olanzapine, risperidone, or quetiapine) or did not (n = 8) discontinue during the follow-up period. Intracranial volume and volumes of total brain, cerebral gray and white matter, cerebellum, third and lateral ventricle, nucleus caudatus, nucleus accumbens, and putamen were obtained. Multiple linear regression analyses were used to assess main effects for group (patient-control) and discontinuation (yes-no) for brain volume (change) while correcting for age, sex, and intracranial volume. Decrease in cerebral gray matter and caudate nucleus volume over time was significantly more pronounced in patients relative to controls. Our data suggest decreases in the nucleus accumbens and putamen volumes during the interval in patients who discontinued antipsychotic medication, whereas increases were found in patients who continued their antipsychotics. We confirmed earlier findings of excessive gray matter volume decrements in patients with schizophrenia compared with normal controls. We found evidence suggestive of decreasing volumes of the putamen and nucleus accumbens over time after discontinuation of medication. This might suggest that discontinuation reverses effects of atypical medication.

▶ These authors studied, in a relatively small sample of 16 patients, the effect on brain volume in various areas, whether patients continued on their second-generation antipsychotic or discontinued it. They studied these patients compared with 20 healthy controls with MRI. They were able to document again that there were decreases in cerebral gray matter and caudate nucleus volume over time in the patients with schizophrenia versus controls. They also found that there were significant decreases in the nucleus accumbens and putamen volumes in the patients who discontinued their antipsychotics, but increases in those who continued their antipsychotics. We have generally assumed that the previously observed and now replicated finding of decreased brain volumes of people with schizophrenia is evidence of a pathological destructive process. In this study, it would suggest (as has been observed in some other studies) that the second-generation antipsychotics appear to, at least in some regions, reverse this process. It presents the dilemma of whether to continue or discontinue the second-generation antipsychotics for this reason alone. However, for clinical reasons, continuation is usually the appropriate choice. These patients had first-episode schizophrenia, making the question a little more complicated but intriguing nonetheless.

J. C. Ballenger, MD

Comparative Mortality Associated With Ziprasidone and Olanzapine in Real-World Use Among 18,154 Patients With Schizophrenia: The Ziprasidone Observational Study of Cardiac Outcomes (ZODIAC)
Strom BL, Eng SM, Faich G, et al (Univ of Pennsylvania School of Medicine, Philadelphia; Pfizer, Inc, NY; United BioSource Corporation, Blue Bell, PA; et al)
Am J Psychiatry 168:193-201, 2011

Objective.—The authors compared 1-year mortality rates associated with ziprasidone and olanzapine in real-world use.

Method.—The Ziprasidone Observational Study of Cardiac Outcomes (ZODIAC) was an open-label, randomized, postmarketing large simple trial that enrolled patients with schizophrenia (N=18,154) in naturalistic practice in 18 countries. The primary outcome measure was nonsuicide mortality in the year after initiation of assigned treatment. Patients were randomly assigned to receive treatment with either ziprasidone or olanzapine and followed for 1 year by unblinded investigators providing usual care. A physician-administered questionnaire was used to collect baseline demographic information, medical and psychiatric history, and concomitant medication use. Follow-up information on hospitalizations and emergency department visits, patients' vital status, and current antipsychotic drug status was collected and reported by treating psychiatrists. Post hoc analyses of sudden death, a secondary endpoint, were also conducted.

Results.—The incidence of nonsuicide mortality within 1 year of initiating pharmacotherapy was 0.91 for ziprasidone (N=9,077) and 0.90 for olanzapine (N=9,077). The relative risk was 1.02 (95% CI=0.76−1.39). This finding was confirmed in numerous secondary and sensitivity analyses.

Conclusions.—Despite the known risk of QTc prolongation with ziprasidone treatment, the findings of this study failed to show that ziprasidone is associated with an elevated risk of nonsuicidal mortality relative to olanzapine in real-world use; the study excludes a relative risk larger than 1.39 with a high probability. However, the study was neither powered nor designed to examine the risk of rare events like torsade de pointes.

▶ In past years, I have followed the issue of whether the second-generation antipsychotics with their attendant metabolic risks have a negative impact on mortality. These authors were able to compare 18154 patients with schizophrenia in naturalistic practices in 18 countries. They primarily followed nonsuicide mortality in the year following treatment with ziprasidone or olanzapine in usual care practices. The nonsuicide mortalities within a year of starting treatment with ziprasidone were 0.91 (n = 9077) and 0.90 (n = 9087), respectively. With a relative risk of 1.02, the authors felt they could say that the known risk of QTc prolongation with ziprasidone did not lead to sudden death in real-world use. This is helpful given all the issues raised with ziprasidone when it was first released about the potential risk with QTc prolongation. It puts in serious doubt our hesitation using it or even the use of electrocardiograms before or during use of ziprasidone.

J. C. Ballenger, MD

Early detection of psychosis: positive effects on 5-year outcome

Larsen TK, Melle I, Auestad B, et al (Stavanger Univ Hosp, Norway; Oslo Univ Hosp, Norway; Univ of Stavanger, Norway; et al)
Psychol Med 41:1461-1469, 2011

Background.—During the last decades we have seen a new focus on early treatment of psychosis. Several reviews have shown that duration of untreated psychosis (DUP) is correlated to better outcome. However, it is still unknown whether early treatment will lead to a better long-term outcome. This study reports the effects of reducing DUP on 5-year course and outcome.

Method.—During 1997−2000 a total of 281 consecutive patients aged >17 years with first episode non-affective psychosis were recruited, of which 192 participated in the 5-year follow-up. A comprehensive early detection (ED) programme with public information campaigns and low-threshold psychosis detection teams was established in one healthcare area (ED-area), but not in a comparable area (no-ED area). Both areas ran equivalent treatment programmes during the first 2 years and need-adapted treatment thereafter.

Results.—At the start of treatment, ED-patients had shorter DUP and less symptoms than no-ED-patients. There were no significant differences in treatment (psychotherapy and medication) for the 5 years. Mixed-effects modelling showed better scores for the ED group on the Positive and Negative Syndrome Scale negative, depressive and cognitive factors and for global assessment of functioning for social functioning at 5-year follow-up. The ED group also had more contacts with friends. Regression analysis did not find that these differences could be explained by confounders.

Conclusions.—Early treatment had positive effects on clinical and functional status at 5-year follow-up in first episode psychosis.

▶ For theoretical and clinical reasons, I have been interested in the issue of whether treating psychosis (or other illnesses) more quickly makes a difference acutely and long term. There have been multiple theoretical and research-based reasons that it might make quite a difference. This study is one of the few to study whether treating psychosis more rapidly (ie, whether having a shorter duration of untreated psychosis) is related to better outcome at 5 years. These authors followed 281 consecutive patients beginning with their first episode of psychosis and kept 192 in the study for 5 years. It appeared at the beginning that the early detection (ED) group did have fewer symptoms, but there was no significant difference in treatment given, either psychotherapy or medications, in the 5 years. Strikingly, they were able to show that the ED group had fewer positive and negative symptoms and better outcomes in depression, cognitive problems, and in their global functioning (especially socially) over the 5 years. I have presented other articles from this year and previous years showing that there are progressive brain changes in schizophrenia, and it is logical that intervening more rapidly to treat the illness should lead to less long-term brain damage, perhaps explaining these results.

J. C. Ballenger, MD

A Double-Blind, Randomized Study Comparing the Efficacy and Safety of Sertindole and Risperidone in Patients With Treatment-Resistant Schizophrenia
Kane JM, Potkin SG, Daniel DG, et al (The Zucker Hillside Hosp, Glen Oaks, NY; Univ of California, Irvine; George Washington Univ, DC; et al)
J Clin Psychiatry 72:194-204, 2011

Objective.—The comparative efficacy of second-generation antipsychotics has yet to be fully elucidated in patients with treatment-resistant schizophrenia. The objective of this study was to examine the efficacy and safety of sertindole, compared to risperidone, in this patient population.

Method.—In this multicenter, phase 3, randomized, double-blind, parallel-group study, only patients with *DSM-IV* schizophrenia who had failed an adequate antipsychotic treatment within the previous 6 months and who had not responded positively to haloperidol during screening were eligible for enrollment. The primary efficacy variable was change in Positive and Negative Syndrome Scale (PANSS) from baseline to final assessment. Weekly assessments included the PANSS, the Brief Psychiatric Rating Scale (BPRS), the Scale for the Assessment of Negative Symptoms (SANS), and the Clinical Global Impressions (CGI) scale. The study was conducted between June 1996 and April 1998.

Results.—Of the 321 patients randomly assigned to double-blind treatment, 217 patients completed the study (sertindole, n/n = 142/216 [66%]; risperidone, n/n = 75/105 [71%]). The main reason for withdrawal in both groups was ineffective therapy. The between-group difference in PANSS total score was not statistically significant and both groups showed improvement, with mean changes of −18.6 in the sertindole group and −20.9 in the risperidone group based on observed cases and −12.0 and −19.0, respectively, based on the last-observation-carried-forward method for imputing missing data. There were no statistically significant differences between the groups in any of the secondary end points: PANSS positive and negative subscales, CGI scores, BPRS total scores and positive symptom subscale scores, and SANS total scores. Patients reported similar levels of adverse events and treatment-emergent adverse events (TEAEs), except for extrapyramidal syndrome-related TEAEs, which were more common in the risperidone-treated group. Prolongation of the QTc interval was observed significantly more frequently with sertindole treatment.

Conclusions.—Sertindole and risperidone are effective and well-tolerated in patients with treatment-resistant schizophrenia. Sertindole offers an alternative treatment option for refractory patients in Europe given its good EPS profile, favorable metabolic profile, and comparable efficacy to risperidone.

▶ These authors studied patients with schizophrenia who failed adequate antipsychotic treatments within the previous 6 months and then who also failed to respond to haloperidol during the screening period. They had 321 patients assigned to double-blind treatment with either sertindole or risperidone. In fact, they found no statistically significant difference in the Positive and Negative Symptoms Scale between the 2 treatments or any of the secondary end points. The patients had similar levels of side effects to the 2 medicines, except there were more extrapyramidal symptoms with risperidone, not surprisingly. Also, not surprisingly, there was prolongation of the QTc interval with sertindole. Sertindole, which is available in Europe, seems to be an effective option with a favorable metabolic profile and extrapyramidal syndrome profile based on this study and many others. The differences between each of the second-generation antipsychotics and differences between them and the first-generation antipsychotics continue to be hotly debated and controversial, and this study adds an important link in that story.

J. C. Ballenger, MD

Assertive Community Treatment as Part of Integrated Care Versus Standard Care: A 12-Month Trial in Patients With First- and Multiple-Episode Schizophrenia Spectrum Disorders Treated With Quetiapine Immediate Release (ACCESS trial)
Lambert M, Bock T, Schöttle D, et al (Univ Centre for Psychosocial Medicine, Martinistr, Hamburg, Germany; et al)
J Clin Psychiatry 71:1313-1323, 2010

Objective.—The ACCESS trial examined the 12-month effectiveness of continuous therapeutic assertive community treatment (ACT) as part of integrated care compared to standard care in a catchment area comparison design in patients with schizophrenia spectrum disorders treated with quetiapine immediate release.

Method.—Two catchment areas in Hamburg, Germany, with similar population size and health care structures were assigned to offer 12-month ACT as part of integrated care (n = 64) or standard care (n = 56) to 120 patients with first- or multiple-episode schizophrenia spectrum disorders (Structured Clinical Interview for *DSM-IV* Axis I Disorders criteria); multiple-episode patients were restricted to those with a history of relapse due to medication nonadherence. The primary outcome was time to service disengagement. Secondary outcomes comprised medication nonadherence, improvements of symptoms, functioning, quality of life, satisfaction with care from patients' and relatives' perspectives, and service use data. The study was conducted from April 2005 to December 2008.

Results.—17 of 120 patients (14.2%) disengaged with service, 4 patients (6.3%) in the ACT and 13 patients (23.2%) in the standard care group. The mean Kaplan-Meier estimated time in service was 50.7 weeks in the ACT group (95% CI, 49.1–52.0) and 44.1 weeks in the standard care group (95% CI, 40.1–48.1). This difference was statistically significant ($P = .0035$). Mixed models repeated measures indicated larger improvements for ACT compared to standard care regarding symptoms ($P < .01$), illness severity ($P < .001$), global functioning ($P < .05$), quality of life ($P < .05$), and client satisfaction as perceived by patients and family (both $P < .05$). Logistic regression analyses revealed that ACT was associated with a higher likelihood of being employed/occupied ($P = .001$), of living independently ($P = .007$), and of being adherent with medication ($P < .001$) and a lower likelihood of persistent substance misuse ($P = .027$).

Conclusions.—Compared to standard care, intensive therapeutic ACT as part of integrated care could improve 1-year outcome. Future studies need to address in which settings these improvements can be sustained.

Trial Registration.—clinicaltrials.gov Identifier: NCT01081418.

▶ This ACCESS study was a 12-month trial in Hamburg, Germany, of continuous therapeutic assertive community treatment (ACT) as part of integrated care and was compared with standard care in patients with schizophrenia spectrum disorders. Both study groups also received the active medication quetiapine immediate release. The primary outcome measure was disengagement with treatment services. Only 17 of 120 patients (14.2%) actually disengaged with service, and there was a distinct advantage for the ACT treatment with only 6% disengaging versus 23.2% in the standard care group. There was also greater symptomatic improvement for the ACT patients in terms of symptoms, illness severity, global functioning, quality of life, and satisfaction by the patients and families. ACT was also associated with better employment and independent living as well as compliance with medication use and lowered substance abuse. I have been a fan of ACT for a long time because it works and seems to address some of the issues that are critical in successfully treating people in the community who have schizophrenia.

J. C. Ballenger, MD

Brain Anatomical Abnormalities in High-Risk Individuals, First-Episode, and Chronic Schizophrenia: An Activation Likelihood Estimation Meta-analysis of Illness Progression

Chan RCK, Di X, McAlonan GM, et al (Chinese Academy of Sciences, Beijing, China; Sun Yat-Sen Univ, Guangzhou, China; Univ of Hong Kong, Hong Kong Special Administrative Region, China; et al)
Schizophr Bull 37:177-188, 2011

Objective.—The present study reviewed voxel-based morphometry (VBM) studies on high-risk individuals with schizophrenia, patients experiencing their first-episode schizophrenia (FES), and those with chronic schizophrenia. We predicted that gray matter abnormalities would show progressive changes, with most extensive abnormalities in the chronic group relative to FES and least in the high-risk group.

Method.—Forty-one VBM studies were reviewed. Eight high-risk studies, 14 FES studies, and 19 chronic studies were analyzed using anatomical likelihood estimation meta-analysis.

Results.—Less gray matter in the high-risk group relative to controls was observed in anterior cingulate regions, left amygdala, and right insula. Lower gray matter volumes in FES compared with controls were also found in the anterior cingulate and right insula but not the amygdala. Lower gray matter volumes in the chronic group were most extensive, incorporating similar regions to those found in FES and high-risk groups but extending to superior temporal gyri, thalamus, posterior cingulate, and parahippocampal gryus. Subtraction analysis revealed less frontotemporal, striatal, and cerebellar gray matter in FES than the high-risk group; the high-risk group had less gray matter in left subcallosal gyrus, left amygdala, and left inferior frontal gyrus compared with FES. Subtraction analysis confirmed lower gray matter volumes through ventral-dorsal anterior cingulate, right insula, left amygdala and thalamus in chronic schizophrenia relative to FES.

Conclusions.—Frontotemporal brain structural abnormalities are evident in nonpsychotic individuals at high risk of developing schizophrenia. The present meta-analysis indicates that these gray matter abnormalities become more extensive through first-episode and chronic illness. Thus, schizophrenia appears to be a progressive cortico-striato-thalamic loop disorder.

▶ These authors examined a large number of studies of voxel-based morphometry (VBM) in high-risk individuals with schizophrenia and first-episode schizophrenia and those with chronic schizophrenia to examine whether the predicted gray matter abnormalities did, in fact, progress over time. They were able to locate 41 appropriate VBM studies and did observe less gray matter in anterior cingulate regions, the left amygdala, and right insula. In the first-episode group, they found decreases only in the anterior cingulate and right insula but not the amygdala. The gray matter decreases were most extensive in the chronic group and were also in the superior gyri, thalamus, posterior cingulate, and parahippocampal gyrus. These results allowed them to document that frontal temporal brain abnormalities were observable in nonpsychotic individuals at high risk of schizophrenia development and that these gray matter abnormalities become more extensive through the first episode and chronic illness. They were able to provide strong evidence that schizophrenia appears to be a progressive cortico-striato-thalamic loop disorder. These findings are consistent with those of a great deal of previous research, but it is a convincing article with findings providing evidence of the conceptualization of schizophrenia as a progressive illness with losses of gray matter progressively increasing from preclinical illness through the first episode and then into chronic condition.

J. C. Ballenger, MD

Preventing breast cancer in women with schizophrenia
Seeman MV (Univ of Toronto, Ontario, Canada)
Acta Psychiatr Scand 123:107-117, 2011

Objective.—To record risk factors for breast cancer in women with schizophrenia and recommend preventive actions.

Method.—A PubMed literature search (from 2005 to 2010) was conducted, using the search terms 'schizophrenia', 'antipsychotics', 'breast cancer' and 'risk factors'.

Results.—Several risk factors of relevance to schizophrenia were identified: obesity, elevated prolactin levels, low participation in mammography screening, high prevalence of diabetes, comparatively low parity, low incidence of breastfeeding, social disadvantage, high levels of smoking and alcohol consumption, low activity levels.

Conclusion.—Awareness of breast cancer risk should lead to more accurate risk ascertainment, stronger linkage with primary care, regular monitoring and screening, judicious choice and low dose of antipsychotic treatment, concomitant use of adjunctive cognitive and psychosocial therapies, referral to diet and exercise programmes as well as smoking and drinking cessation programmes, avoidance of hormonal treatment and discussion with patient and family about the pros and cons of preventive measures in high-risk women. Psychiatrists are in a position to reverse many of the identified risk factors.

▶ Dr Seeman is a leading Canadian psychiatrist who has dedicated her career to women's issues among patients with schizophrenia. She is best known for her work on estrogen and schizophrenia, specifically for her hypothesis that the later onset of illness, the better outcome and responsivity to treatment among females with schizophrenia, noting that this might be related to estrogen-induced downregulation of dopamine receptors. So in this elegant review, she ties together several aspects of neurobiology with clinical and service issues to address the risk of breast cancer among females with schizophrenia. There has long been a concern that prolactin-elevating antipsychotic medications might increase the risk of breast cancer. Indeed, some reports speculated at this, and there was initial concern regarding tumors in rodents receiving risperidone. These findings do not appear to have come about, and antipsychotic medications do not appear as balanced to raise the risk. Dr Seeman does point out that obesity, smoking, and lifestyle—concerns that are typical among both females and males with schizophrenia—are of themselves risk factors for breast cancer. Thus, as in all other instances, females with schizophrenia need to take care of themselves and seek preventative breast cancer screenings.

P. F. Buckley, MD

Substance Abuse

Cannabis and First-Episode Psychosis: Different Long-Term Outcomes Depending on Continued or Discontinued Use

González-Pinto A, Alberich S, Barbeito S, et al (Univ of the Basque Country, Vitoria, Spain; et al)
Schizophr Bull 37:631-639, 2011

Objective.—To examine the influence of cannabis use on long-term outcome in patients with a first psychotic episode, comparing patients who have never used cannabis with (*a*) those who used cannabis before the first episode but stopped using it during follow-up and (*b*) those who used cannabis both before the first episode and during follow-up.

Methods.—Patients were studied following their first admission for psychosis. They were interviewed at years 1, 3, and 5. At follow-up after 8 years, functional outcome and alcohol and drug abuse were recorded. Patients were classified according to cannabis use: 25 had cannabis use before their first psychotic episode and continuous use during follow-up (CU), 27 had cannabis use before their first episode but stopped its use during follow-up (CUS), and 40 never used cannabis (NU).

Results.—The 3 groups did not differ significantly in symptoms or functional outcome at baseline or during short-term follow-up. The CUS group exhibited better long-term functional outcome compared with the other 2 groups and had fewer negative symptoms than the CU group, after adjusting for potential confounders. For the CUS group, the effect size was 1.26 (95% confidence interval [CI] = 0.65 to 1.86) for functional outcome and −0.72 (95% CI = −1.27 to −0.14) for negative symptoms. All patients experienced improvements in positive symptoms during long-term follow-up.

Conclusion.—Cannabis has a deleterious effect, but stopping use after the first psychotic episode contributes to a clear improvement in outcome. The positive effects of stopping cannabis use can be seen more clearly in the long term.

▶ In past years, we have followed the issue of what we should tell patients about the use of marijuana. We have followed articles documenting that patients who smoke marijuana are more likely to have psychiatric problems, specifically psychosis. These authors provide data on a very critical issue: what advice we should give psychotic patients using marijuana, which is common. They followed 25 users who used marijuana before their first psychotic episode and continued to use it during follow-up and compared them with 27 patients who stopped its use during follow-up and 40 patients who never used. Although the 3 groups did not differ significantly at baseline or at short-term follow-up, the group that stopped exhibited significantly better long-term functional outcome and had fewer negative symptoms. The effect size was 1.26, a reasonably large effect for functional outcome, and −0.72 for negative symptoms. It just seems clear that we should strongly advise our patients to stop marijuana use, especially our psychotic patients.

J. C. Ballenger, MD

Comorbidity and risk indicators for alcohol use disorders among persons with anxiety and/or depressive disorders: Findings from the Netherlands Study of Depression and Anxiety (NESDA)
Boschloo L, Vogelzangs N, Smit JH, et al (VU Univ Med Ctr, Amsterdam, The Netherlands; et al)
J Affect Disord 131:233-242, 2011

Introduction.—This study examines comorbidity of alcohol abuse and alcohol dependence as well as its risk indicators among anxious and/or depressed persons, also considering temporal sequencing of disorders.

Methods.—Baseline data from the Netherlands Study of Depression and Anxiety (NESDA) were used, including 2329 persons with lifetime DSM-IV anxiety (social phobia, generalized anxiety disorder, panic disorder, and agoraphobia) and/or depressive (major depressive disorder and dysthymia) disorders and 652 controls. Lifetime diagnoses of DSM-IV alcohol abuse and dependence were established, as well as information about socio-demographic, vulnerability, addiction-related and anxiety/depression-related characteristics. Temporal sequencing of disorders was established retrospectively, using age of onset.

Results.—Of persons with combined anxiety/depression 20.3% showed alcohol dependence versus 5.5% of controls. Prevalence of alcohol abuse was similar across groups (±12%). Independent risk indicators for alcohol dependence among anxious and/or depressed persons were male gender, vulnerability factors (family history of alcohol dependence, family history of anxiety/depression, openness to experience, low conscientiousness, being single, and childhood trauma), addiction-related factors (smoking and illicit drug use) and early anxiety/depression onset. Persons with secondary alcohol dependence were more neurotic, more often single and lonelier, while persons with primary alcohol dependence were more often male and more extravert.

Discussion.—Alcohol dependence, but not abuse, is more prevalent in anxious and/or depressed persons. Persons with comorbid alcohol dependence constitute a distinct subgroup of anxious and/or depressed persons, characterized by addiction-related habits and vulnerability. However, considerable variation in characteristics exists depending on temporal sequencing of disorders. This knowledge may improve identification and treatment of those anxious and/or depressed patients who are additionally suffering from alcohol dependence.

▶ These authors used a large dataset from the Netherlands Study of Depression and Anxiety (NESDA) including 2329 persons with lifetime DSM-IV anxiety diagnoses or depressive disorders and compared them with 652 controls. Of the individuals with combined anxiety and depression, 20.3% showed alcohol dependence versus 5.5% of controls. Alcohol abuse was higher among the anxious or depressed individuals who were male, had vulnerability factors like a family history of alcohol dependence or anxiety or depression, had an openness to experience, had low conscientiousness, were single, and had childhood trauma and addiction-related factors (eg, smoking and illicit drug use as well as earlier onset of anxiety or depression). The authors hope that this subgrouping could allow better identification and treatment of these individuals with comorbid substance abuse problems.

J. C. Ballenger, MD

Gabapentin Combined With Naltrexone for the Treatment of Alcohol Dependence

Anton RF, Myrick H, Wright TM, et al (Med Univ of South Carolina, Charleston)
Am J Psychiatry 168:709-717, 2011

Objective.—Naltrexone, an efficacious medication for alcohol dependence, does not work for everyone. Symptoms such as insomnia and mood instability that are most evident during early abstinence might respond better to a different pharmacotherapy. Gabapentin may reduce these symptoms and help prevent early relapse. This clinical trial evaluated whether the combination of naltrexone and gabapentin was better than naltrexone alone and/or placebo during the early drinking cessation phase (first 6 weeks), and if so, whether this effect persisted.

Method.—A total of 150 alcohol-dependent individuals were randomly assigned to a 16-week course of naltrexone alone (50 mg/day [N=50]), naltrexone (50 mg/day) with gabapentin (up to 1,200 mg/day [N=50]) added for the first 6 weeks, or double placebo (N=50). All participants received medical management.

Results.—During the first 6 weeks, the naltrexone-gabapentin group had a longer interval to heavy drinking than the naltrexone-alone group, which had an interval similar to that of the placebo group; had fewer heavy drinking days than the naltrexone-alone group, which in turn had more than the placebo group; and had fewer drinks per drinking day than the naltrexone-alone group and the placebo group. These differences faded over the remaining weeks of the study. Poor sleep was associated with more drinking in the naltrexone-alone group but not in the naltrexone-gabapentin group, while a history of alcohol withdrawal was associated with better response in the naltrexone-gabapentin group.

Conclusions.—The addition of gabapentin to naltrexone improved drinking outcomes over naltrexone alone during the first 6 weeks after cessation of drinking. This effect did not endure after gabapentin was discontinued.

▶ My former colleagues at the Medical University of South Carolina Institute of Psychiatry continue to do excellent work developing treatments for substance abuse—in this case, alcoholism. They studied combined treatment of the Food and Drug Administration—approved naltrexone with gabapentin, which works through an entirely different mechanism (eg, gamma-aminobutyric acid). They followed 150 patients with alcohol dependence for a 16-week course, comparing naltrexone alone or naltrexone plus gabapentin for 6 weeks compared with double placebo. Importantly, during the first 6 weeks, the naltrexone plus gabapentin group did much better than the naltrexone alone group. The effect was lost after gabapentin was discontinued, and this promises to be an important addition in this area of research.

J. C. Ballenger, MD

Pharmacogenetic Approach at the Serotonin Transporter Gene as a Method of Reducing the Severity of Alcohol Drinking
Johnson BA, Ait-Daoud N, Seneviratne C, et al (Univ of Virginia, Charlottesville; Univ of Texas Health Science Ctr at San Antonio; Univ of Maryland, Baltimore)
Am J Psychiatry 168:265-275, 2011

Objective.—Severe drinking can cause serious morbidity and death. Because the serotonin transporter (5-HTT) is an important regulator of neuronal 5-HT function, allelic differences at that gene may modulate the severity of alcohol consumption and predict therapeutic response to the 5-HT_3 receptor antagonist, ondansetron.

Method.—The authors randomized 283 alcoholics by genotype in the 5'-regulatory region of the 5-HTT gene (LL/LS/SS), with additional genotyping for another functional single-nucleotide polymorphism (T/G), rs1042173, in the 3'-untranslated region, in a double-blind controlled trial. Participants received either ondansetron (4 µg/kg twice daily) or placebo for 11 weeks, plus standardized cognitivebehavioral therapy.

Results.—Individuals with the LL genotype who received ondansetron had a lower mean number of drinks per drinking day (−1.62) and a higher percentage of days abstinent (11.27%) than those who received placebo. Among ondansetron recipients, the number of drinks per drinking day was lower (−1.53) and the percentage of days abstinent higher (9.73%) in LL compared with LS/SS individuals. LL individuals in the ondansetron group also had a lower number of drinks per drinking day (−1.45) and a higher percentage of days abstinent (9.65%) than all other genotype and treatment groups combined. For both number of drinks per drinking day and percentage of days abstinent, 5'-HTTLPR and rs1042173 variants interacted significantly. LL/TT individuals in the ondansetron group had a lower number of drinks per drinking day (−2.63) and a higher percentage of days abstinent (16.99%) than all other genotype and treatment groups combined.

Conclusions.—The authors propose a new pharmacogenetic approach using ondansetron to treat severe drinking and improve abstinence in alcoholics.

▶ These authors randomized 283 alcoholics by genotype in the regulatory region of the serotonin transporter (5-HTT) gene (LL/LS/SS). They compared subjects' response to ondansetron (4 µg/kg twice daily) versus placebo for 11 weeks combined with cognitive-behavioral therapy. Interestingly, those with the LL genotype receiving ondansetron had a lower mean number drinks and higher days abstinent than those who received placebo. The ondansetron effect was greater in the LL group versus the LL/SS individuals on multiple parameters. In particular, those within the LL group and the LL/TT group at the single-nucleotide polymorphism (T/G) rs1042173 in the 3'-untranslated region had the greatest effect with ondansetron. This is not only a new pharmacological treatment for severe drinking and alcoholism but also a fascinating step in using pharmacogenetics to predict who will respond.

J. C. Ballenger, MD

General Psychiatry

Antidepressants and Body Weight: A Comprehensive Review and Meta-Analysis
Serretti A, Mandelli L (Univ of Bologna, Viale Carlo Pepoli, Italy)
J Clin Psychiatry 71:1259-1272, 2010

Objective.—Psychotropic drugs often induce weight gain, leading to discomfort and discontinuation of treatment and, more importantly, increasing the risk of obesity-related illnesses such as diabetes mellitus, hypertension, and coronary heart disease. There is evidence that antidepressant drugs may induce a variable amount of weight gain, but results are sparse and often contradictory.

Data Sources.—We performed a literature search using the MEDLINE, ISI Web of Knowledge, and Cochrane research databases for all publications available to January 2009. We used the following keywords: *antidepressant, psychotropic drugs, body weight, weight gain, obesity, overweight, adverse event, side effects, SSRIs, tricyclic antidepressants,* and the name of each antidepressant active compound together with *body weight* or other keywords. Studies reporting body weight changes during treatment with different antidepressants were selected for eligibility. Finally, 116 studies were included in the analysis.

Data Extraction.—Weight change mean and standard deviation and size of each group were recorded. Missing means and standard deviations were directly calculated by using information available in the article when possible. Non—placebo-controlled studies were compared to a virtual placebo sample, whose mean and standard deviation were derived by the weighted mean of means and standard deviations of all placebo samples. Methodological quality of studies, heterogeneity, publication bias, and effect of treatment duration were systematically controlled.

Data Synthesis.—Quantitative results evidenced that amitriptyline, mirtazapine, and paroxetine were associated with a greater risk of weight gain. In contrast, some weight loss occurs with fluoxetine and bupropion, although the effect of fluoxetine appears to be limited to the acute phase of treatment. Other compounds have no transient or negligible effect on body weight in the short term. However, the effect of each antidepressant may vary greatly depending on an individual's characteristics and generally became more evident in the long term to a variable degree across compounds.

Conclusions.—Despite the fact that some analyses were done on only a few studies due to the difficulty of finding reliable information in literature, to our knowledge, this is the first comprehensive meta-analysis to allow comparison of different antidepressants as regards their impact on body weight. Data presented may be helpful for a more accurate treatment selection in patients at risk of obesity or related medical illness.

▶ Perhaps no topic gets more attention in patients' minds when I talk with them about using antidepressants than the issue of potential weight gain "caused" by them. I end up dealing with it almost on a daily basis. These authors reviewed the literature and ultimately included 16 studies in their analysis of this issue. They used placebo trials when possible, and in those that were not placebo controlled, they compared them with a virtual placebo sample. The results were interesting. They found that amitriptyline, mirtazapine, and paroxetine were associated with a greater risk for weight gain. However, there was some weight loss with fluoxetine and bupropion, although the fluoxetine effects appeared to be limited to acute treatment. In their analysis, other antidepressants had little or no effect on body weight in the short term. In my experience (and in the literature), this is a highly individual issue, and some patients gain weight when others don't. The authors believe that this is the "first comprehensive meta-analysis" allowing a comparison between different antidepressants effects on weight gain. Even limited, this is a useful and not surprising result. Mirtazapine is actually used on purpose to cause weight gain in some individuals, and paroxetine has been known for some time to have a higher risk of weight gain. I think what is most interesting is the relative lack of effects on weight from the remaining antidepressants. At some level, this "first comprehensive meta-analysis" can allow us to be more reassuring to patients that in general, the use of antidepressants is not associated with weight gain as much as they perhaps are thought to be.

J. C. Ballenger, MD

Antidepressant Medicine Use and Risk of Developing Diabetes During the Diabetes Prevention Program and Diabetes Prevention Program Outcomes Study

Rubin RR, for the Diabetes Prevention Program Research Group (The Johns Hopkins Univ School of Medicine, Baltimore, MD; et al)
Diabetes Care 33:2549-2551, 2010

Objective.—To assess the association between antidepressant medicine use and risk of developing diabetes during the Diabetes Prevention Program (DPP) and Diabetes Prevention Program Outcomes Study (DPPOS).

Research Design and Methods.—DPP/DPPOS participants were assessed for diabetes every 6 months and for antidepressant use every 3 months in DPP and every 6 months in DPPOS for a median 10.0-year follow-up.

Results.—Controlled for factors associated with diabetes risk, continuous antidepressant use compared with no use was associated with diabetes risk in the placebo (adjusted hazard ratio 2.34 [95% CI 1.32–4.15]) and lifestyle (2.48 [1.45–4.22]) arms, but not in the metformin arm (0.55 [0.25–1.19]).

Conclusions.—Continuous antidepressant use was significantly associated with diabetes risk in the placebo and lifestyle arms. Measured confounders and mediators did not account for this association, which could represent a drug effect or reflect differences not assessed in this study between antidepressant users and nonusers.

▶ I included this article because it concerns 2 very common occurrences: continuous antidepressant use and diabetes. This study used excellent samples and was able to demonstrate that continuous antidepressant use was associated with a significant increased risk of developing diabetes (hazard ratio 2.34). Interestingly, this was not seen in the metformin arm. There are so many people on long-term antidepressants, and diabetes is so common, that this association might not be noticeable except in a study like this. This is an important issue to which we need to give significant thought.

In another article,[1] the authors again had a huge sample size of 151 347 in which they were able to demonstrate a higher risk of diabetes in the 9197 participants taking continuous antidepressants. They observed a similar increase in diabetes, representing essentially a doubling from 1.1 in nonusers to as high as 2.3 in those who took more than 400 daily doses a year.

J. C. Ballenger, MD

Reference

1. Kivimaki M, Hamer M, Batty GD, et al. Antidepressant medication use, weight gain, and risk of type 2 diabetes: a population-based study. *Diabetes Care.* 2010; 33:2611-2616.

Antidepressants and Fracture Risk in Older Adults: A Comparative Safety Analysis

Gagne JJ, Patrick AR, Mogun H, et al (Brigham and Women's Hosp and Harvard Med School, Boston, MA)
Clin Pharmacol Ther 89:880-887, 2011

We examined variations in fracture rates among patients initiated on antidepressant drug treatment as identified from Medicare data in two US states and assessed whether the observed variation could be explained by affinity for serotonin transport receptors. We used Cox proportional hazards models to compare fracture rates of the hip, humerus, pelvis, wrist, and a composite of these, among propensity score—matched cohorts of users of secondary amine tricyclics, tertiary amine tricyclics, selective serotonin reuptake inhibitors (SSRIs), and atypical antidepressants. As compared with secondary amine tricyclics, SSRIs showed the highest association with composite fracture rate (hazard ratio 1.30; 95% confidence interval (CI) 1.12—1.52), followed by atypical antidepressants (hazard ratio 1.12; 95% CI 0.96—1.31) and tertiary amine tricyclics (hazard ratio 1.01; 95% CI 0.87—1.18). The results were robust to sensitivity analyses. Although SSRI use was associated with the highest rate of fractures, variation in fracture risk across specific antidepressant medications did not depend on affinity for serotonin transport receptors.

▶ These authors used Medicare data in 2 US states and compared fractures of hip, humerus, pelvis, wrists, and a composite of these in patients recently started on antidepressants. It was somewhat surprising to me that it was the selective serotonin reuptake inhibitors (SSRIs) that showed the highest association with composite fracture rate (hazard ratio [HR], 1.30) followed by atypical antidepressants (HR, 1.12). I grew up in this field worried by Sandy Glassman's data about hypotensive falls and fractures while taking tricyclics and am frankly surprised that they were more common with SSRIs than even tricyclics.

J. C. Ballenger, MD

Association of Cerebrovascular Events With Antidepressant Use: A Case-Crossover Study

Wu C-S, Wang S-C, Cheng Y-C, et al (Far Eastern Memorial Hosp, Taipei, Taiwan; Natl Taiwan Univ Hosp, Taipei; Natl Health Res Insts, Taipei; et al)
Am J Psychiatry 168:511-521, 2011

Objective.—The authors sought to assess the risk of cerebrovascular events associated with use of antidepressant medications.

Method.—The authors conducted a case-crossover study of 24,214 patients with stroke enrolled in the National Health Insurance Research Database in Taiwan from 1998 to 2007. The authors compared the rates of antidepressant use during case and control time windows of 7, 14, and 28 days. Adjustments were made for time-dependent variables, such as health system utilization and proposed confounding medications. Stratified analyses were performed for valuing the interaction between the stroke risk of antidepressant use and age, sex, presence of mood disorder, stroke type, severity of chronic illness, and duration of antidepressant treatment. A conditional logistic regression model was used to determine the odds of antidepressant use during case time windows.

Results.—The adjusted odds ratio of stroke risk with antidepressant exposure was 1.48 (95% confidence interval=1.37−1.59) using 14-day time windows. Stroke risk was negatively associated with the number of antidepressant prescriptions reported. Use of antidepressants with high inhibition of the serotonin transporter was associated with a greater risk of stroke than use of other types of antidepressants.

Conclusions.—These findings suggest that antidepressant use may be associated with an increased risk of stroke. However, the underlying mechanisms remain unclear.

▶ We have followed the cardiovascular risk with and without depression and with and without antidepressants for some time. These authors used a case crossover study of 24 214 patients with stroke in the Taiwanese National Health Insurance Research database. Remarkably, they demonstrated that the adjusted odds ratio for risk of having a stroke after antidepressant exposure was 1.48, a marked increase. Surprisingly, the selective serotonin reuptake inhibitors were associated with a greater risk of stroke than other types of antidepressants.

J. C. Ballenger, MD

Atypical antipsychotic drugs

Mackin P, Thomas SHL (Newcastle Univ, Newcastle upon Tyne, UK; Newcastle Hosps NHS Foundation Trust, UK)
BMJ 342:d1126, 2011

Background.—Antipsychotics produce their effects through their role as D2 dopamine receptor antagonists. "Typical" or first-generation antipsychotic drugs have been used to manage schizophrenia since the 1950s, but "atypical" or second-generation agents have been in use just since the 1990s. The therapeutic effects of atypical antipsychotics are related to their 5-HT2A antagonism and/or 5-HT1A agonism. Both generations are used for acute schizophrenia and related psychoses, long-term maintenance, and relapse prevention. The adverse effects of the typical drugs, such as haloperidol, chlorpromazine, and trifluoperazine, include extrapyramidal features such as dystonia, parkinsonism, akathisia, and tardive dyskinesia. The atypical agents are less likely to cause these effects but more likely to cause adverse metabolic symptoms. These adverse effects appear to be dose related and reflect their action at histaminergic, cholinergic, alpha-adrenergic, and other receptor sites.

Efficacy.—Evidence comparing the efficacy of antipsychotics can be difficult to interpret because of methodological heterogeneity. A meta-analysis of 150 randomized controlled trials (RCTs) covering 21,533 subjects with schizophrenia and related disorders found that the atypical agents amisulpride, clozapine, olanzapine, and risperidone were more effective than some typical drugs (specifically haloperidol) for overall symptom improvement. Effect sizes were modest; numbers needed to treat ranged from 6 to 15. Two other RCTs found no significant differences in overall efficacy, but olanzapine improved symptoms more rapidly. Clozapine is the prototype atypical antipsychotic and may be more effective for treatment-resistant schizophrenia than other atypical agents. It should only be given by specialists because of its adverse effects, especially agranulocytosis. Overall, except for clozapine, the evidence does not support any recommendation for one antipsychotic over the others.

Safety.—The dose-related adverse effects found most often with atypical antipsychotics are sedation, anticholinergic effects (eg, dry mouth, constipation, and blurred vision), dizziness, and postural hypotension. The atypical agents clozapine, olanzapine, and risperidone are significantly less often linked to extrapyramidal symptoms than low-potency typical antipsychotics. However, some atypical agents cause significant metabolic effects. Olanzapine is more likely to cause weight gain than perphenazine, quetiapine, risperidone, and ziprasidone, leading to its discontinuation. Substantial weight gain, dyslipidemia, and hyperglycemia are associated with clozapine, olanzapine, and quetiapine. Some atypical drugs, especially risperidone and amisulpride, can cause hyperprolactinemia, leading to gynecomastia, galactorrhea, menstrual cycle disruption, impotence, and osteoporosis. Atypical agents are less often associated with QT interval prolongation, which can be clinically significant when typical agents are used, leading to the ventricular arrhythmia torsade de pointes. Both typical and atypical agents can provoke seizures in susceptible patients, with the highest risk among atypical agents involving the use of clozapine and the lowest for risperidone.

Patients must be monitored for adverse effects. Because clozapine can provoke agranulocytosis, white blood cell count is monitored to detect this complication early and reduce mortality. Clozapine can also produce sialorrhea, ileus, tachycardia, and myocarditis. The weight gain and other metabolic disturbances associated with clozapine, olanzapine, and quetiapine can increase cardiovascular morbidity, so weight, glycemic status, and lipid levels must be monitored regularly, especially if the patient has cardiovascular disease. Increased cardiovascular risk is managed according to national guidelines. If the person has a prolonged QT interval on electrocardiography (ECG), antipsychotic agents should be used at the lowest effective dose and those with more marked ECG effect avoided. ECG effects should be monitored closely, especially at the beginning of treatment or when a dose is increased. Patients with epilepsy should be encouraged to adhere to their anticonvulsant therapy; seizure frequency is monitored. For patients who are pregnant or breastfeeding, the benefits and possible risks of effective treatment for both mother and child should be considered, since little evidence exists regarding the use of atypical agents in these situations. The lowest effective dose of antipsychotic is advised. Exposure in utero to atypical antipsychotic drugs can increase infant birth weight and the risk of an infant who is large for gestational age and the accompanying complications. Although antipsychotic drugs are detected in breast milk, no adverse effects have occurred, with the benefits of treatment probably outweighing any risks. Elderly patients with dementia are given antipsychotic agents only for compelling indications because of the small but increased risk of mortality and the risk of stroke and transient ischemic attack.

Cost-Effectiveness.—Atypical antipsychotics are being prescribed more often than previously, with a corresponding fall in typical antipsychotic drugs. Increased costs reflect the higher prices of the newer agents. Comparisons of agents based on cost-effectiveness have not yielded consistent findings, but overall, olanzapine and risperidone may be more cost effective than haloperidol.

Administration.—Patients who have difficulty with compliance or swallowing can be given orodispersible tablets or oral solutions rather than tablets. Parenteral medication may be needed to control the acute behavioral disturbances that accompany psychosis. Patients who require long-term treatment and prefer this mode of administration and patients who tend to be noncompliant can be given long-acting (depot) preparations.

Conclusions.—Evidence supports the use of antipsychotic agents, showing consistent efficacy against the core symptoms of schizophrenia and schizophrenia-like illness. No atypical agent was consistently found to be more efficacious or cost-effective than the typical antipsychotics. For some atypical drugs the substantial metabolic disturbances and increased cardiovascular risk must be weighed against the reduced extrapyramidal adverse effects compared to typical drugs. Overall, choosing the most appropriate drug and formulation should be tailored to the individual rather than relying on a specific drug group for all patients.

▶ This article is from one of the online publications of the *British Medical Journal*, which addresses in review form very important topics in a very usable form for doctors. These authors tackle many of the critical issues doctors and patients had about atypical antipsychotics. Although not an extensive scientific article, it is a useful brief summary of this complex area.

J. C. Ballenger, MD

Neuroanatomical Abnormalities That Predate the Onset of Psychosis: A Multicenter Study
Mechelli A, Riecher-Rössler A, Meisenzahl EM, et al (King's College London, UK; Univ Hosp Basel, Switzerland; Ludwig-Maximilians-Univ, Munich, Germany; et al)
Arch Gen Psychiatry 68:489-495, 2011

Context.—People experiencing possible prodromal symptoms of psychosis have a very high risk of developing the disorder, but it is not possible to predict, on the basis of their presenting clinical features, which individuals will subsequently become psychotic. Recent neuroimaging studies suggest that there are volumetric differences between individuals at ultra-high risk (UHR) for psychosis who later develop psychotic disorder and those who do not. However, the samples examined to date have been small, and the findings have been inconsistent.

Objective.—To assess brain structure in individuals at UHR for psychosis in a larger and more representative sample than in previous studies by combining magnetic resonance imaging data from 5 different scanning sites.

Design.—Case-control study.

Setting.—Multisite.

Participants.—A total of 182 individuals at UHR and 167 healthy controls. Participants were observed clinically for a mean of 2 years. Forty-eight individuals (26.4%) in the UHR group developed psychosis and 134 did not.

Main Outcome Measures.—Magnetic resonance images were acquired from each participant. Group differences in gray matter volume were examined using optimized voxel-based morphometry.

Results.—The UHR group as a whole had less gray matter volume than did controls in the frontal regions bilaterally. The UHR subgroup who later developed psychosis had less gray matter volume in the left parahippocampal cortex than did the UHR subgroup who did not.

Conclusions.—Individuals at high risk for psychosis show alterations in regional gray matter volume regardless of whether they subsequently develop the disorder. In the UHR population, reduced left parahippocampal volume was specifically associated with the later onset of psychosis. Alterations in this region may, thus, be crucial to the expression of illness. Identifying abnormalities that specifically predate the onset of psychosis informs the development of clinical investigations designed to predict which individuals at high risk will subsequently develop the disorder.

▶ This excellent study in the *Archives of General Psychiatry* provides much better data of brain structure in patients who were at ultra-high risk (UHR) for psychosis, who do become psychotic subsequently, compared with those who do not. The authors were able to combine MRI data from 5 different scanning sites comparing a total of 182 individuals at UHR and 167 healthy controls. These individuals were observed clinically for a mean of 2 years. In fact, 48 individuals (26.4%) in the UHR group developed psychosis. There were 2 interesting findings; the UHR as a group had less gray matter volume in the frontal regions bilaterally than did controls. Secondly, the UHR group who did become psychotic had less gray matter volume in the left parahippocampal cortex than the group that did not become psychotic. Certainly, this finding of a reduced left parahippocampal volume in the high-risk individuals who became psychotic is certainly an intriguing finding and will direct research attention to this critical area.

J. C. Ballenger, MD

A pharmaco-epidemiological study of migraine and antidepressant medications: Complete one year data from the Norwegian population
Oedegaard KJ, Riise T, Dilsaver SC, et al (Haukeland Univ Hosp, Norway; Univ of Bergen, Norway; Comprehensive Doctors Med Group, Arcadia, CA; et al)
J Affect Disord 129:198-204, 2011

Background.—Migraine, depression and anxiety disorders have been associated with one another in several epidemiological studies. However, it is not known if or how these associations are reflected in the concurrent use of medications for migraine and depressive/anxiety disorders in the general population. The purpose of the present study was to identify groups of patients particularly likely to receive clinical treatment for both conditions.

Methods.—Data from the Norwegian Prescription Database for 2006 were analysed for the purpose of ascertaining concurrence of prescriptions for migraine and depression/anxiety disorders. Data were subjected to analysis testing deviation from unity for the OR performed by a chi-square test.

Results.—In the total Norwegian population ($N = 4640219$) migraine drugs were prescribed to 81225 persons (1.8% of the population), antidepressant drugs to 257700 persons (5.6% of the population), and 11269 persons were prescribed both types of drugs. The prescription of antidepressants was significantly increased in patients receiving a prescription for a medication used to treat migraine (OR $= 2.82$ (95% CI $= 2.76-2.88$); chi-square $p < 0.001$), and this association was stronger for men than for women. Teenage women carried the highest risk for this co-morbid constellation (OR $= 3.89$ CI $= 3.17-4.77$); chi-square $p < 0.001$).

Conclusion.—This study revealed a strong positive association between the prescription of migraine and antidepressant medications, and this association was generally most pronounced in men. However, teenage girls carried the highest risk of receiving both kinds of prescriptions, suggesting particular attentiveness is required in the clinical management of these patients.

▶ These Norwegian investigators were able to use their prescription database to analyze the potential relationship between migraine and depression and anxiety disorders. They found that in the total Norwegian population (N = 4 640 219), migraine drugs were prescribed for 1.8% and antidepressants for 5.6% of the population. Approximately 0.2% received both types of medications. It appeared that prescriptions of antidepressants increased the chance of migraine treatment prescription 2.82-fold and that this association was stronger in men than in women. However, teenage girls carried the highest risk for this comorbidity. This is an interesting and not entirely surprising association, although one we do not understand.

J. C. Ballenger, MD

A randomized clinical trial of cognitive behavioural therapy *versus* short-term psychodynamic psychotherapy *versus* no intervention for patients with hypochondriasis
Sørensen P, Birket-Smith M, Wattar U, et al (Copenhagen Univ Hosp, Denmark; Kognitivt Psykolog Centre, Copenhagen, Denmark; et al)
Psychol Med 41:431-441, 2011

Background.—Hypochondriasis is common in the clinic and in the community. Cognitive behavioural therapy (CBT) has been found to be effective in previous trials. Psychodynamic psychotherapy is a treatment routinely offered to patients with hypochondriasis in many countries, including Denmark. The aim of this study was to test CBT for hypochondriasis in a centre that was not involved in its development and compare both CBT and short-term psychodynamic psychotherapy (STPP) to a waiting-list control and to each other. CBT was modified by including mindfulness and group therapy sessions, reducing the therapist time required. STPP consisted of individual sessions.

Method.—Eighty patients randomized to CBT, STPP and the waiting list were assessed on measures of health anxiety and general psychopathology before and after a 6-month treatment period. Waiting-list patients were subsequently offered one of the two active treatments on the basis of re-randomization, and assessed on the same measures post-treatment. Patients were again assessed at 6- and 12-month follow-up points.

Results.—Patients who received CBT did significantly better on all measures relative to the waiting-list control group, and on a specific measure of health anxiety compared with STPP. The STPP group did not significantly differ from the waiting-list group on any outcome measures. Similar differences were observed between CBT and STPP during follow-up, although some of the significant differences between groups were lost.

Conclusions.—A modified and time-saving CBT programme is effective in the treatment of hypochondriasis, although the two psychotherapeutic interventions differed in structure.

▶ These authors actually examined a difficult treatment concern, hypochondriasis. They developed a modified cognitive-behavioral therapy (CBT) program and compared it with psychodynamic psychotherapy; both treatments were compared with a wait-list control group. CBT had been modified to include mindfulness and group therapy sessions, making it less therapist-intensive. Psychodynamic psychotherapy was administered in individual sessions. The authors randomized 80 patients and followed up at 6 and 12 months. Strikingly, the CBT was effective, and the psychodynamic psychotherapy was not, suggesting that this modified CBT could be used effectively in practice.

J. C. Ballenger, MD

Abnormal metabolic brain networks in Tourette syndrome

Pourfar M, Feigin A, Tang CC, et al (The Feinstein Inst for Med Res, Manhasset, NY; et al)
Neurology 76:944-952, 2011

Objectives.—To identify metabolic brain networks that are associated with Tourette syndrome (TS) and comorbid obsessive-compulsive disorder (OCD).

Methods.—We utilized [^{18}F]-fluorodeoxyglucose and PET imaging to examine brain metabolism in 12 unmedicated patients with TS and 12 age-matched controls. We utilized a spatial covariance analysis to identify 2 disease-related metabolic brain networks, one associated with TS in general (distinguishing TS subjects from controls), and another correlating with OCD severity (within the TS group alone).

Results.—Analysis of the combined group of patients with TS and healthy subjects revealed an abnormal spatial covariance pattern that completely separated patients from controls ($p < 0.0001$). This TS-related pattern (TSRP) was characterized by reduced resting metabolic activity of the striatum and orbitofrontal cortex associated with relative increases in premotor cortex and cerebellum. Analysis of the TS cohort alone revealed the presence of a second metabolic pattern that correlated with OCD in these patients. This OCD-related pattern (OCDRP) was characterized by reduced activity of the anterior cingulate and dorsolateral prefrontal cortical regions associated with relative increases in primary motor cortex and precuneus. Subject expression of OCDRP correlated with the severity of this symptom ($r = 0.79$, $p < 0.005$).

Conclusion.—These findings suggest that the different clinical manifestations of TS are associated with the expression of 2 distinct abnormal metabolic brain networks. These, and potentially other disease-related spatial covariance patterns, may prove useful as biomarkers for assessing responses to new therapies for TS and related comorbidities.

▶ This is a study published in *Neurology* of the Tourette syndrome with or without comorbid obsessive-compulsive disorder (OCD). They studied 12 unmedicated patients with Tourette syndrome and matched them to 12 age-matched controls. Using positron emission tomography imaging, they were able to identify 2 metabolic brain networks that were distinctly different in these patients. They were able to demonstrate a very abnormal spatial covariance pattern separating Tourette patients from controls ($P < .0001$). This pattern included reduced resting metabolic activity in the striatum and orbitofrontal cortex with relative increases in premotor cortex and cerebellum. Those Tourette patients who also had OCD had a second pattern characterized by reduced activity in the anterior cingulate and dorsal lateral prefrontal cortical areas and relative increases in primary motor cortex and precuneus. This is consistent with previous findings and a definitive study. It seems that our field, perhaps with assistance from the National Institutes of Health, needs to make the general public more aware of the clear brain pathways that are associated with these 2 disorders, as well as others, in an effort to change public attitudes about these conditions.

J. C. Ballenger, MD

Body dysmorphic disorder and other psychiatric morbidity in aesthetic rhinoplasty candidates
Alavi M, Kalafi Y, Dehbozorgi GR, et al (Shiraz Univ of Med Sciences, Iran)
J Plast Reconstr Aesth Surg 64:738-741, 2011

Background.—Body dysmorphic disorder (BDD) is a psychiatric disorder characterised by the patient's preoccupation with an imagined defect in his or her physical appearance. Subjects with BDD often seek cosmetic surgery; however, the outcome of surgery is usually not satisfactory. The aim of current study was to investigate the prevalence of BDD among the patients seeking cosmetic surgery.

Method.—In a cross-sectional study, 306 patients referred to cosmetic surgery clinics were recruited. Two psychiatrists detected BDD by interviewing the patients using Diagnostic and Statistical Manual of Mental Disorders fourth edition Text Revision (DSM IV-TR) criteria. Data analysis was done in Statistical Package for Social Sciences (SPSS) using the *t*-test and the Mann—Whitney test for numeral variables and the chi-square and Fisher's exact tests for nominal variables.

Results.—Data analysis of demographics showed that 80% of patients were female. Analysis on disease-related variables showed that 126 (41%) of patients had an associated psychiatric disorder. Moreover, 75 patients (24.5%) fulfilled the DSM IV criteria for BDD.

Conclusion.—Findings from this study support earlier studies, which found that BDD is a relatively common disorder among individuals seeking aesthetic surgery, in particular in rhinoplasty patients. Preoperative psychiatry assessment recommends avoiding subsequent risk for both patients and surgeons.

▶ As I have mentioned before, if you look at the psychiatric issues of people seeking cosmetic surgery, there is a surprising number who have psychiatric problems. These problems often lead to a lack of satisfaction of the results of surgery. I was close to one dramatic example from my old medical school, Duke, where the Chairman of Plastic Surgery was tragically killed by a dissatisfied surgery patient. In this study, they examined 306 patients referred for cosmetic surgery and strikingly found that 41% have an associated psychiatric disorder. Even more worrisome was the fact that 75 patients (24.5%) actually met the criteria for body dysmorphic disorder. Operating on someone with body dysmorphic disorder would certainly lead to a high likelihood of a dissatisfied patient, and fully a quarter of patients asking for surgery, particularly rhinoplasty, were found to have that disorder in this study.

J. C. Ballenger, MD

Current Concepts in the Pharmacotherapy of Paraphilias

Garcia FD, Thibaut F (Rouen Univ Hosp, France; Rouen Univ, France)
Drugs 71:771-790, 2011

Concerns about paraphilia and its treatment have grown in the past few years. Although the aetiology of paraphilia disorder is still not completely understood, pharmacological treatments have been proposed for this disorder. Paraphilias are a major burden for patients and society; nevertheless, only a few individuals with paraphilias voluntarily seek treatment. Antidepressants have been used in the treatment of certain types of mild (e.g. exhibitionism) and juvenile paraphilias. Antilibidinal hormonal treatments, such as steroidal antiandrogens and gonadotrophin-releasing hormone (GnRH) analogues, have also been studied and they seem to be effective in paraphilic disorders, although caution should be taken in the prescription of these treatments in order to avoid or minimize adverse effects and the risk of victimization. The combination of psychotherapy and pharmacological therapy is associated with better efficacy compared with either treatment as monotherapy. Paraphilia is a chronic disorder and a minimal duration of treatment of 3–5 years is highly recommended for severe paraphilia with a high risk of sexual violence. In conclusion, this review of the literature provides suggestive evidence that paraphilias are well characterized disorders marked by pathological dimensions. Although further research is necessary to confirm treatment efficacy and to improve our knowledge of long-term tolerance, available data on the use of selective serotonin reuptake inhibitors, steroidal antiandrogens and GnRH analogues strongly suggest the efficacy of these treatments for paraphilic disorders.

▶ This article reviews the current pharmacologic treatments for this important set of disorders and makes it clear that they are now well characterized and dangerous, very long-term (lifelong) disorders that need treatment for 35 years or more in each patient. They review that antidepressants have been found to be useful in milder and juvenile paraphilias. However, the antilibidinal hormonal treatments, such as steroidal antiandrogens and gonadotropin-releasing hormone analogues, do seem to be effective. They recommend a combination of pharmacotherapy and psychotherapy. Given the increased recognition of these disorders, clinically coupled with the accompanying increase in interest by society and the legal system, this area is one that will not go away. It's clear that increasingly many of these patients will come to the attention of not just specialists in this field but to the rank-and-file psychiatrist. I know that my practice has started to include patients with some of these issues.

J. C. Ballenger, MD

Electroconvulsive Therapy in the Spotlight
Goodman WK (Mount Sinai School of Medicine, NY)
N Engl J Med 364:1785-1787, 2011

Background.—Electroconvulsive therapy (ECT) involves the therapeutic application of electricity to the scalp to induce a seizure. It is used for patients with depression, schizophrenia, bipolar mania, and catatonia who have not responded to pharmacotherapy, those whose symptoms are severe, and those with geriatric depression. In January 2011 the Food and Drug Administration (FDA) convened the Neurological Devices Advisory Panel to review the classification of ECT devices, which are currently class III devices, indicating the highest risk. They were grandfathered in through a regulatory pathway where no premarket approval application (PMA) was required. If they remain in class III, PMA would be required, whereas reclassification into class II (intermediate-risk devices) would require establishing measures to mitigate risk. Safety, efficacy, and controls that could mitigate risk were considered. Most members recommended these devices remain in class III. The issues associated with ECT devices were reviewed.

Safety and Efficacy.—First used in 1938, ECT has been made safer through the use of general anesthesia, cardiopulmonary support, muscle relaxation, waveform and energy dosing, electroencephalographic monitoring, and various electrode placements. Usually 6 to 12 treatments are given two or three times a week. It is helpful for severe depression and other severe mental disorders, but significantly affects cognitive function, with the degree and duration of adverse effects both domain-specific and related to ECT settings. Disorientation is common but usually resolves within minutes of treatment. Anterograde amnesia, the inability to form new memories, usually disappears within days, but the inability to recall events before the ECT, known as retrograde amnesia, can persist.

Problems.—Should ECT devices remain in class III, PMAs will be required for each indication, possibly requiring more randomized, sham-controlled trials. Acceptable applications must be submitted within 30 months of the issuance of the PMA requirements. The costs for these trials may be prohibitive for the two small US manufacturers of ECT devices. The ethics and feasibility of sham-controlled studies for conditions such as severe depression, which has a high risk of suicide, are questionable. Reviews of ECT's effectiveness have been based on randomized controlled trials using sham-procedure, pill-placebo, or active-drug controls. These found that active ECT was more effective than sham ECT, placebo, and some antidepressants during acute treatment (up to 4 weeks) but not beyond that. Clinically, ECT is used when rapid onset of action is critical, then followed by antidepressant therapy. Safety reviews indicated risks for cognitive and memory dysfunction. Settings associated with greater cognitive and memory impairment are bilateral and dominant-hemisphere electrode placement, sine-wave stimulus, and high-energy doses. Persistent disorientation has not been found, and anterograde memory disturbances usually clear in 2 weeks. Global cognitive function tends to be unimpaired or improved from baseline within 3 to 6 months, which may reflect a response to treatment, since major depression often causes reversible cognitive impairment. The most troubling issue is the possible persistence of impaired retrieval of personal memories (retrograde autobiographical memory) compared to retrograde impersonal memories, which are regained in 6 months. Personal memory deficits are difficult to characterize and measure, with challenges in authenticating the memories because of the patient's underlying mental illness and the personal nature of the events. The primary instrument used to measure autobiographical memory also has limitations, including the inability to verify baseline information. Objective measures and subjective accounts of personal memory deficits often do not agree, with geriatric patients presenting particular problems differentiating the effects of cerebrovascular or degenerative brain disease from the effects of ECT.

Conclusions.—The uncertain risk of memory loss with ECT must be considered in the context of the patient's grave mental illness and the effectiveness of ECT in improving severe mental conditions. More research is needed, including the development of safer alternatives that can be compared to ECT without ethical compromise.

▶ In this perspective article in the *New England Journal of Medicine*, one of our distinguished psychiatric colleagues, Wayne Goodman, wrote of his experience being on the Neurological Devices Advisory Panel that considered the US Food and Drug Administration's (FDA) classification of electroconvulsive therapy (ECT) machines. The panel concluded that there were moderating effects of various ECT techniques and summarized that right unilateral placement with brief or ultrabrief pulses was associated with fewer cognitive or memory problems compared with bilateral, high-dose, and more frequent (3 vs 2 times a week) treatments. The panel tried to tackle the most troubling worry in the ECT field, which is permanent memory loss reported by a small number of patients. The panel concluded that there was no evidence of persistent disorientation, and the anterograde memory disturbance usually cleared within 2 weeks, and global cognitive function was either unchanged or actually improved 3 to 6 months after ECT. What they term as the "most troubling finding" was impaired retrieval of personal memories, ie, biographical memory. Whereas there was no evidence of impairment of impersonal memories by ECT, there is some evidence that autobiographical memory is changed in some patients, perhaps permanently. However, the panel failed to reach complete agreement about this issue because of the tremendous difficulty in having objective measures of baseline personal and family history prior to ECT, much less prior to the depression that interferes significantly with personal memory. They conclude that these isolated cases cannot be ignored and called for significant research into this issue, but research in this area will be extremely difficult. They remind us that these issues need to be thought about in the clinical context in which ECT is proposed, ie, in serious depression that has usually failed to respond to other treatments. I fear that they have not changed the situation much, but this is a good review in a very authoritative place that can be used in the more extended informed consent process that this FDA review now will require.

J. C. Ballenger, MD

Relationship Between Household Income and Mental Disorders: Findings From a Population-Based Longitudinal Study
Sareen J, Afifi TO, McMillan KA, et al (Univ of Manitoba, Winnipeg, Canada; Univ of Regina, Saskatchewan, Canada)
Arch Gen Psychiatry 68:419-427, 2011

Context.—There has been increasing concern about the impact of the global economic recession on mental health. To date, findings on the relationship between income and mental illness have been mixed. Some studies have found that lower income is associated with mental illness, while other studies have not found this relationship.

Objective.—To examine the relationship between income, mental disorders, and suicide attempts.

Design.—Prospective, longitudinal, nationally representative survey.

Setting.—United States general population.

Participants.—A total of 34 653 noninstitutionalized adults (aged ≥20 years) interviewed at 2 time points 3 years apart.

Main Outcomes.—Lifetime *DSM-IV* Axis I and Axis II mental disorders and lifetime suicide attempts, as well as incident mental disorders and change in income during the follow-up period.

Results.—After adjusting for potential confounders, the presence of most of the lifetime Axis I and Axis II mental disorders was associated with lower levels of income. Participants with household income of less than $20 000 per year were at increased risk of incident mood disorders during the 3-year follow-up period in comparison with those with income of $70 000 or more per year. A decrease in household income during the 2 time points was also associated with an increased risk of incident mood, anxiety, or substance use disorders (adjusted odds ratio, 1.30; 99% confidence interval, 1.06-1.60) in comparison with respondents with no change in income. Baseline presence of mental disorders did not increase the risk of change in personal or household income in the follow-up period.

Conclusions.—Low levels of household income are associated with several lifetime mental disorders and suicide attempts, and a reduction in household income is associated with increased risk for incident mental disorders. Policymakers need to consider optimal methods of intervention for mental disorders and suicidal behavior among low-income individuals.

▶ These authors examined the often controversial relationship between mental illness and income. They had data available from 34 653 noninstitutionalized adults interviewed twice 3 years apart. They were able to find that the Diagnostic and Statistical Manual of Mental Disorders-IV mental disorders and suicide attempts were significantly higher in households in which household income was less than $20 000 a year compared with $70 000 or more. Not surprisingly, a decrease in household income during the 2 time periods was also associated with new mood, anxiety, and substance abuse disorders when compared with those who had no change in their income. I'm not sure what to actually do with these data except it clearly alerts us to lower income individuals who are at greater risk for serious psychiatric problems.

J. C. Ballenger, MD

Sleep Problems and Disability Retirement: A Register-Based Follow-up Study
Lallukka T, Haaramo P, Lahelma E, et al (Univ of Helsinki, Helsinki, Finland)
Am J Epidemiol 173:871-881, 2011

Among aging employees, sleep problems are prevalent, but they may have serious consequences that are poorly understood. This study examined whether sleep problems are associated with subsequent disability retirement. Baseline questionnaire survey data collected in 2000–2002 among employees of the city of Helsinki, Finland, were linked with register data on disability retirement diagnoses by the end of 2008 ($n = 457$) for those with written consent for such linkages (74%; $N = 5,986$). Sleep problems were measured by the Jenkins Sleep Questionnaire. Cox regression analysis was used to calculate hazard ratios and 95% confidence intervals for disability retirement. Gender- and age-adjusted frequent sleep problems predicted disability retirement due to all causes (hazard ratio (HR) = 3.22,

95% confidence interval (CI): 2.26, 4.60), mental disorders (HR = 9.06, 95% CI: 3.27, 25.10), and musculoskeletal disorders (HR = 3.27, 95% CI: 1.91, 5.61). Adjustments for confounders, that is, baseline sociodemographic factors, work arrangements, psychosocial working conditions, and sleep duration, had negligible effects on these associations, whereas baseline physical working conditions and health attenuated the associations. Health behaviors and obesity did not mediate the examined associations. In conclusion, sleep problems are associated with subsequent disability retirement. To prevent early exit from work, sleep problems among aging employees need to be addressed.

▶ These authors used a large sample of Danish employed individuals and were able to demonstrate that sleep problems significantly predicted disability retirement for all causes. They were actually able to tease this effect apart from many potential confounders, and they were able to clearly document that sleep problems led to a much higher rate of disability retirement. As it is with so much of the sleep literature, this is yet another poorly recognized association between sleep problems and dysfunction.

J. C. Ballenger, MD

The Clinical Course of Body Dysmorphic Disorder in the Harvard/Brown Anxiety Research Project (HARP)

Bjornsson AS, Dyck I, Moitra E, et al (Rhode Island Hosp, Providence; Warren Alpert Med School of Brown Univ, Providence, RI)
J Nerv Ment Dis 199:55-57, 2011

This report prospectively examines the course of body dysmorphic disorder (BDD) for up to 8 years in a sample of 514 participants in the Harvard/Brown Anxiety Research Project, a naturalistic, longitudinal study of anxiety disorders. Diagnostic and Statistical Manual of Mental Disorders (4th ed.) BDD was assessed with a reliable semi-structured measure. For participants with BDD, severity of BDD symptoms was assessed with the Longitudinal Interval Follow-up Evaluation Psychiatric Status Rating scale. At the initial assessment, 17 participants (3.3%; 95% confidence interval = 1.8%−4.8%) had current BDD; 22 (4.3%; 95% confidence interval = 2.6%−6.1%) had lifetime BDD. Participants with BDD had significantly lower Global Assessment Scale scores than those without BDD, indicating poorer functioning. The probability of full recovery from BDD was 0.76, and probability of recurrence, once remitted, was 0.14 over the 8 years. In conclusion, among individuals ascertained for anxiety disorders, the probability of recovering from BDD was relatively high and probability of BDD recurrence was low.

▶ Body dysmorphic disorder (BDD) is becoming increasingly well recognized and characterized. These authors followed 515 participants in the Harvard/ Brown Anxiety Research Project, a naturalistic longitudinal study of the anxiety disorders. At initial assessment, 3.3% of the 514 participants had current BDD and 4.3% had lifetime BDD. The percentage with full recovery over the 8 years from BDD was 76% and recurrence after they had remitted occurred in 14%. This is a surprisingly high recovery rate and low relapse rate for BDD. These data are more encouraging than what many would have predicted.

J. C. Ballenger, MD

Antibiotic-induced serotonin syndrome
Miller DG, Lovell EO (Advocate Christ Med Ctr, Oak Lawn, IL)
J Emerg Med 40:25-27, 2011

Due to its broad spectrum of clinical presentations and to the large number of available serotonergic medications, serotonin syndrome (SS) remains an elusive diagnosis to many clinicians. SS results from the over-stimulation of serotonin receptors by a variety of mechanisms. New medications with the potential to cause SS are released regularly, and among them is the antibiotic linezolid. We present a case of SS in a 36-year-old woman that occurred after linezolid was added to a drug regimen that included lithium, venlafaxine, and imipramine.

▶ Serotonin syndrome is one of the severe side effects that occurs in psychiatry. Various medications that lead to the overstimulation of serotonin receptors have been observed to cause it. These authors present a case in which the new antibiotic linezolid led to the serotonin syndrome when it was added to lithium, venlafaxine, and imipramine in a 36-year-old woman. The authors make a compelling case that we should be more on the alert for this severe complication, which may seem to come out of left field, often caused by medications prescribed by another physician.

J. C. Ballenger, MD

Neurosurgeons' perspectives on psychosurgery and neuroenhancement: a qualitative study at one center
Mendelsohn D, Lipsman N, Bernstein M (Univ of Toronto, Ontario, Canada)
J Neurosurg 113:1212-1218, 2010

Object.—Advances in the neurosciences are stirring debate regarding the ethical issues surrounding novel neurosurgical interventions. The application of deep brain stimulation (DBS) for treating refractory psychiatric disease, for instance, has introduced the prospect of altering disorders of mind and behavior and the potential for neuroenhancement. The attitudes of current and future providers of this technology and their position regarding its possible future applications are unknown. The authors sought to gauge the opinions of neurosurgical staff and trainees toward various uses of neuromodulation technology including psychosurgery and neuroenhancement.

Methods.—The authors conducted a qualitative study involving in-depth interviews with 47 neurosurgery staff, trainees, and other neuroclinicians at a quaternary care center.

Results.—Several general themes emerged from the interviews. These included universal support for psychosurgery given adequate informed consent and rigorous scientific methodology, as well as a relative consensus regarding the priority given to patient autonomy and the preservation of personal identity. Participants' attitudes toward the future use of DBS and other means of neuromodulation for cognitive enhancement and personality alteration revealed less agreement, although most participants felt that alteration of nonpathological traits is objectionable.

Conclusions.—There is support in the neurosurgical community for the surgical management of refractory psychiatric disease. The use of neuromodulation for the alteration of nonpathological traits is morally and ethically dubious when it is out of sync with the values of society at large. Both DBS and neuromodulation will have far-reaching and profound public health implications.

▶ This is a fun read. The brief case vignettes are intriguing. They are provocative, and in some instances, one might consider them forceful. The authors kind of set up a strong man argument against neuromodulation of unusual conditions not readily associated with deep brain stimulation. Thus, the authors seem to reinforce their own beliefs and research focus. Moreover, while they rightly acknowledge that their sample comes from within their own program, that does not hold their generalization in the discussion of this work. Nor are the breaks put on by the absence of our effort at anonymity among interviewers and interviewees.

P. F. Buckley, MD

Miscellaneous

Seasonality patterns in postpartum depression
Sylvén SM, Papadopoulos FC, Olovsson M, et al (Uppsala Univ, Sweden)
Am J Obstet Gynecol 204:413.e1-413.e6, 2011

Objective.—To investigate the possible association between postpartum depressive symptoms and season of delivery.

Study Design.—During 1 year, delivering women in the Uppsala University Hospital were asked to participate in the study by filling out 3 postpartum questionnaires containing the Edinburgh Postnatal Depression scale and questions assessing life style, medical history, breastfeeding, and social support.

Results.—Two thousand three hundred eighteen women participated. Women delivering in the last 3 months of the year had a significantly higher risk of self-reported depressive symptomatology both at 6 weeks (odds ratio, 2.02, 95% confidence interval, 1.32–3.10) and at 6 months after delivery (odds ratio, 1.82, 95% confidence interval, 1.15–2.88), in comparison to those delivering April-June, both before and after adjustment for possible confounders.

Conclusion.—Women delivering during the last quartile of the year had a significantly higher risk for depressive symptoms 6 weeks and 6 months postpartum and would thus benefit from a closer support and follow-up after delivery.

▶ These Swedish investigators followed 2318 pregnant women and their depressive difficulties relative to the season of the year they delivered. In fact, women who delivered in the last 3 months of the year did have a significantly higher risk of depressive symptomatology both at 6 weeks and 6 months after delivery compared with those who delivered between April and June. This is just another of the many alerting factors for clinicians working with this high-risk group.

J. C. Ballenger, MD

Reliability and Comparability of Psychosis Patients' Retrospective Reports of Childhood Abuse
Fisher HL, Craig TK, Fearon P, et al (King's College London, UK; et al)
Schizophr Bull 37:546-553, 2011

An increasing number of studies are demonstrating an association between childhood abuse and psychosis. However, the majority of these rely on retrospective self-reports in adulthood that may be unduly influenced by current psychopathology. We therefore set out to explore the reliability and comparability of first-presentation psychosis patients' reports of childhood abuse. Psychosis case subjects were drawn from the Aetiology and Ethnicity of Schizophrenia and Other Psychoses (ÆSOP) epidemiological study and completed the Childhood Experience of Care and Abuse Questionnaire to elicit abusive experiences that occurred prior to 16 years of age. High levels of concurrent validity were demonstrated with the Parental Bonding Instrument (antipathy: $r_s = 0.35–0.737$, $P < .001$; neglect: $r_s = 0.688–0.715$, $P < .001$), and good convergent validity was shown with clinical case notes (sexual abuse: $\kappa = 0.526$, $P < .001$; physical abuse: $\kappa = 0.394$, $P < .001$). Psychosis patients' reports were also reasonably stable over a 7-year period (sexual abuse: $\kappa = 0.590$, $P < .01$; physical abuse: $\kappa = 0.634$, $P < .001$; antipathy: $\kappa = 0.492$, $P < .01$; neglect: $\kappa = 0.432$, $P < .05$). Additionally, their reports of childhood abuse were not associated with current severity of psychotic symptoms (sexual abuse: $U = 1768.5$, $P = .998$; physical abuse: $U = 2167.5$, $P = .815$; antipathy: $U = 2216.5$, $P = .988$; neglect: $U = 1906.0$, $P = .835$) or depressed mood (sexual abuse: $\chi^2 = 0.634$, $P = .277$; physical abuse: $\chi^2 = 0.159$, $P = .419$; antipathy: $\chi^2 = 0.868$, $P = .229$; neglect: $\chi^2 = 0.639$, $P = .274$).

These findings provide justification for the use in future studies of retrospective reports of childhood abuse obtained from individuals with psychotic disorders.

▶ This article provides evidence that reports of childhood abuse from now adult psychotic patients probably should be believed and not widely doubted as is often the case. They found good evidence that these reports were stable over a 7-year period and had good convergent validity with clinical case notes and other measures. The authors found that these reports were not in any way associated with the severity of psychosis. This result gives validity to our use of childhood reports of abuse by psychotic patients both in clinical practice and in research.

J. C. Ballenger, MD

Distinguishing Between Major Depressive Disorder and Obsessive-Compulsive Disorder in Children by Measuring Regional Cortical Thickness
Fallucca E, MacMaster FP, Haddad J, et al (Wayne State Univ, Detroit, MI)
Arch Gen Psychiatry 68:527-533, 2011

Context.—Cortical abnormalities have been noted in previous studies of major depressive disorder (MDD).

Objective.—To hypothesize differences in regional cortical thickness among children with MDD, children with obsessive-compulsive disorder (OCD), and healthy controls.

Design.—Cross-sectional study of groups.

Setting.—Children's Hospital of Michigan in Detroit.

Participants.—A total of 24 psychotropic drug—naive pediatric patients with MDD (9 boys and 15 girls), 24 psychotropic drug—naive pediatric outpatients with OCD (8 boys and 16 girls), and 30 healthy controls (10 boys and 20 girls).

Intervention.—Magnetic resonance imaging.

Main Outcome Measure.—Cortical thickness.

Results.—In the right hemisphere of the brain, the pericalcarine gyrus was thinner in patients with MDD than in outpatients with OCD ($P = .002$) or healthy controls ($P = .04$), the postcentral gyrus was thinner in patients with MDDthan in outpatients with OCD ($P = .002$) or healthy controls ($P = .02$), and the superior parietal gyrus was thinner in patients with MDD than in outpatients with OCD ($P = .008$) or healthy controls ($P = .03$). The outpatients with OCD and the healthy controls did not differ in these regions of the brain. The temporal pole was thicker in patients with MDD than in outpatients with OCD ($P < .001$) or healthy controls ($P = .01$), both of which groups did not differ in temporal pole thickness. The cuneus was thinner in patients with MDD than in outpatients with OCD ($P = .008$), but it did not differ from that in healthy controls. In the left hemisphere, the supramarginal gyrus was thinner in both patients with MDD ($P = .04$) and outpatients with OCD ($P = .01$) than in healthy controls, and the temporal pole was thicker in patients with MDD than in both healthy controls and outpatients with OCD ($P < .001$).

Conclusions.—To our knowledge, this is the first study to explore cortical thickness in pediatric patients with MDD. Although differences in some regions of the brain would be expected given neurobiological models of MDD, our study highlights some unexpected regions (ie, supramarginal and superior parietal gyri) that merit further investigation. These results underscore the need to expand exploration beyond the frontal-limbic circuit.

▶ These authors compared 24 drug-naïve pediatric patients with major depressive disorder (MDD) with 24 drug-naïve pediatric outpatients with obsessive-compulsive disorder (OCD) and 30 healthy controls. On magnetic resonance imaging, the patients with MDD had thinner cortical thickness in the pericalcarine gyrus, postcentral gyrus, and superior parietal gyrus than both patients with OCD and healthy controls, which did not differ from each other. The temporal pole was thicker in patients with MDD and the cuneus was thinner (although not when compared with healthy controls). In the left hemisphere, the supramarginal gyrus was thinner in both patients with MDD and OCD than in controls, and the temporal pole was thicker in patients with MDD than both comparison groups. This well-done study in the *Archives* joins the large documentation that our psychiatric disorders are related to differing brain development. Again, this is the type of research that we certainly hope will allow us to ultimately better treat our patients as well as to reduce the stigma associated with their illnesses.

J. C. Ballenger, MD

Association Between Traumatic Injury and Psychiatric Disorders and Medication Prescription to Youths Aged 10–19

Zatzick DF, Grossman DC (Univ of Washington Harborview Med Ctr, Seattle; Univ of Washington School of Medicine, Seattle)
Psychiatr Serv 62:264-271, 2011

Objective.—Few clinical epidemiologic investigations have assessed whether youths exposed to a traumatic injury demonstrate elevations in the full spectrum of provider-recognized psychiatric disorders compared with unexposed, noninjured youths.

Methods.—In a population-based prospective cohort study, data for children and adolescents aged ten to 19 who were enrolled in the Group Health Cooperative health plan were screened for injury visits in the index year of 2001 (N=20,507). Psychiatric diagnoses, including anxiety and acute stress, depressive, substance use, and disruptive behavior disorders, given to these youths over the next three years (2002–2004) were documented, as were psychotropic medication prescriptions. Regression analyses assessed for an independent association between injury and psychiatric disorders and prescription of psychotropic medication.

Results.—In adjusted regression analyses, injury in the index year was independently associated with significantly increased odds of receiving a diagnosis of anxiety or acute stress (odds ratio [OR]=1.21, 95% confidence interval [CI]=1.02−1.44), depression (OR=1.30, CI=1.10−1.53), and a substance use disorder (OR=1.56, CI=1.21−2.00) and of receiving a psychotropic medication prescription (OR=1.37, CI=1.20−1.57). Youths with traumatic brain injuries also were significantly more likely to receive psychotropic medication prescriptions.

Conclusions.—Traumatic injury was independently associated with an increased risk of receiving a full spectrum of anxiety, depressive, and substance use diagnoses among youths aged ten to 19. Population-based surveillance procedures that incorporate screening and stepped-care interventions targeting the spectrum of postinjury emotional disturbances have the potential to improve the quality of mental health care for youths treated in general medical settings.

▶ This study explored an understudied area of what happens to children and adolescents who are 10 to 19 years old after a traumatic brain injury (TBI). These authors used the Group Health Cooperative Plan database of 20 507 individuals and then followed them over the next 3 years. Interestingly, they were able to document that a TBI was associated with an increased risk of a diagnosis of anxiety, depression, or a substance abuse disorder, and also for receiving a psychotropic medication prescription. This is another approach that documents the importance of TBI in our society and an article that certainly those of us who see children should be well aware of.

J. C. Ballenger, MD

BREATHE: A Pilot Study of a One-Day Retreat to Reduce Burnout Among Mental Health Professionals
Salyers MP, Hudson C, Morse G, et al (Indiana Univ−Purdue Univ Indianapolis; Roudebush Dept of Veterans Affairs Med Ctr, Indianapolis, IN; Community Alternatives, St Louis, MO; et al)
Psychiatr Serv 62:214-217, 2011

Objective.—Staff burnout is a frequent problem for mental health providers and may be associated with negative outcomes for providers, consumers, and organizations. This study tested an intervention to reduce staff burnout.

Methods.—Community mental health providers were invited to participate in a day-long training session to learn methods to reduce burnout. A Web-based survey was given at time of registration, before the intervention, and again six weeks later.

Results.—Eighty-four providers participated in the training, and follow-up data were available for 74. Six weeks after the day-long training, staff reported significant decreases in emotional exhaustion and depersonalization and significant increases in positive views toward consumers. There were no significant changes in providers' sense of personal accomplishment, job satisfaction, or intention to leave their position. Ninety-one percent of the staff reported the training to be helpful.

Conclusions.—This brief intervention is feasible, is acceptable to staff, and may improve burnout and staff attitudes.

▶ This was an interesting study of a 1-day retreat for mental health providers that attempted to teach methods to reduce burnout. Interestingly, 84 providers participated, and there were follow-up data from 74 providers 6 weeks later. At that point, they did report significant decreases in emotional exhaustion and depersonalization and significant increases in positive views towards their consumers. Ninety-one percent found the training to be helpful. This is an interesting attempt to try to help us as we do our very difficult jobs. More power to them.

J. C. Ballenger, MD

Cognitive Effects of Atypical Antipsychotic Medications in Patients With Alzheimer's Disease: Outcomes From CATIE-AD

Vigen CLP, Mack WJ, Keefe RSE, et al (Univ of Southern California, Los Angeles, CA; Duke Univ, Durham, NC; Mount Sinai School of Medicine, NY; et al)
Am J Psychiatry 168:1-9, 2011

Objective.—The impact of the atypical antipsychotics olanzapine, quetiapine, and risperidone on cognition in patients with Alzheimer's disease is unclear. The authors assessed the effects of time and treatment on neuropsychological functioning during the Clinical Antipsychotic Trials of Intervention Effectiveness—Alzheimer's Disease study (CATIE-AD).

Method.—CATIE-AD included 421 outpatients with Alzheimer's disease and psychosis or agitated/aggressive behavior who were randomly assigned to receive masked, flexible-dose olanzapine, quetiapine, risperidone, or placebo. Based on their clinicians' judgment, patients could discontinue the originally assigned medication and receive another randomly assigned medication. Patients were followed for 36 weeks, and cognitive assessments were obtained at baseline and at 12, 24, and 36 weeks. Outcomes were compared for 357 patients for whom data were available for at least one cognitive measure at baseline and one follow-up assessment that took place after they had been on their prescribed medication or placebo for at least 2 weeks.

Results.—Overall, patients showed steady, significant declines over time in most cognitive areas, including in scores on the Mini-Mental State Examination (MMSE; −2.4 points over 36 weeks) and the cognitive subscale of the Alzheimer's Disease Assessment Scale (−4.4 points). Cognitive function declined more in patients receiving antipsychotics than in those given placebo on multiple cognitive measures, including the MMSE, the cognitive subscale of the Brief Psychiatric Rating Scale, and a cognitive summary score summarizing change on 18 cognitive tests.

Conclusions.—In CATIE-AD, atypical antipsychotics were associated with worsening cognitive function at a magnitude consistent with 1 year's deterioration compared with placebo. Further cognitive impairment is an additional risk of treatment with atypical antipsychotics that should be considered when treating patients with Alzheimer's disease.

▶ There are some disturbing but inconsistent studies that the use of antipsychotics in elderly patients with Alzheimer disease to treat their delusions or aggressive behavior may be associated with an increased death rate. This has led to a black box warning on the antipsychotics, particularly because the antipsychotics are only marginally helpful in these patients, but clinicians have few other treatment options. This remains an important research issue. These authors also followed up the research, suggesting that use of atypical antipsychotics also leads to cognitive worsening in these patients. These authors used the Clinical Antipsychotic Trials of Intervention Effectiveness—Alzheimer's Disease study of 421 outpatients with Alzheimer disease and psychosis, agitation, or aggression who were randomly assigned to receive flexible doses of olanzapine, quetiapine, risperidone, or placebo. They were followed up for 36 weeks, and strikingly, the patients showed significant declines in several cognitive areas. They likened the decrease in cognitive function to the same order of magnitude as the beneficial effects of Aricept in these patients. However, there are few other medicines that are approved or effective in this particularly important clinical indication. However, this research strongly suggests that clinicians must try hard to find other ways to treat these patients, because antipsychotics obviously appear to have significant effects on cognitive function as well as other potential increases in death, stroke, and the metabolic syndrome.

J. C. Ballenger, MD

Counter-transference in Eating Disorder Treatment: A Systematic Review
Forget K, Marussi DR, Corff YL (Université d'Ottawa, Ontario, Canada; Université de Sherbrooke, Québec, Canada)
Can J Psychiatry 56:303-310, 2011

Objective.—To identify counter-transference occurrences and causes in therapists treating patients with eating disorders, and to present suggested solutions to overcome counter-transference's negative aspects and to enhance treatment quality.

Method.—Using the major health science and psychology databases, we have identified studies dealing with counter-transference in eating disorder treatment.

Results.—Many counter-transference occurrences are identified. It seems that therapists often feel negative affects while treating patients with eating disorders. Counter-transference seems to be affected by factors related to both the disorder and to the patient and therapist. Further, negative counter-transference can lead to consequences interfering with proper conduct of treatment. The main solutions identified to deal with counter-transference are supervision, consulting with colleagues, and teamwork.

Conclusions.—Many factors involved in counter-transference seem hardly modifiable; hence it is important to implement efficient solutions allowing overcoming its negative aspects. Moreover, few empirical studies have focused on counter-transference in eating disorder treatment. That research field is highly pertinent but very rarely exploited, and it deserves the scientific community's attention.

▶ Anyone who treats patients with eating disorders knows that it is hard, difficult work and work that is often avoided by many practitioners. These authors review the evidence of the counter-transference difficulties therapists of these patients frequently have and the resultant negative consequences. They propose countermeasures, including supervision and consultation with colleagues, as well as working as a team, to help deal with this as a practical matter. This is a good review article that any practitioner treating or thinking about treating these patients should read.

J. C. Ballenger, MD

Risk of placental abruption in relation to maternal depressive, anxiety and stress symptoms

de Paz NC, Sanchez SE, Huaman LE, et al (Univ of Washington, Seattle; Hospital Nacional dos de Mayo, Peru; Instituto Especializado Materno Perinatal, Lima, Peru; et al)
J Affect Disord 130:280-284, 2011

Background.—Little is known about the influence of psychiatric factors on the etiology of placental abruption (PA), an obstetrical condition that complicates 1—2% of pregnancies. We examined the risk of PA in relation to maternal psychiatric symptoms during pregnancy.

Methods.—This case—control study included 373 PA cases and 368 controls delivered at five medical centers in Lima, Peru. Depressive, anxiety and stress symptoms were assessed using the Patient Health Questionnaire (PHQ-9) and the Depression Anxiety Stress Scales (DASS-21). Multivariable logistic regression models were fit to calculate odds ratios (aOR) and 95% confidence intervals (CI) adjusted for confounders.

Results.—Depressive symptoms of increasing severity (using the DASS depression subscale) was associated with PA (p for trend = 0.02). Compared with women with no depressive symptoms, the aOR (95%CI) for PA associated with each level of severity of depression symptoms based on the DASS assessment were as follows: mild 1.84 (0.91—3.74); moderate 1.25 (0.67—2.33); and severe 4.68 (0.98—22.4). The corresponding ORs for mild, moderate, and moderately severe depressive symptoms based on the PHQ assessment were 1.10 (0.79—1.54), 3.31 (1.45—7.57), and 5.01 (1.06—23.6), respectively. A positive gradient was observed for the odds of PA with severity of anxiety (p for trend $= 0.002$) and stress symptoms (p for trend $= 0.002$).

Limitations.—These cross-sectionally collected data may be subject to recall bias.

Conclusions.—Maternal psychiatric disorders may be associated with an increased occurrence of AP. Larger studies that allow for more precise evaluations of maternal psychiatric health in relation to PA risk are warranted.

▶ We have followed the issues of depression and pregnancy for the past few years. These authors approach it from a different direction, that is, whether depressive symptoms were associated with placental abruption (PA). They stated that they in fact did find that PA was associated with severe depression with an odds ratio of 5.01, a striking increase. There was also a positive relationship with the severity of anxiety that was significant. At the very least, this adds to the large database for those who manage pregnant women, indicating that they should be concerned about the impact of depression during this critical period.

J. C. Ballenger, MD

The Delivery of Behavioral Sleep Medicine to College Students

Kloss JD, Nash CO, Horsey SE, et al (Drexel Univ, Philadelphia, PA; et al)
J Adolesc Health 48:553-561, 2011

College students are vulnerable to a variety of sleep disorders, which can result in sleep deprivation and a variety of other consequences. The delivery of behavioral sleep medicine is particularly relevant for the college student population, as the early intervention on their sleep problems might prevent lifelong consequences. This article critically reviews the efficacy of relevant behavioral sleep medicine interventions and discusses special considerations for using them with college students who have unique sleep patterns and lifestyles. Recommendations are also given regarding ways to disseminate these empirically supported treatments into this environment. Finally, recommendations regarding future research directions are discussed in the present study.

▶ As a parent and clinician, I am often confronted with the remarkable sleep issues in college students given their almost reversal of day/night many nights of the week. This article is a nice review of the many issues and also makes suggestions about how to disseminate empirically supported treatments in this particular population. I would recommend this article to those readers who have to deal with these issues.

J. C. Ballenger, MD

The Long-Term Effect of Insomnia on Primary Headaches: A Prospective Population-Based Cohort Study (HUNT-2 and HUNT-3)

Ødegård SS, Sand T, Engstrøm M, et al (Norwegian Univ of Science and Technology, Trondheim, Norway; et al)
Headache 51:570-580, 2011

Objective.—Few prospective studies have evaluated the relationship between insomnia and headache. We aimed to analyze the influence of insomnia at baseline on the risk for headache 11 years later.

Methods.—This longitudinal cohort study included subjects who participated in 2 consecutive surveys of the Nord-Trøndelag Health Study (HUNT-2 and HUNT-3). Among the invited individuals aged 20 years or more in HUNT-2 (n = 92,566) and HUNT-3 (n = 94,194), a total of 26,197 completed the headache section of both surveys. A proxy insomnia diagnosis based on DSM-IV at baseline and ICDH-2-based headache diagnoses at follow-up were derived from questionnaires. Headache-free individuals in HUNT-2 (n = 15,268) were selected for analysis. The relative risks (RRs) for headache in insomniacs were calculated with logistic regression.

Results.—The presence of baseline insomnia was associated with a 40% increased risk for headache in HUNT-3 (RR = 1.4, 95% CI = 1.2-1.7). Similar results were found for tension-type headache (TTH), migraine, and non-classified headache. Subjects with insomnia-related working disability had a 60% increased headache risk (RR = 1.6, 95% CI = 1.3-2.1). The RR was larger for migraine (RR = 2.0, 95% CI = 1.3-3.1) than for TTH (RR = 1.5, 95% CI = 1.1-2.1). Insomnia at baseline was related to headache frequency at follow-up for both migraine (*P* trend = 0.02) and TTH (*P* trend < 0.001).

Conclusion.—In headache-free subjects, insomnia was associated with an increased risk of headache 11 years later. The association was particularly strong for chronic headache.

▶ This is another study of the increasing knowledge base of the effect of poor sleep on symptoms and function. They were able to use 2 huge databases of more than 90 000 individuals. They were able to study a total of 26 197 individuals who filled out the insomnia and headache sections of the questionnaire. They studied the 15 268 headache-free individuals to demonstrate that, in the presence of baseline insomnia, there was a 40% increased risk for headache 11 years later. The insomnia-related working disability had a 60% increased headache rate, and the risk was even higher for migraine and tension headaches. This association was particularly strong for chronic headaches. This is yet another effect of poor sleep.

J. C. Ballenger, MD

Transition from military to VHA care: Psychiatric health services for Iraq/Afghanistan combat-wounded

Copeland LA, Zeber JE, Bingham MO, et al (Veterans Affairs: Central Texas Veterans Health Care System Temple; South Texas Veterans Health Care System, San Antonio; et al)
J Affect Disord 130:226-230, 2011

Objective.—Veterans from the wars in Afghanistan and Iraq (OEF/OIF) report high rates of mental distress especially affective disorders. Ensuring continuity of care across institutions is a priority for both the Department of Defense (DoD) and the Veterans Health Administration (VHA), yet this process is not monitored nor are medical records integrated. This study assessed transition from DoD to VHA and subsequent psychiatric care of service members traumatically injured in OEF/OIF.

Methods.—Inpatients at a DoD trauma treatment facility discharged in FY02-FY06 (n = 994) were tracked into the VHA via archival data (n = 216 OEF/OIF veterans). Mental health utilization in both systems was analyzed.

Results.—VHA users were 9% female, 15% Hispanic; mean age 32 (SD = 10; range 19—59). No DoD inpatients received diagnoses of post-traumatic stress disorder (PTSD); 21% had other mental health diagnoses, primarily drug abuse. In the VHA, 38% sought care within 6 months of DoD discharge; 75% within 1 year. VHA utilization increased over time, with 88—89% of the transition cohort seeking care in FY07—FY09. Most accessed VHA mental health services (81%) and had VHA psychiatric diagnoses (71%); half met criteria for depression (27%) or PTSD (38%). Treatment retention through FY09 was significantly greater for those receiving psychiatric care: 98% vs 62% of those not receiving psychiatric care ($x^2 = 53.3$; p<.001).

Limitations.—DoD outpatient data were not available. The study relied on administrative data.

Conclusions.—Although physical trauma led to hospitalization in the DoD, high rates of psychiatric disorders were identified in subsequent VHA care, suggesting delay in development or recognition of psychiatric problems.

▶ Perhaps for the first time in our history, we are paying greater attention to the issue of psychiatric problems in our war veterans after they have come home. Although continuity of care is so important, it is striking that the Department of Defense (DoD) records are not integrated with the medical records of Veterans Health Administration (VHA). In general, with each of the past wars, we have underappreciated the impact of posttraumatic stress disorder (PTSD). In this large sample, none of the DoD patients received a diagnosis of PTSD, although 21% had other mental health diagnoses, mostly drug abuse. However, in the VHA, 38% sought care within 6 months of DoD discharge, and 75% sought care after 1 year. The VHA services increased over time, the greatest increase being for mental health services (81%). Almost half met the criteria for depression or PTSD (now at 38%). Although in many ways we appear to be doing better, these data would suggest that we are still very slow in recognizing psychiatric problems, particularly PTSD, in our returning veterans.

J. C. Ballenger, MD

"A Disease Like Any Other"? A Decade of Change in Public Reactions to Schizophrenia, Depression, and Alcohol Dependence
Pescosolido BA, Martin JK, Long JS, et al (Indiana Univ, Bloomington; Columbia Univ, NY)
Am J Psychiatry 167:1321-1330, 2010

Objective.—Clinicians, advocates, and policy makers have presented mental illnesses as medical diseases in efforts to overcome low service use, poor adherence rates, and stigma. The authors examined the impact of this approach with a 10-year comparison of public endorsement of treatment and prejudice.

Method.—The authors analyzed responses to vignettes in the mental health modules of the 1996 and 2006 General Social Survey describing individuals meeting DSM-IV criteria for schizophrenia, major depression, and alcohol dependence to explore whether more of the public 1) embraces neurobiological understandings of mental illness; 2) endorses treatment from providers, including psychiatrists; and 3) reports community acceptance or rejection of people with these disorders. Multivariate analyses examined whether acceptance of neurobiological causes increased treatment support and lessened stigma.

Results.—In 2006, 67% of the public attributed major depression to neurobiological causes, compared with 54% in 1996. High proportions of respondents endorsed treatment, with general increases in the proportion endorsing treatment from doctors and specific increases in the proportions endorsing psychiatrists for treatment of alcohol dependence (from 61% in 1996 to 79% in 2006) and major depression (from 75% in 1996 to 85% in 2006). Social distance and perceived danger associated with people with these disorders did not decrease significantly. Holding a neurobiological conception of these disorders increased the likelihood of support for treatment but was generally unrelated to stigma. Where associated, the effect was to increase, not decrease, community rejection.

Conclusions.—More of the public embraces a neurobiological understanding of mental illness. This view translates into support for services but not into a decrease in stigma. Reconfiguring stigma reduction strategies may require providers and advocates to shift to an emphasis on competence and inclusion.

▶ I have long been interested in issues concerning the stigma around the illnesses we treat and have been heartened by improvements over my almost 40 years in psychiatry. This particular study compared responses in 1996 to 2006 about public understanding that these illnesses are neurobiological;

whether they believe psychiatrists should treat these illnesses; and ultimately, in issues of stigmatization and rejection of people with these disorders. We, in fact, have observed some improvement in this time period. The understanding that depression is a neurobiological issue increased from 54% in 1996 to 67% in 2006. In the alcohol field, the proportion who feel that patients should be treated by doctors and psychiatrists for alcohol dependence increased from 61% in 1996 to 79% in 2006; and major depression increased from 75% in 1996 to 85% in 2006. However, distressingly, the social distance and perceived danger associated with people with these disorders did not decrease significantly, and it appears that having a neurobiological conception of these disorders did not help with reducing stigma. It appears that we will require other strategies to improve things on the stigma front.

J. C. Ballenger, MD

Sleep Disturbances and Cause-Specific Mortality: Results From the GAZEL Cohort Study
Rod NH, Vahtera J, Westerlund H, et al (Univ of Copenhagen, Denmark; Univ of Turku and Turku Univ Hosp, Finland; Univ of Stockholm, Sweden; et al)
Am J Epidemiol 173:300-309, 2011

Poor sleep is an increasing problem in modern society, but most previous studies on the association between sleep and mortality rates have addressed only duration, not quality, of sleep. The authors prospectively examined the effects of sleep disturbances on mortality rates and on important risk factors for mortality, such as body mass index, hypertension, and diabetes. A total of 16,989 participants in the GAZEL cohort study were asked validated questions on sleep disturbances in 1990 and were followed up until 2009, with <1% loss to follow-up. Body mass index, hypertension, and diabetes were measured annually through self-reporting. During follow-up, a total of 1,045 men and women died. Sleep disturbances were associated with a higher overall mortality risk in men ($P = 0.005$) but not in women ($P = 0.33$). This effect was most pronounced for men <45 years of age (≥ 3 symptoms vs. none: hazard ratio $= 2.03$, 95% confidence interval: 1.24, 3.33). There were no clear associations between sleep disturbances and cardiovascular mortality rates, although men and women with sleep disturbances were more likely to develop hypertension and diabetes ($P < 0.001$). Compared with people with no sleep disturbances, men who reported ≥ 3 types of sleep disturbance had an almost 5 times' higher risk of committing suicide (hazard ratio $= 4.99$, 95% confidence interval: 1.59, 15.7). Future strategies to prevent premature deaths may benefit from assessment of sleep disturbances, especially in younger individuals.

▶ I have been interested in the evolving education of the general public and the clinical treatment population about the association of sleep problems with mortality. In the GAZEL study, 16 989 individuals were asked questions about their sleep disturbances, and this was correlated with their body mass index, diabetes, and hypertension. In fact, the authors did observe that sleep disturbances were associated with a higher overall mortality risk in men but not in women. This was most pronounced in men aged more than 45 years. What they observed was an association between sleep disturbances and the development of hypertension and diabetes and, strikingly, a 5 times higher risk of suicide. The authors strongly suggest that we may prevent premature deaths if we pay greater attention to sleep disturbances, especially in younger individuals and, I think, in men. This study is consistent with the whole advance of sleep-disorder medicine correlating sleep disturbances, both in length and quality of sleep, with medical conditions (eg, hypertension, diabetes) and higher mortality rates. The sleep disturbance field has had a champion, Bill Dement from Stanford, who has been preaching these lessons ahead of the data for many years to Congress and even on the "David Letterman Show." The data have finally caught up with him and are leading to better public understanding of these issues.

J. C. Ballenger, MD

Psychiatry in General Medicine

Antidepressant medication use and future risk of cardiovascular disease: the Scottish Health Survey

Hamer M, David Batty G, Seldenrijk A, et al (Univ College London, UK; Vrije Universiteit Med Ctr, Amsterdam, The Netherlands)
Eur Heart J 32:437-442, 2011

Aims.—The association between antidepressant use and risk of cardiovascular disease (CVD) remains controversial, particularly in initially healthy samples. Given that antidepressants such as selective serotonin reuptake inhibitors (SSRIs) are now prescribed not only for depression, but also for a wide range of conditions, this issue has relevance to the general population. We assessed the association between antidepressant medication use and future risk of CVD in a representative sample of community-dwelling adults without known CVD.

Methods and Results.—A prospective cohort study of 14 784 adults (aged 52.4 ± 11.9 years, 43.9% males) without a known history of CVD was drawn from the Scottish Health Surveys. Of these study participants, 4.9% reported the use of antidepressant medication. Incident CVD events (comprising CVD death, non-fatal myocardial infarction, coronary surgical procedures, stroke, and heart failure) over 8-year follow-up were ascertained by a linkage to national registers; a total of 1434 events were recorded. The use of tricyclic antidepressants (TCAs) was associated with elevated risk of CVD [multivariate-adjusted hazard ratio (HR) = 1.35, 95% confidence interval (CI), 1.03—1.77] after accounting for a range of covariates. There was a non-significant association between TCA use and coronary heart disease events (969 events, multivariate-adjusted HR = 1.24, 95% CI, 0.87—1.75). The use of SSRIs was not associated with CVD. Neither class of drug was associated with all-cause mortality risk.

Conclusion.—Although replication is required, the increased risk of CVD in men and women taking TCAs was not explained by existing mental illness, which suggests that this medication is associated with an excess disease burden.

▶ These authors used a large sample of 14 740 adults without a history of cardiovascular disease (CVD) in Scotland to study use of antidepressant medication and CVD. In this trial, 4.9% reported the use of antidepressant medications, and using the Scottish Health Registry, the authors reviewed an 8-year follow-up and observed 1434 cardiovascular events. They observed that the use of tricyclic antidepressants (TCAs) was associated with an elevated risk of CVD (hazard ratio [HR] = 1.35) and also found a nonsignificant association with TCA use and coronary heart disease events (HR = 1.24). Interestingly, the use of selective serotonin reuptake inhibitors (SSRIs) was not associated with increased CVD, and neither class of drug led to a significant increase in all-cause mortality. The authors were able to factor out the portion of deaths related to mental illness and taking TCAs and laid the burden of this increased risk squarely on the TCAs. This is an interesting study but one that has less relevance today because the SSRIs are much more frequently prescribed, particularly in developed nations. However, in the developing world, TCAs are often recommended and used preferentially because they are less expensive. This study certainly adds complexity to that issue.

J. C. Ballenger, MD

Azithromycin-Induced Agitation and Choreoathetosis
Farooq O, Memon Z, Stojanovski SD, et al (Women and Children's Hosp of Buffalo, NY)
Pediatr Neurol 44:311-313, 2011

We report a child who developed agitation and choreoathetoid movements with azithromycin therapy on 2 separate occasions. In both instances, the symptoms resolved when the antibiotic was discontinued. By means of the Naranjo adverse drug reaction probability scale, we classified this event as a probable adverse drug reaction (score of 6 points). To our knowledge, this is the first published case of azithromycin-induced agitation with choreoathetosis. Because this is a widely used medication for many common infectious conditions, including otitis media and pneumonia, this potential serious adverse reaction should be considered.

▶ I thought we should include this article, which is pertinent to every psychiatrist and every physician for that matter. The authors report a case of a child who developed agitation and choreoathetoid movements after being treated with azithromycin (Z-pack) on 2 separate occasions. The symptoms resolved when the antibiotic was discontinued, and the authors are fairly convinced that it was secondary to the commonly used Z-pack. We should think about this and every similar kind of case and ask if these patients are currently taking a Z-pack. This is such a commonly used antibiotic that I think we will see this, even if it's a very rare side effect.

J. C. Ballenger, MD

The Blind Spot in the Drive for Childhood Obesity Prevention: Bringing Eating Disorders Prevention Into Focus as a Public Health Priority
Austin SB (Children's Hosp Boston, MA)
Am J Public Health 101:e1-e4, 2011

Public health attention to childhood obesity has increased in tandem with the growing epidemic, but despite this intense focus, successes in prevention have lagged far behind. There is a blind spot in our drive for childhood obesity prevention that prevents us from generating sufficiently broad solutions.

Eating disorders and the constellation of perilous weight-control behaviors are in that blind spot. Evidence is mounting that obesity and eating disorders are linked in myriad ways, but entrenched myths about eating disorders undermine our ability to see the full range of leverage points to target in obesity preventive intervention studies.

Our efforts to prevent childhood obesity can no longer afford to ignore eating disorders and the assemblage of related behaviors that persist unabated.

▶ My readers will recognize a familiar theme: that ignoring traditional psychiatric knowledge in nonpsychiatric settings is foolish. Here again, the authors point out that part of our failure to effectively target childhood obesity is an apparent "blind spot" in this area in which we fail to pay attention to the eating disorders and related behaviors that seem to have such an important impact.

J. C. Ballenger, MD

A Western Diet Increases Serotonin Availability in Rat Small Intestine
Bertrand RL, Senadheera S, Markus I, et al (Univ of New South Wales, Sydney, Australia)
Endocrinology 152:36-47, 2011

Diet-induced obesity is associated with changes in gastrointestinal function and induction of a mild inflammatory state. Serotonin (5-HT) containing enterochromaffin (EC) cells within the intestine respond to nutrients and are altered by inflammation. Thus, our aim was to characterize the uptake and release of 5-HT from EC cells of the rat ileum in a physiologically relevant model of diet-induced obesity. In chow-fed (CF) and Western diet–fed (WD) rats electrochemical methods were used to measure compression evoked (peak) and steady state (SS) 5-HT levels with fluoxetine used to block the serotonin reuptake transporter (SERT). The levels of mRNA for tryptophan hydroxylase 1 (TPH1) and SERT were determined by quantitative PCR, while EC cell numbers were determined immunohistochemically. In WD rats, the levels of 5-HT were significantly increased (SS: 19.2 ± 3.7 μM; peak: 73.5 ± 14.1 μM) compared with CF rats (SS: 12.3 ± 1.8 μM; peak: 32.2 ± 7.2 μM), while SERT-dependent uptake of 5-HT was reduced (peak WD: 108% of control versus peak CF: 212% control). In WD rats, there was a significant increase in TPH1 mRNA, a decrease in SERT mRNA and protein, and an increase in EC cells. In conclusion, our data show that foods typical of a Western diet are associated with an increased 5-HT availability in the rat ileum. Increased 5-HT availability is driven by the up-regulation of 5-HT synthesis genes, decreased re-uptake of 5-HT, and increased numbers and/or 5-HT content of EC cells which are likely to cause altered intestinal motility and sensation *in vivo*.

▶ We are what we eat! This is a very cool article. It basically describes the effect of a western diet on the intestine such that it also affects serotonin function in the gut. There is, of course, the proposition that altering serotonin in the gut might also affect central serotonin function, especially in the hypothalamus area, so I was surprised that this study did not include some subsequent postmortem autoradiography of the rat brains. This would have really made it even more interesting than it already is. This is the kind of hard science article that gets taken up by CNN and the world media. It's easy to understand why. Great work.

P. F. Buckley, MD

Pain Documentation and Predictors of Analgesic Prescribing for Elderly Patients During Emergency Department Visits

Iyer RG (CVS|Caremark Inc, Northbrook, IL)
J Pain Symptom Manage 41:367-373, 2011

Context.—Inappropriate pain documentation is likely to be an important contributor to the poor management of pain in elderly patients in the emergency department (ED). Failure to assess pain limits ability to treat pain.

Objectives.—The objectives of this study were to examine the relationship between visit characteristics of elderly patients and pain score documentation in the ED, and to determine predictors of analgesic use in the ED.

Methods.—This was a cross-sectional analysis of documented ED visits by elderly patients from the National Hospital Ambulatory Medical Care Survey (2003–2006). The study included 5661 ED visits by patients aged 65 years and older, representing an estimated 18 million ED visits during the four-year study period. Univariate logistic regression was used to analyze associations among independent variables and documentation of pain. Multivariate logistic regression was used to determine whether non-opioid and opioid analgesic prescribing disparities existed and were associated with pain level.

Results.—Pain score documentation was found to be suboptimal in the elderly population in this study, with only 75% of visits having documented pain scores. Older age, self-pay, patients residing in the Western region of the United States, and emergent ED visits were associated with decreased pain score documentation. Documentation of pain score was associated with increased odds of an analgesic prescription and opioid analgesic prescription. Odds of prescribing an opioid increased significantly with increasing level of pain severity.

Conclusion.—ED pain score documentation is suboptimal in the elderly population. Disparity in the use of analgesic prescriptions and opioid analgesics exists and may result in patients not receiving analgesics. Improving pain assessment and documentation, changes in attitude toward analgesic prescribing, and recognition of ethnic, racial, and age differences in patients with pain have the potential to contribute to effective management of pain in the ED.

▶ This article highlights the strengths and weaknesses of using national databases to study medication practices. On the plus side, the database is very large, clearly defined, and circumscribed. It appears to represent well the population of interest. Additionally, the availability of the assessment list is an asset. On the negative side, the lack of clinical information to inform the research findings severely curtails the conclusions that can be drawn from this work. Additionally, there are concerns regarding the available data, especially reasons for use of opioids. Notwithstanding these important caveats, this study does give us a realistic glimpse at the extent and pattern of analgesic use among elderly attendees at emergency departments. The magnitude of the effect is certainly noteworthy.

P. F. Buckley, MD

7 Biological Psychiatry

Introduction

This year's selection of articles has a strong emphasis on how genetics and neuroscience inform our understanding of illness. Several articles address emergent data on genetics, brain neurotrophins, and serotonin receptors. This work is complex and evolving as our field is also evolving. There are also several articles regarding pain—often considered the "fifth vital sign"—that should be of interest to readers.

I hope you find this year's selection of articles to be both topical and interesting.

Peter F. Buckley, MD

Schizophrenia

Prenatal and Neonatal Brain Structure and White Matter Maturation in Children at High Risk for Schizophrenia

Gilmore JH, Kang C, Evans DD, et al (Univ of North Carolina at Chapel Hill; Columbia Univ, NY; Univ of Utah, Salt Lake City)

Am J Psychiatry 167:1083-1091, 2010

Objective.—Schizophrenia is a neurodevelopmental disorder associated with abnormalities of brain structure and white matter, although little is known about when these abnormalities arise. This study was conducted to identify structural brain abnormalities in the prenatal and neonatal periods associated with genetic risk for schizophrenia.

Method.—Prenatal ultrasound scans and neonatal structural magnetic resonance imaging (MRI) and diffusion tensor imaging were prospectively obtained in the offspring of mothers with schizophrenia or schizoaffective disorder (N=26) and matched comparison mothers without psychiatric illness (N=26). Comparisons were made for prenatal lateral ventricle width and head circumference, for neonatal intracranial, CSF, gray matter, white matter, and lateral ventricle volumes, and for neonatal diffusion properties of the genu and splenium of the corpus callosum and corticospinal tracts.

Results.—Relative to the matched comparison subjects, the offspring of mothers with schizophrenia did not differ in prenatal lateral ventricle width or head circumference. Overall, the high-risk neonates had nonsignificantly larger intracranial, CSF, and lateral ventricle volumes. Subgroup analysis revealed that male high-risk infants had significantly larger intracranial, CSF, total gray matter, and lateral ventricle volumes; the female high-risk neonates were similar to the female comparison subjects. There were no group differences in white matter diffusion tensor properties.

Conclusions.—Male neonates at genetic risk for schizophrenia had several larger than normal brain volumes, while females did not. To the authors' knowledge, this study provides the first evidence, in the context of its limitations, that early neonatal brain development may be abnormal in males at genetic risk for schizophrenia.

▶ This is a really cool study and an extension of a fascinating line of research by Dr John Gilmore and colleagues at the University of North Carolina. They have been examining the early neurodevelopmental trajectories of children who later went on to develop schizophrenia. Their provocative finding here is that children who later developed schizophrenia actually had larger fetal brain size compared with fetal brains of normal children when the mothers had fetal ultrasound examinations. This is interesting because one usually thinks of autism as the condition where brain size is larger. It is also interesting to note that this effect was predominantly observed in male rather than female brains in utero in accordance with other neurodevelopmental abnormalities in schizophrenia (eg, obstetric complications), which occur more in male than female patients.

P. F. Buckley, MD

Psychosis Susceptibility Gene *ZNF804A* and Cognitive Performance in Schizophrenia
Walters JTR, Corvin A, Owen MJ, et al (Cardiff Univ, Wales, UK; Trinity College, Dublin, Ireland; et al)
Arch Gen Psychiatry 67:692-700, 2010

Context.—The Zinc Finger Protein 804A gene (*ZNF804A*) has been implicated in schizophrenia susceptibility by several genome-wide association studies. *ZNF804A* is brain expressed but of unknown function.

Objective.—To investigate whether the identified risk allele at the disease-associated single nucleotide polymorphism rs1344706 is associated with variation in neuropsychological performance in patients and controls.

Design.—Comparison of cases and controls grouped according to *ZNF804A* genotype (*AA* vs *AC* vs *CC*) on selected measures of cognition in 2 independent samples.

Setting.—Unrelated patients from general adult psychiatric inpatient and outpatient services and unrelated healthy participants from the general population were ascertained.

Participants.—Patients with *DSM-IV*–diagnosed schizophrenia and healthy participants from independent samples of Irish (297 cases and 165 controls) and German (251 cases and 1472 controls) nationality.

Main Outcome Measures.—In this 2-stage study, we tested for an association between *ZNF804A* rs1344706 and cognitive functions known to be impaired in schizophrenia (IQ, episodic memory, working memory, and attention) in an Irish discovery sample. We then tested significant results in a German replication sample.

Results.—In the Irish samples, the *ZNF804A* genotype was associated with differences in episodic and working memory in patients but not in controls. These findings replicated in the same direction in the German samples. Furthermore, in both samples, when patients with a lower IQ were excluded, the association between *ZNF804A* and schizophrenia strengthened.

Conclusions.—In a disorder characterized by heterogeneity, a risk variant at *ZNF804A* seems to delineate a patient subgroup characterized by relatively spared cognitive ability. Further work is required to establish whether this represents a discrete molecular pathogenesis that differs from that of other patient groups and whether this also has consequences for nosologic classification, illness course, or treatment.

▶ This is another important genetics study. Here, the authors found abnormalities selective to the Zinc Finger Protein 804A (*ZNF804A*) gene. In contrast to most studies that report negative functional impact of abnormalities, they found that the single-nucleotide polymorphism in *ZNF804A* was seen in those patients who performed better on cognitive tests. These results are unusual. There is a huge effort to find cognitive enhancement drugs and techniques to improve treatment for patients with schizophrenia. This study is important because it may identify a genetic vulnerability that could be a candidate or target for future drug design in the search for cognitive enhancers. Although this idea seems fanciful at present, it is sobering and exciting to note that similar strategies are now guiding cancer chemotherapy.

P. F. Buckley, MD

Microdeletions of 3q29 Confer High Risk for Schizophrenia

Mulle JG, Dodd AF, McGrath JA, et al (Emory Univ School of Medicine, Atlanta, GA; Johns Hopkins School of Medicine, Baltimore, MD; et al)
Am J Hum Genet 87:229-236, 2010

Schizophrenia (SZ) is a severe psychiatric illness that affects ∼1% of the population and has a strong genetic underpinning. Recently, genome-wide analysis of copy-number variation (CNV) has implicated rare and de novo events as important in SZ. Here, we report a genome-wide analysis of 245 SZ cases and 490 controls, all of Ashkenazi Jewish descent. Because many studies have found an excess burden of large, rare deletions in cases, we limited our analysis to deletions over 500 kb in size. We observed seven large, rare deletions in cases, with 57% of these being de novo. We focused on one 836 kb de novo deletion at chromosome 3q29 that falls within a 1.3–1.6 Mb deletion previously identified in children with intellectual disability (ID) and autism, because increasing evidence suggests an overlap of specific rare copy-number variants (CNVs) between autism and SZ. By combining our data with prior CNV studies of SZ and analysis of the data of the Genetic Association Information Network (GAIN), we identified six 3q29 deletions among 7545 schizophrenic subjects and one among 39,748 controls, resulting in a statistically significant association with SZ (p = 0.02) and an odds ratio estimate of 17 (95% confidence interval: 1.36−1198.4). Moreover, this 3q29 deletion region contains two linkage peaks from prior SZ family studies, and the minimal deletion interval implicates 20 annotated genes, including *PAK2* and *DLG1*, both paralogous to X-linked ID genes and now strong candidates for SZ susceptibility.

▶ The scientific focus on the copy number variant (CNV) abnormalities in schizophrenia has been a major focus of research. This is an intriguing collaboration study evaluating CNVs in a large sample of Ashkenazi Jewish patients with schizophrenia. In line with other CNV studies, they found an excess of large, rare CNVs in patients on chromosome 3. This was a robust finding with an odds ratio of 16.98. The CNV microdeletion was specific to chromosome 3Q29 site. This finding adds to the growing literature on CNVs in schizophrenia. Moreover, it extends the power of research and the pathophysiological significance, especially given that 2 genes within that region are known to be associated with mental retardation.

P. F. Buckley, MD

Metabolome in schizophrenia and other psychotic disorders: a general population-based study
Orešič M, Tang J, Seppänen-Laakso T, et al (VTT Technical Res Centre of Finland, Tietotie, Espoo; et al)
Genome Med 3:19, 2011

Background.—Persons with schizophrenia and other psychotic disorders have a high prevalence of obesity, impaired glucose tolerance, and lipid abnormalities, particularly hypertriglyceridemia and low high-density lipoprotein. More detailed molecular information on the metabolic abnormalities may reveal clues about the pathophysiology of these changes, as well as about disease specificity.

Methods.—We applied comprehensive metabolomics in serum samples from a general population-based study in Finland. The study included all persons with DSM-IV primary psychotic disorder (schizophrenia, $n = 45$; other nonaffective psychosis (ONAP), $n = 57$; affective psychosis, $n = 37$) and controls matched by age, sex, and region of residence. Two analytical platforms for metabolomics were applied to all serum samples: a global lipidomics platform based on ultra-performance liquid chromatography coupled to mass spectrometry, which covers molecular lipids such as phospholipids and neutral lipids; and a platform for small polar metabolites based on two-dimensional gas chromatography coupled to time-of-flight mass spectrometry (GC × GC-TOFMS).

Results.—Compared with their matched controls, persons with schizophrenia had significantly higher metabolite levels in six lipid clusters containing mainly saturated triglycerides, and in two small-molecule clusters containing, among other metabolites, (1) branched chain amino acids, phenylalanine and tyrosine, and (2) proline, glutamic, lactic and pyruvic acids. Among these, serum glutamic acid was elevated in all psychoses ($P = 0.0020$) compared to controls, while proline upregulation ($P = 0.000023$) was specific to schizophrenia. After adjusting for medication and metabolic comorbidity in linear mixed models, schizophrenia remained independently associated with higher levels in seven of these eight clusters ($P < 0.05$ in each cluster). The metabolic abnormalities were less pronounced in persons with ONAP or affective psychosis.

Conclusions.—Our findings suggest that specific metabolic abnormalities related to glucoregulatory processes and proline metabolism are specifically associated with schizophrenia and reflect two different disease-related pathways. Metabolomics, which is sensitive to both genetic and environmental variation, may become a powerful tool in psychiatric research to investigate disease susceptibility, clinical course, and treatment response.

▶ Metabolomics is a hot new field. It may be particularly of advantage in deciphering potential biomarkers, of either disease or its treatment. It already has been widely applied to the study of several medical conditions. We have also used metabolomics to study biochemical patterns in patients with first-episode psychosis. Accordingly, I was intrigued when I saw this article appear in the literature. This study shows highly significant perturbations in 6 lipid clusters. The overexpression of proline metabolites seen only in patients with schizophrenia is of interest. Although the influence of medications could not be entirely discounted here, the authors did report that, in adjusting for both medication status and physical comorbidities, these abnormal findings prevailed and, therefore, may represent additional evidence of fundamental disturbances of glucose/lipid regulation in schizophrenia. Additionally, it suggests a perhaps less appreciated—and perhaps more specific—abnormality of the serum amino acid proline in patients with schizophrenia. The study also highlights the potential role of metabolomics as a tool in the search for a biomarker for schizophrenia.

P. F. Buckley, MD

Oral versus depot antipsychotic drugs for schizophrenia—A critical systematic review and meta-analysis of randomised long-term trials
Leucht C, Heres S, Kane JM, et al (Klinikum rechts der Isar der Technischen Universität München, Ismaningerstr, Germany; North Shore—Long Island Jewish Health System, Glen Oaks, NY; et al)
Schizophr Res 127:83-92, 2011

Objective.—Non-adherence is a major problem in the treatment of schizophrenia. Depot antipsychotic drugs are thought to reduce relapse rates by improving adherence, but a systematic review of long-term studies in outpatients is not available.

Method.—We searched the Cochrane Schizophrenia Group's register, ClinicalTrials.gov, Cochrane reviews on depot medication, and the reference sections of included studies for randomised controlled trials lasting at least 12 months in outpatients that compared depot with oral antipsychotics in schizophrenia. Data on relapse (primary outcome), rehospitalisation, nonadherence, and dropout due to any reason, inefficacy of treatment and adverse events were summarised in a meta-analysis using a random-effects model. Study quality was assessed with the Cochrane collaboration's risk of bias tool, and publication bias with funnel plots.

Results.—Ten studies with 1700 participants met the inclusion criteria. Depot formulations significantly reduced relapses with relative and absolute risk reductions of 30% and 10%, respectively (RR 0.70, CI 0.57−0.87, NNT 10, CI 6−25, P = 0.0009), and dropout due to inefficacy (RR 0.71, CI 0.57−0.89). Limited data on non-adherence, rehospitalisation and dropout due to any reason and adverse events revealed no significant differences. There were several potential sources of bias such as limited information on randomisation methods, problems of blinding and different medications in the depot and oral groups. Other studies reduced a potential superiority of depot by excluding non-adherent patients.

Discussion.—Depot antipsychotic drugs significantly reduced relapse. Due to a number of methodological problems in the single trials the evidence is, nonetheless, subject to possible bias.

▶ This is an important meta-analysis of the role of injectable medications in the treatment of schizophrenia. Although it includes both early and more recent studies, it is important to appreciate that not all available studies are represented here. This is particularly relevant to considering new studies of second-generation antipsychotic injectable medications. Obviously, this is the information that is of most appeal to clinicians. The meta-analysis suggests a substantial advantage of long-acting injectables (LAIs), in fact, the relative risk of relapse in schizophrenia is reported to be 30% lower than the rate with oral medications. The meta-analysis also points out that there is substantial variation regarding efficacy against relapse rates across studies. The report also highlights how the sample chosen for study also powerfully influences the results of the study: the advantage of LAIs is most pronounced in studies that focus on patient samples characterized by repeated nonadherence to oral medications.

P. F. Buckley, MD

Long-Acting Risperidone and Oral Antipsychotics in Unstable Schizophrenia
Rosenheck RA, for the CSP555 Research Group (VA Connecticut Healthcare System, West Haven; et al)
N Engl J Med 364:842-851, 2011

Background.—Long-acting injectable risperidone, a second-generation antipsychotic agent, may improve adherence to treatment and outcomes in schizophrenia, but it has not been tested in a long-term randomized trial involving patients with unstable disease.

Methods.—We randomly assigned patients in the Veterans Affairs (VA) system whoı had schizophrenia or schizoaffective disorder and who had been hospitalized within the previous 2 years or were at imminent risk for hospitalization to 25 to 50 mg of long-acting injectable risperidone every two weeks or to a psychiatrist's choice of an oral antipsychotic. All patients were followed for up to 2 years. The primary end point was hospitalization in a VA or non-VA psychiatric hospital. Symptoms, quality of life, and functioning were assessed in blinded videoconference interviews.

Results.—Of 369 participants, 40% were hospitalized at randomization, 55% were hospitalized within the previous 2 years, and 5% were at risk for hospitalization. The rate of hospitalization after randomization was not significantly lower among patients who received long-acting injectable risperidone than among those who received oral antipsychotics (39% after 10.8 months vs. 45% after 11.3 months; hazard ratio, 0.87; 95% confidence interval, 0.63 to 1.20). Psychiatric symptoms, quality of life, scores on the Personal and Social Performance scale of global functioning, and neurologic side effects were not significantly improved with long-acting injectable risperidone as compared with control treatments. Patients who received long-acting injectable risperidone reported more adverse events at the injection site and more extrapyramidal symptoms.

Conclusions.—Long-acting injectable risperidone was not superior to a psychiatrist's choice of oral treatment in patients with schizophrenia and schizoaffective disorder who were hospitalized or at high risk for hospitalization, and it was associated with more local injection-site and extrapyramidal adverse effects. (Supported by the VA Cooperative Studies Program and Ortho-McNeil Janssen Scientific Affairs; ClinicalTrials.gov number, NCT00132314.)

▶ The use of long-acting injectable (LAI) formulations of antipsychotic medications has been limited in part by the availability of only first-generation antipsychotics (FGAs). This is particularly interesting when you compare US usage with European usage, which is more common. However, this study of these drugs given to reduce relapse rates in patients with schizophrenia estimated that relapse rates are reduced by 30% on LAI therapy. This important study is the first major well-conducted study to test whether this advantage also is seen in second-generation antipsychotic (SGAs) treatment. Many were surprised that Rosenheck and colleagues found that hospitalization was similar (37% vs 45%, a nonsignificant difference) between the group receiving LAI risperidone and the group treated with oral SGAs. It is possible that the sample drawn from the Veteran's Administration was different from other samples. Also, patients were followed closely, which may have mitigated differences.

P. F. Buckley, MD

Using Computational Patients to Evaluate Illness Mechanisms in Schizophrenia

Hoffman RE, Grasemann U, Gueorguieva R, et al (Yale Univ School of Medicine, New Haven, CT; Univ of Texas at Austin; et al)
Biol Psychiatry 69:997-1005, 2011

Background.—Various malfunctions involving working memory, semantics, prediction error, and dopamine neuromodulation have been hypothesized to cause disorganized speech and delusions in schizophrenia. Computational models may provide insights into why some mechanisms are unlikely, suggest alternative mechanisms, and tie together explanations of seemingly disparate symptoms and experimental findings.

Methods.—Eight corresponding illness mechanisms were simulated in DISCERN, an artificial neural network model of narrative understanding and recall. For this study, DISCERN learned sets of autobiographical and impersonal crime stories with associated emotion coding. In addition, 20 healthy control subjects and 37 patients with schizophrenia or schizoaffective disorder matched for age, gender, and parental education were studied using a delayed story recall task. A goodness-of-fit analysis was performed to determine the mechanism best reproducing narrative breakdown profiles generated by healthy control subjects and patients with schizophrenia. Evidence of delusion-like narratives was sought in simulations best matching the narrative breakdown profile of patients.

Results.—All mechanisms were equivalent in matching the narrative breakdown profile of healthy control subjects. However, exaggerated prediction-error signaling during consolidation of episodic memories, termed hyperlearning, was statistically superior to other mechanisms in matching the narrative breakdown profile of patients. These simulations also systematically confused autobiographical agents with impersonal crime story agents to model fixed, self-referential delusions.

Conclusions.—Findings suggest that exaggerated prediction-error signaling in schizophrenia intermingles and corrupts narrative memories when incorporated into long-term storage, thereby disrupting narrative language and producing fixed delusional narratives. If further validated by clinical studies, these computational patients could provide a platform for developing and testing novel treatments.

▶ This is a very interesting and provocative study by Dr Ralph Hoffman and his colleagues evaluating artificial neural networks in patients with chronic schizophrenia. They used an artificial neural network that they called DISCERN to evaluate recall as well disorganized speech pattern in 20 healthy control subjects and 37 patients with schizophrenia or schizoaffective disorder. Their results replicate and extend many of the other studies of thought disorder in schizophrenia in that patients had excessive neural activation with unorganized delusional themes. These effects were more pronounced as the artificial system was exaggerated, demonstrating stress on the system. The study is a fascinating read and opens the door to applications of this approach to other aspects of schizophrenia research.

P. F. Buckley, MD

Understanding Schizoaffective Disorder: From Psychobiology to Psychosocial Functioning
Correll CU (Zucker Hillside Hosp, Glen Oaks, NY)
J Clin Psychiatry 71:8-13, 2010

Psychobiologic evidence and psychosocial functioning in patients with schizoaffective disorder suggest that the disease may be a distinct disorder, a variant of schizophrenia or affective disorders, the comorbidity of schizophrenia and a mood disorder, or an intermediate disorder on a spectrum that ranges from schizophrenia to mood disorders. These data, although inconclusive, contribute to clinicians' understanding of the etiology of the disorder. Further research may lead to an increased understanding of the disorder, improved treatment, and, ultimately, better outcomes (Fig 1).

▶ I really like this succinct and thoughtful review. This is an easy-to-read review of a complex and vexing topic. Although the article has more neurobiological emphasis on genetics than other putative markers of phenotypic distinction, it does cover other areas, including phenomenology. The bottom line is anticipated: "schizoaffective disorder patients occupy an intermediate position between more severely disturbed schizophrenia and less severely impaired affective disorder patients...additional research into biomarkers of the illness and treatment course and response is needed." This summation does not bode well for the *Diagnostic and Statistical Manual of Mental Disorders* (Fifth Edition). Time will tell how all this plays out.

P. F. Buckley, MD

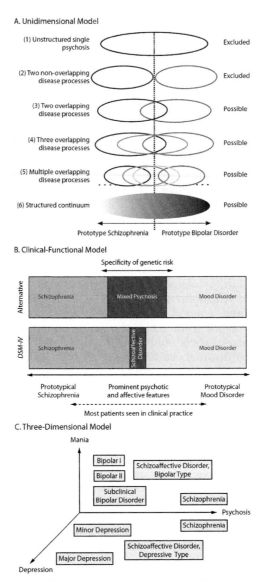

FIGURE 1.—Model of Possible Biologic-Genetic Overlap Between Schizophrenia and Bipolar Disorder[a]. A. Unidimensional Model. B. Clinical-Functional Model. C. Three-Dimensional Model. [a]Reprinted with permission from Craddock et al.[2] *Abbreviation: DSM-IV = Diagnostic and Statistical Manual of Mental Disorders*, Fourth Edition. (Reprinted from Correll CU. Understanding schizoaffective disorder: from psychobiology to psychosocial functioning. *J Clin Psychiatry.* 2010;71:8-13. Copyright 2010, Physicians Postgraduate Press. Adapted or Reprinted with Permission.)

Clinical Features Associated With Poor Pharmacologic Adherence in Bipolar Disorder: Results From the STEP-BD Study

Perlis RH, Ostacher MJ, Miklowitz DJ, et al (Massachusetts General Hosp and Harvard Med School, Boston; Univ of Colorado, Boulder; et al)
J Clin Psychiatry 71:296-303, 2010

Background.—Poor medication adherence is common among bipolar patients.

Method.—We examined prospective data from 2 cohorts of individuals from the Systematic Treatment Enhancement Program for Bipolar Disorder (STEP-BD) study (1999—2005) with bipolar disorder. Clinical and sociodemographic features associated with missing at least 25% of doses of at least 1 medication were assessed using logistic regression, and a risk stratification model was developed and validated.

Results.—Of 3,640 subjects with 48,287 follow-up visits, 871 (24%) reported nonadherence on 20% or more study visits. Clinical features significantly associated ($P < .05$) with poor adherence included rapid cycling, suicide attempts, earlier onset of illness, and current anxiety or alcohol use disorder. Nonadherence during the first 3 months of follow-up was associated with less improvement in functioning at 12-month follow-up ($P < .03$). A risk stratification model using clinical predictors accurately classified 80.6% of visits in an independent validation cohort.

Conclusion.—Risk for poor medication adherence can be estimated and may be useful in targeting interventions (Table 1).

▶ To a certain extent, there is no new news in this study. It shows that patients with bipolar disorder don't take their medications and that patients who don't take their medications fare poorer over time. Patients with an earlier age of onset of illness, with comorbid anxiety symptoms and particularly with comorbid substance abuse are the patients who are the least likely to take their medications (Tables 1A and 1B). All of this is well known and well replicated in previous studies. What this study adds is the robust and meticulous methodology of this longitudinal treatment study in bipolar disorder—Systematic Treatment Enhancement Program for Bipolar Disorder. The study also well quantifies the degree of functional impairment, based upon both symptomatic and quality of life measures taken repeatedly over time, associated with nonadherence with medications among people with bipolar disorder. Of course, it's never as simple as saying just take your medications, but these data and lots of other studies sure emphasize the detrimental impact of not taking medications as prescribed.

P. F. Buckley, MD

TABLE 1.—

Variable	STEP-2000[a] Crude Odds Ratio	95% CI	Adjusted Odds Ratio	95% CI	STEP-2[b] Adjusted Odds Ratio	95 %CI
A. Clinical Features Associated With Poor Adherence at Any Given Follow-Up Visit in 2 Cohorts of Individuals With Bipolar Disorder						
Socioeconomic						
Ethnicity: Hispanic	1.48	1.00−2.19*	1.51	1.01−2.24*	1.79	1.36−2.36*
Household income <$50,000/y	1.45	1.23−1.71*	1.43	1.22−1.68*	1.47	1.25−1.72*
Currently married	0.80	0.68−0.95*	0.80	0.68−0.94*	0.81	0.70−0.95*
Male sex	0.83	0.71−0.97*	0.86	0.73−1.00	0.91	0.79−1.05
White (vs all others)	0.88	0.66−1.17	0.87	0.66−1.15	NA	
Age (per 10 y)	0.89	0.84−0.94*	0.89	0.84−0.95*	0.86	0.82−0.91*
At least some college (vs none)	0.95	0.78−1.17	0.99	0.81−1.21	NA	
Currently unemployed	1.01	0.83−1.23	0.99	0.82−1.20	NA	
Clinical (study entry)						
Alcohol use disorder (current)	1.68	1.35−2.09*	1.63	1.32−2.03*	1.42	1.17−1.73*
Anxiety disorder (current)	1.47	1.26−1.72*	1.35	1.16−1.57*	1.31	1.13−1.51*
Rapid cycling, lifetime	1.40	1.17−1.68*	1.32	1.11−1.58*	1.34	1.14−1.57*
Rapid cycling, year prior to entry	1.37	1.17−1.60*	1.30	1.11−1.51*	1.26	1.09−1.45*
History of suicide attempt, lifetime	1.32	1.12−1.54*	1.21	1.04−1.42*	1.20	1.03−1.39*
Onset age (per 10 y)	0.77	0.70−0.83*	0.78	0.72−0.85*	0.84	0.77−0.92*
Manic symptoms (*DSM-IV*), count	1.23	1.18−1.27*	1.17	1.13−1.22*	1.22	1.18−1.27*
History of psychosis, lifetime	0.90	0.77−1.06	0.93	0.79−1.10	NA	
Bipolar 1disorder (vs bipolar II disorder or NOS)	1.11	0.94−1.30	1.11	0.95−1.31	NA	
Depressive symptoms (*DSM-IV*), count	1.10	1.08−1.12*	1.07	1.05−1.10*	1.07	1.05−1.10*
Bipolar II disorder (vs bipolar I disorder or NOS)	0.93	0.79−1.09	0.92	0.78−1.08	NA	
Days depressed, past year (per 105)	1.06	1.03−1.08*	1.04	1.01−1.07*	1.06	1.03−1.08*
Days irritable, past year (per 10%)	1.05	1.03−1.07*	1.03	1.01−1.06*	1.04	1.01−1.06*
Days elevated, past year (10%)	1.05	1.01−1.08*	1.03	1.00−1.07	NA	
Days anxious, past year (per 10%)	1.03	1.01−1.05*	1.01	0.99−1.03	NA	
Clinical (each visit)						
Days irritable, past 2 weeks (per 10%)	1.09	1.07−1.10*	1.06	1.03−1.08*	1.04	1.01−1.06*
Days elevated, past 2 weeks (per 10%)	1.05	1.01−1.08*	1.03	1.00−1.06	NA	
Days depressed, past 2 weeks (per 10%)	1.04	1.02−1.05*	1.00	0.98−1.01	NA	
Days anxious, past 2 weeks (per 10%)	1.04	1.02−1.05*	1.01	0.99−1.02	NA	
Personality (NEO-FFI)						
Agreeableness (*t* score)	0.98	0.97−0.99*	0.98	0.97−0.99*	1.00	0.98−1.02
Openness (*t* score)	1.02	1.01−1.03*	1.02	1.01−1.03*	1.02	1.00−1.04*
Conscientiousness (*t* score)	1.02	1.01−1.03*	1.02	1.01−1.02*	1.00	0.99−1.02
Neuroticism (*t* score)	1.01	0.99−1.02	1.00	0.99−1.02	NA	
Extraversion (*t* score)	1.00	0.99−1.01	1.00	0.99−1.01	NA	
B. Adverse Effects and Other Aspects of Treatment Associated With Poor Adherence						
Adverse Effect						
Memory impairment	1.21	10.02−1.44*	1.08	0.90−1.29	NA	
Extrapyramidal symptoms	1.20	0.83−1.73	1.11	0.77−1.60	NA	
Increase in appetite	1.12	0.96−1.31	1.04	0.89−1.21	NA	
Sexual dysfunction	1.11	0.88−1.39	1.05	0.83−1.33	NA	
Dry mouth	1.10	0.93−1.29	1.00	0.85−1.17	NA	
Constipation	1.10	0.83−1.45	1.00	0.76−1.33	NA	
Sedation	1.02	0.88−1.18	0.94	0.80−1.09	NA	
Tremors	1.00	0.86−1.16	0.93	0.80−1.09	NA	
Cumulative no. of clinicians	0.98	0.95−1.01	0.99	0.96−1.02	NA	
No. of psychotropic medications	1.04	1.01−1.07*	1.02	0.99−1.06	NA	

Abbreviations: NA = not applicable, NOS = not otherwise specified.

[a]The STEP-2000 subsample was derived from the 3,640 completing the Systematic Treatment Enhancement Program for Bipolar Disorder (STEP-BD) study with at least 1 follow-up visit being divided based on study protocol into the 1,771 subjects with at least 1 follow-up visit who were among the first 2,000 to enter the STEP-BD study.

[b]STEP-2 refers to the 1,869 subjects remaining from the cohort of 3,640 completing the STEP-BD study with at least 1 follow-up visit.

*Nominal P < .05 (ie, 95% CI excludes 1).

Serotonin transporter and BDNF genetic variants interact to predict cognitive reactivity in healthy adults

Wells TT, Beevers CG, McGeary JE (Univ of Texas at Austin; Brown Univ, RI)
J Affect Disord 126:223-229, 2010

Background.—Cognitive theory and empirical evidence both suggest that cognitive reactivity (the tendency to think more negatively when in a sad mood) is an important marker of depression vulnerability. Research has not yet determined whether genetic factors contribute to the expression of cognitive reactivity.

Methods.—The present study examined associations between the 5-HTTLPR polymorphism of the SLC6A4 gene, the Val66Met polymorphism of the brain-derived neurotrophic factor (BDNF) gene, and cognitive reactivity in a never depressed, unmedicated, young adult sample ($N = 151$).

Results.—The interaction between 5-HTTLPR and Val66Met polymorphisms significantly predicted change in dysfunctional thinking from before to after a standardized sad mood provocation. Cognitive reactivity increased among S/L$_G$ 5-HTTLPR homozygotes if they were also homozygous for the Val Val66Met allele. In contrast, presence of a Met Val66Met allele was associated with attenuated cognitive reactivity among S/L$_G$ 5-HTTLPR homozygotes.

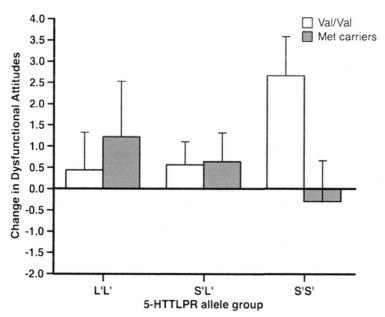

FIGURE 1.—Change in Dysfunctional Attitudes Scale-Short Form (DAS-SF) score from pre to post-mood provocation as a function of allele grouping. Error bars represent the standard error of the mean. (Reprinted from Wells TT, Beevers CG, McGeary JE. Serotonin transporter and BDNF genetic variants interact to predict cognitive reactivity in healthy adults. *J Affect Disord.* 2010;126:223-229, The International Society for Affective Disorders.)

Limitations.—The sample size of the current study is relatively small for modern genetic association studies. However, results are consistent with previous research demonstrating biological epistasis between SLC6A4 and BDNF for predicting connectivity among neural structures involved in emotion regulation.

Conclusions.—The BDNF Met allele may protect S/L$_G$ 5-HTTLPR homozygotes from increased dysfunctional thinking following a sad mood provocation. Study results are the first to demonstrate an epistatic genetic relationship predicting cognitive reactivity and suggest the need for more complex and integrative models of depression vulnerability (Fig 1).

▶ Although this study was conducted in a relatively small sample of 151 young adults without depression, the methodology and results are of interest and potentially have broad generalization. The results illustrate the genetic vulnerability to sad mood—based upon polymorphisms of the serotonin transporter gene—and how this is also influenced by genetic variants of the brain-derived neurotropic factor (*BDNF*) gene. Both genetic variants have independently been associated in various prior studies with a heightened risk for depression. Here, the associations between the 2 are illustrated (Fig 1), such that it appears that possession of the Met allele for the *BDNF* gene may be protective on S/L$_G$ homozygotes of the *5HTTR* gene. This is interesting stuff. However, as the authors admirably point out, these associations explain only 5% of the variance As in most instances, we are only seeing a tiny portion of a huge landscape.

P. F. Buckley, MD

Interactive Effects of *DAOA* (G72) and Catechol-*O*-Methyltransferase on Neurophysiology in Prefrontal Cortex
Nixon DC, Prust MJ, Sambataro F, et al (Natl Inst of Mental Health, Bethesda, MD)
Biol Psychiatry 69:1006-1008, 2011

Background.—Accumulating evidence indicates that genetic polymorphisms of D-amino acid oxidase activator (*DAOA*) (M24; rs1421292; T-allele) and catechol-O-methyltransferase (*COMT*) (Val[158]Met; rs4680) likely enhance susceptibility to schizophrenia. Previously, clinical association between *DAOA* M24 (T-allele) and a functionally inefficient 3-marker *COMT* haplotype (that included *COMT* Val[158]Met) uncovered epistatic effects on risk for schizophrenia. Therefore, we projected that healthy control subjects with risk genotypes for both *DAOA* M24 (T/T) and *COMT*Val[158]Met (Val/Val) would produce prefrontal inefficiency, a critical physiological marker of the dorsolateral prefrontal cortex (DLPFC) in schizophrenic patients influenced by both familial and heritable factors.

Methods.—With 3T blood oxygen level dependent functional magnetic resonance imaging data, we analyzed in SPM5 the proposed interaction of

DAOA and *COMT* in 82 healthy volunteers performing an N-back executive working memory paradigm (2-back > 0-back).

Results.—As predicted, we detected a functional gene × gene interaction between *DAOA* and *COMT* in the DLPFC.

Conclusions.—The neuroimaging findings here of inefficient information processing in the prefrontal cortex seem to echo prior statistical epistasis between risk alleles for *DAOA* and *COMT,* albeit within a small sample. These in vivo results suggest that deleterious genotypes for *DAOA* and *COMT* might contribute to the pathophysiology of schizophrenia, perhaps through combined glutamatergic and dopaminergic dysregulation.

▶ This report is from the National Institute of Mental Health group led by Dr Weinberger. This is an interactive refinement of original and seminal experiments concerning catechol-*O*-methyltransferase (COMT) and frontal lobe functioning. They showed a linear relationship between COMT polymorphism and cortical efficiency. However, when several other groups attempted to replicate these findings, they could do so only partially or not at all. This suggests that either the effect was overestimated or that the mechanism of action here might be more complex. This report provides some evidence for the latter proposition. This study shows an interaction between COMT activity and D-amino acid and oxidase activator and cortical efficiency in healthy subjects. This provocative and interesting report suggests a complex interaction between dopaminergic and glutamatergic function that influences cortical activity.

P. F. Buckley, MD

Research Review: The neurobiology and genetics of maltreatment and adversity
McCrory E, De Brito SA, Viding E, et al (Univ College London (UCL), UK)
J Child Psychol Psychiatry 51:1079-1095, 2010

The neurobiological mechanisms by which childhood maltreatment heightens vulnerability to psychopathology remain poorly understood. It is likely that a complex interaction between environmental experiences (including poor caregiving) and an individual's genetic make-up influence neurobiological development across infancy and childhood, which in turn sets the stage for a child's psychological and emotional development. This review provides a concise synopsis of those studies investigating the neurobiological and genetic factors associated with childhood maltreatment and adversity. We first provide an overview of the neuroendocrine findings, drawing from animal and human studies. These studies indicate an association between early adversity and atypical development of the hypothalamic-pituitary-adrenal (HPA) axis stress response, which can predispose to psychiatric vulnerability in adulthood. We then review the neuroimaging findings of structural and functional brain differences in children and adults who have experienced childhood maltreatment. These studies offer evidence of several structural differences associated with early stress, most notably in the corpus callosum in children and the hippocampus in adults; functional studies have reported atypical activation of several brain regions, including decreased activity of the prefrontal cortex. Next we consider studies that suggest that the effect of environmental adversity may be conditional on an individual's genotype. We also briefly consider the possible role that epigenetic mechanisms might play in mediating the impact of early adversity. Finally we consider several ways in which the neurobiological and genetic research may be relevant to clinical practice and intervention.

▶ This is a highly readable and very useful article on the risks and neurobiological vulnerability to developing mental illness as a (later) consequence of childhood (maltreatment) adversity. Although the focus is on childhood and attendant manifestations, the neurobiological pathways and illness trajectories apply equally well to several adult mental illnesses, most notably to depression and posttraumatic stress disorder. The review of the relevant literature is timely and succinct. The authors have managed to put the various risk factors nicely in context. Overall, an excellent article and a great contribution to the literature in what is otherwise an extremely complex area of current neurobiological and environmental research.

P. F. Buckley, MD

Serotonin Transporter Polymorphism Moderates Effects of Prenatal Maternal Anxiety on Infant Negative Emotionality

Pluess M, Velders FP, Belsky J, et al (Birkbeck Univ of London, UK; Erasmus Univ Med Ctr, Rotterdam, Netherlands; et al)
Biol Psychiatry 69:520-525, 2011

Background.—Consistent with the fetal programming hypothesis, effects of maternal prenatal anxiety have been found to predict various measures of infant temperament in the early postnatal period. In recent years, a polymorphism in the serotonin transporter gene (5-HTTLPR) emerged as a moderator of diverse environmental influences on different outcomes, with individuals carrying the short allele being generally more vulnerable to adversity.

Methods.—We tested whether the association between self-reported maternal anxiety at 20 weeks gestation (Brief Symptom Inventory) and mother-rated infant negative emotionality at 6 months after birth (Infant Behavior Questionnaire-Revised) would be moderated by the 5-HTTLPR in a large Dutch cohort sample ($n = 1513$). We hypothesized that infants carrying the 5-HTTLPR short allele would be more susceptible and therefore more affected by both low and high prenatal maternal anxiety vis-á-vis negative emotionality than other genotypes.

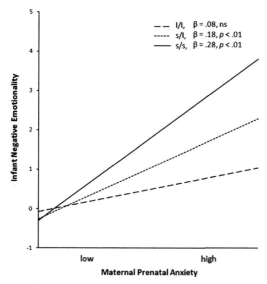

FIGURE 1.—Linear relations between maternal reports of anxiety during pregnancy and infant emotional negativity at 6 months after birth as a function of the serotonin transporter polymorphism, 5-HTTLPR. (Reprinted from Biological Psychiatry, Pluess M, Velders FP, Belsky J, et al. Serotonin transporter polymorphism moderates effects of prenatal maternal anxiety on infant negative emotionality. *Biol Psychiatry*. 2011;69:520-525. Copyright 2011, with permission from Society of Biological Psychiatry.)

Results.—Findings of a significant gene × environment interaction ($B = .65$, $p = .01$) were supportive of a vulnerability model, with infants carrying the short allele being more negatively emotional when mothers reported anxiety during pregnancy, whereas there was no difference between genotypes on negative emotionality when maternal anxiety was low.

Conclusions.—The association between maternal anxiety during pregnancy and negative emotionality in early infancy was significant in infants carrying one or more copies of the short allele but not in those homozygous for the long allele. The 5-HTTLPR short allele might increase vulnerability to adverse environmental influences as early as the fetal period.

▶ This is an analysis from an ongoing, large Dutch study of the effects of maternal anxiety upon their offspring (Table 1). Interestingly, the authors report an effect for the short allele of the serotonin transporter gene polymorphism that is associated with greater maternal anxiety and a negative emotional impact on the infant over time (Fig 1). This is consistent with the notion that serotonin polymporphisms may modulate sensitivity to stress and anxiety, even early in infant life, even during the prenatal period. If this finding held up and was a robust marker for neonatal stress, one could imagine (in a kind of Star Trek

TABLE 1.—Demographic Characteristics of the Sample

Variables	n (%)
Age at First Contact (yrs)	mean = 31.81, SD = 4.03 (range: 17–43)
Educational Level	
No education	20 (1.3%)
Low (12 yrs or less)	129 (8.5%)
Mid-low (13–15 yrs)	369 (24.4%)
Mid-high (16–17 yrs)	399 (26.4%)
High (18 yrs or more)	596 (39.4%)
Living Situation	
Living with partner	1443 (95.3%)
Living without partner	70 (4.6%)
Income	
< €1200	69 (4.6%)
€1200–2200	261 (17.3%)
> €2200	1183 (78.2%)
Smoking During Pregnancy	174 (11.5%)
Alcohol During Pregnancy	861 (56.9%)
Anxiety During Pregnancy	mean = .18, SD = .31
Anxiety at 6 Months Postnatal	mean = .22, SD = .36
Depression at 6 Months Postnatal	mean = .16, SD = .35
Child Gender	
Boy	761 (50.3%)
Girl	752 (49.7%)
Child Gestational Age at Birth (weeks)	mean = 40.16, SD = 1.44
Child Birth Weight (g)	mean = 3552.40, SD = 508.28
Child 5-HTTLPR	
l/l	497 (32.8%)
s/l	738 (48.8%)
s/s	278 (18.4%)
Child Negative Emotionality at 6 Months	
Fear	mean = .33, SD = .27
Distress to limitations	mean = .62, SD = .30
Recovery of distress	mean = 1.56, SD = .28
Negative emotionality composite (standardized)	mean = .00, SD = 2.18

$N = 1513$.
5-HTTLPR, serotonin transporter polymorphism.

way) how this test would be added to fetal ultrasound as a measure of fetal integrity. Dream on!

P. F. Buckley, MD

The Neurobiology of the Switch Process in Bipolar Disorder: A Review
Salvadore G, Quiroz JA, Machado-Vieira R, et al (Natl Inst of Mental Health, Bethesda, MD; Roche Pharmaceuticals, NY; et al)
J Clin Psychiatry 71:1488-1501, 2010

Objective.—The singular phenomenon of switching from depression to its opposite state of mania or hypomania, and vice versa, distinguishes bipolar disorder from all other psychiatric disorders. Despite the fact that it is a core aspect of the clinical presentation of bipolar disorder, the neurobiology of the switch process is still poorly understood. In this review, we summarize the clinical evidence regarding somatic interventions associated with switching, with a particular focus on the biologic underpinnings presumably involved in the switch process.

Data Sources.—Literature for this review was obtained through a search of the MEDLINE database (1966-2008) using the following keywords and phrases: *switch, bipolar disorder, bipolar depression, antidepressant, SSRIs, tricyclic antidepressants, norepinephrine, serotonin, treatment emergent affective switch, mania, hypomania, HPA-axis, glucocorticoids, amphetamine, dopamine, and sleep deprivation.*

Study Selection.—All English-language, peer-reviewed, published literature, including randomized controlled studies, naturalistic and open-label studies, and case reports, were eligible for inclusion.

Data Synthesis.—Converging evidence suggests that certain pharmacologic and nonpharmacologic interventions with very different mechanisms of action, such as sleep deprivation, exogenous corticosteroids, and dopaminergic agonists, can trigger mood episode switches in patients with bipolar disorder. The switch-inducing potential of antidepressants is unclear,

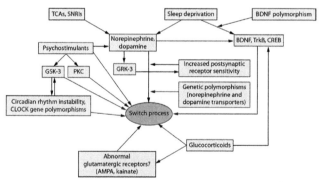

FIGURE 1.—Neurobiology of the Switch Process: A Comprehensive Overview of the Current Evidence[a]. [a]Several factors have been associated with the switch process in bipolar disorder, but little is known about how these neurobiological variables are interconnected. Psychostimulants, TCAs, SNRIs, and sleep deprivation, 4 interventions that trigger manic switches in a significant proportion of individuals with bipolar disorder, are all known to increase catecholamine levels. Increased catecholamine levels lead to upregulation of factors involved in neurosplasticity cascades and to increased postsynaptic receptor sensitivity, which might ultimately increase the liability to switch. Psychostimulants also act by activating GSK-3 and PKC, 2 major proteins whose inhibition is important in he mechanism of action of mood stabilizers. GSK-3 and PKC, 2 major proteins whose inhibition is important in the mechanism of action of mood stabilizers. Other major determinants of this complex phenomenon include glucocorticoids, which increase cellular vulnerability to different physiologic stressors (eg, glutamatergic-mediated excitoxicity), abnormal glutamatergic transmission, and circadian rhythm instability. Some genetic polymorphisms that regulate catecholaminergic transmission (norepinephrine and dopamine transporters), neuroplasticity (BDNF), circadian period length (GSK-3), and GRK-3 may also be important mediators of the switch phenomenon. *Abbreviations*: AMPA = α-amino-3-hydroxy-5-methyl-4-isoxazole propionic acid, BDNF = brain-derived neurotrophic factor, CREB = cyclic AMP response element-binding protein, GRK-3 = G protein receptor kinase 3, GSK-3 = glycogen synthase kinase 3, PKC = protein kinase C, SNRI = serotonin-norepinephrine reuptake inhibitor, TCA = tricyclic antidepressant, TrkB = tyrosine receptor kinase B. (Reprinted from Salvadore G, Quiroz JA, Machado-Vieira R, et al. The neurobiology of the switch process in bipolar disorder: a review. *J Clin Psychiatry.* 2010;71:1488-1501. Copyright 2010, Physicians Postgraduate Press. Adapted or Reprinted with Permission.)

TABLE 1.—Operational Criteria Defining *Switch* Applied in Different Pharmacologic Studies

Study	Time From Start of Antidepressant Required to Define Treatment-Emergent Affective Switch	Type of Study	Definition of Switch and Treatment-Emergent Switch
Lewis and Winokur,[38] 1982	None required	Retrospective	*DSM-III* mania while hospitalized or within 6 mo of discharge
Cohn et al,[42] 1989	6 wk	RCT	Not specified
Himmelhoch et al,[40] 1991	6 wk	RCT	Mania, research diagnostic criteria
Peet,[33] 1994	Not specified	Retrospective	Not specified
Sachs et al,[43] 1994	8 wk	RCT	*DSM-III*-R mania or hypomania
Altshuler et al,[15] 1995	8 wk	Retrospective	Mania within 8 wk of the initiation of antidepressant treatment
Boerlin et al,[34] 1998	Within 2 mo after a depressive episode	Retrospective	*DSM-IV* mania/hypomania
Bottlender et al,[37] 2001	None required	Retrospective	Mania/hypomania according to the physician's assessment based on *DSM-IV* criteria
Henry et al,[21] 2001	6 wk	Naturalistic	*DSM-IV* mania/hypomania or mixed episode within 6 wk of initiation of antidepressant/treatment
Mundo et al,[9] 2001	None required	Retrospective	*DSM-IV* mania/hypomania while being treated with SSRIs for depression
Nemeroff et al,[39] 2001	10 wk	RCT	*DSM-IV* mania
Silverstone,[41] 2001	8 wk	RCT	YMRS score ≥ 10, or study discontinuation for manic symptoms
Joffe et al,[49] 2002	Not specified; switch attributed to an antidepressant based on clinical judgment	Naturalistic	*DSM-IV* mania or hypomania
McIntyre et al,[48] 2002	8 wk	RCT	Not specified
Maj et al,[14] 2002	None required	Naturalistic	One episode of mania or hypomania and 1 episode of depression (research diagnostic criteria) with an intervening period of < 1 mo
Vieta et al,[50] 2002	6 wk	RCT	YMRS score > 11 and fulfilling *DSM-IV* criteria for mania or hypomania
Rousseva et al,[56] 2003	None required/90 d	Retrospective	Broad definition: self-report of mood elevation at any time after the introduction of an antidepressant; Narrow definition: self-report of mood elevation within 90 d from the beginning of treatment
Serretti et al,[20] 2003	None required	Retrospective	*DSM-IV* mania/hypomania while being treated with SSRIs for depression
Tohen et al,[53] 2003	8 wk	RCT	YMRS score < 15 at baseline and > 15 at any time thereafter
Serrettic et al,[57] 2004	4 wk	Retrospective	*DSM-IV* mania/hypomania while being treated with antidepressants for depression
Tamada et al,[24] 2004	None required	Naturalistic	*DSM-IV* hospitalized mania or mixed state; YMRS score ≥ 12 and at least 3 d of antidepressant treatment within 2 wk of hospital admission
Amsterdam and Shults,[52] 2005	8 wk	RCT	YMRS score > 8 at any visit
Fonseca et al,[54] 2006	12 wk	Open label	YMRS > 12 and DSM-IV criteria for manic switch; DSM-IV criteria for hypomania for hypomanic switch

(Continued)

TABLE 1.—(*Continued*)

Study	Time From Start of Antidepressant Required to Define Treatment-Emergent Affective Switch	Type of Study	Definition of Switch and Treatment-Emergent Switch
Post et al,[25] 2006	10 wk	RCT	Two-point increase on the CGI-BP, CGI-BP score of at least 3, or YMRS score > 13
Schaffer et al,[55] 2006	12 wk	RCT	Not specified
Carlson et al,[23] 2007	None required	Retrospective	*DSM-IV* mania/hypomania while being treated with antidepressants or within 30 d of stopping treatment
Nolen et al,[45] 2007	10 wk	RCT	At least "much worse" on the CGI-BP rating of change in mania as baseline and/or YMRS score ≥ 14
Sachs et al,[19] 2007	16 wk	RCT	*DSM-IV* criteria for mania or hypomania or clinically significant mood elevation needing clinical intervention within 16 wk or before reaching durable recovery (up to 26 wk)
Truman et al,[22] 2007	12 wk	Retrospective	Non-*DSM-IV* report of mania, hypomania, or mixed episode
Amsterdam and Shults,[51] 2008	12 wk	Open label	Two different criteria: YMRS ≥ 8 or YMRS ≥ 12 at any visit

Abbreviations: CGI-BP = Clinical Global Impressions scale-Bipolar Version, DSM = *Diagnostic and Statistical Manual of Mental Disorders*, RCT = randomized controlled trial, SSRI = selective serotonin reuptake inhibitor, YMRS = Young Mania Rating Scale.
Editor's Note: Please refer to original journal article for full references.

although tricyclic antidepressants, which confer higher risk of switching than other classes of antidepressants, are a possible exception. Several neurobiological factors appear to be associated with both spontaneous and treatment-emergent mood episode switches; these include abnormalities in catecholamine levels, upregulation of neurotrophic and neuroplastic factors, hypothalamic-pituitary-adrenal axis hyperactivity, and circadian rhythms.

Conclusions.—There is a clear need to improve our understanding of the neurobiology of the switch process; research in this field would benefit from the systematic and integrated assessment of variables associated with switching.

▶ This is a very interesting and topical review of a clinically relevant issue that all of us grapple with: when you have to use an antidepressant in somebody with bipolar disorder (or as yet undetected bipolar disorder), which antidepressant should you stay away from because it is more likely to induce mania. Table 1 details the studies that are cited in this review; many are of short duration and several are of limited sample size. They also span a considerable duration of years in psychopharmacology, possibly also reflecting other potential influences upon the risk for mania. Fig 1 is broad and all encompassing. I do not really share the authors' conclusion that the best data exist for brain-derived neurotrophic factor. This is still a pretty murky area of research and the true value for clinical guidance of the extent literature is modest at best.

P. F. Buckley, MD

Looking on the Bright Side of Serotonin Transporter Gene Variation
Homberg JR, Lesch K-P (Radboud Univ Nijmegen Med Ctr, The Netherlands; Univ of Wuerzburg, Germany)
Biol Psychiatry 69:513-519, 2011

Converging evidence indicates an association of the short (s), low-expressing variant of the repeat length polymorphism, serotonin transporter-linked polymorphic region (5-HTTLPR), in the human serotonin transporter gene (*5-HTT, SERT, SLC6A4*) with anxiety-related traits and increased risk for depression in interaction with psychosocial adversity across the life span. However, genetically driven deficient serotonin transporter (5-HTT) function would not have been maintained throughout evolution if it only exerted negative effects without conveying any gain of function. Here, we review recent findings that humans and nonhuman

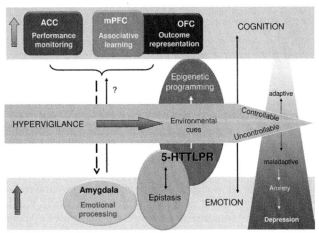

FIGURE 1.—The short variant of the serotonin transporter-linked polymorphic region is associated with hyperreactivity of prefrontal cortical regions (anterior cingulate cortex, medial prefrontal cortex, orbitofrontal cortex) and the amygdala, which contribute to hypervigilance, i.e., an increased sensitivity to motivationally relevant environmental cues. Under stable or uncontrollable conditions, the outcome is generally emotional, leading to maladaptive responses and increased risk for mood disorders. However, when there are stimuli that divert attention from adversity or reward, hypervigilance may confer increased processing and integration of (task) relevant stimuli, increased associative (new) learning, and altered use of outcome representations. The outcome is adaptive, expressed as improved cognition and social conformity. These brain phenotypes and behavioral responses can be modified by epigenetic modifications, induced by environmental stimuli, as well as gene by gene interactions (epistasis). 5-HTTLPR, serotonin transporter-linked polymorphic region; ACC, anterior cingulate cortex; mPFC, medial prefrontal cortex; OFC, orbitofrontal cortex. (Reprinted from Biological Psychiatry, Homberg JR, Lesch K-P. Looking on the bright side of serotonin transporter gene variation. *Biol Psychiatry.* 2011;69:513-519. Copyright 2011, with permission from Society of Biological Psychiatry.)

TABLE 1.—The Effect of the 5-HTTLPR s-Allele in Humans and Rhesus Macaques on Positive and Negative Emotions and (Social) Cognition

Increased Emotionality	Improved Cognition
• Psychosocial stressors (1,4,5,35−37,44−47,49)	• Decision making (17,50,54,57)
• Fear conditioning (16)	• Response inhibition (51)
• Startle response (9)	• Passive avoidance (53)
• Viewing happy/sad pictures (11−15,26,27,50)	• Risk aversion (17,50,55,56)
• Attentional bias for anxious words (10)	• Motivationally speeded action (52)
• Autonomic reactivity (17,23)	• Attentional set-shifting (58)
• Increased HPA axis reactivity (18−21,47)	• Reversal learning (68)
• Increased levels of inflammatory cytokines (22)	• Delayed matching-to-sample (68)
• Smoking, drinking, gambling (30−32,46)	• Probability discounting task (68)
• Excessive internet use (28)	• Delay discounting (68)
• Social blushing (38)	
• Social aggression (48)	
• Creative dancing (39)	
• Social support (40−42)	

5-HTTLPR, serotonin transporter-linked polymorphic region; HPA, hypothalamic-pituitary-adrenal.
Editor's Note: Please refer to original journal article for full references.

primates carrying the s variant of the 5-HTTLPR outperform subjects carrying the long allele in an array of cognitive tasks and show increased social conformity. In addition, studies in 5-HTT knockout rodents are included that provide complementary insights in the beneficial effects of the 5-HTTLPR s-allele. We postulate that hypervigilance, mediated by hyperactivity in corticolimbic structures, may be the common denominator in the anxiety-related traits and (social) cognitive superiority of s-allele carriers and that environmental conditions determine whether a response will turn out to be negative (emotional) or positive (cognitive, in conformity with the social group). Taken together, these findings urge for a conceptual change in the current deficit-oriented connotation of the 5-HTTLPR variants. In fact, these factors may counterbalance or completely offset the negative consequences of the anxiety-related traits. This notion may not only explain the modest effect size of the 5-HTTLPR and inconsistent reports but may also lead to a more refined appreciation of allelic variation in 5-HTT function.

▶ This is an excellent and current review on the evolutionary and neurobiological consequences of serotonin transporter gene receptor polymorphisms. It reviews the extant literature on polymorphism-conferred susceptibility to anxiety disorders. In addition, it overviews (Table 1) both preclinical studies (mostly on monkeys) and clinical studies and several functional MRI (fMRI) studies examining the relationships between serotonin transporter gene variation and cortical (mainly amygdalar region) arousal on fMRI. A model linking genetic liability, emotional arousal, and cognition to brain function is proposed (Fig 1). This is a very complex yet really exciting aspect of current neurobiological research.

P. F. Buckley, MD

Further exploration of the possible influence of polymorphisms in *HTR2C* and *5HTT* on body weight

Bah J, Westberg L, Baghaei F, et al (The Sahlgrenska Academy at Göteborg Univ, Sweden)
Metab Clin Exp 59:1156-1163, 2010

Receptors of the 5-HT2C subtype are of importance for the influence of serotonin on food intake, and 2 single nucleotide polymorphisms in this gene (*HTR2C*)—Cys23Ser (*rs6318*) and −759C>T (*rs3813929*)—have been reported to be associated with weight and/or antipsychotic-induced weight gain. The present study aimed to replicate these associations; in addition, the 5-HTTLPR polymorphism in the promoter region of the serotonin transporter

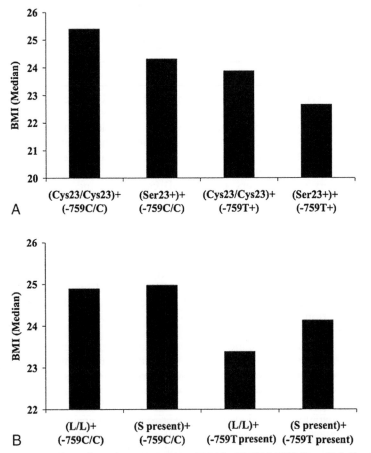

FIGURE 1.—Additive effects of *HTR2C*-Cys23Ser, *HTR2C*−759C/T, 5-HTTLPR on BMI. Two-locus genotype analysis of *HTR2C*-Cys23Ser, *HTR2C*−759C/T and BMI (A); and 5-HTTLPR, *HTR2C*−759C/T and BMI (B). Ser23+ = Ser23/Ser23 + Cys23/Ser23; −759T+ = T/T+ C/T; S+ = S/S+L/S. (Reprinted from Bah J, Westberg L, Baghaei F, et al. Further exploration of the possible influence of polymorphisms in HTR2C and 5HTT on body weight. *Metabolism*. 2010;59:1156-1163, with permission from Elsevier.)

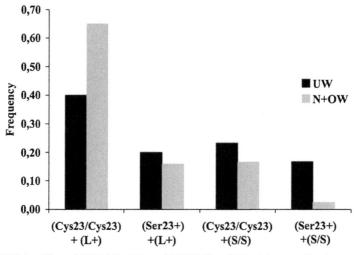

FIGURE 2.—Effects of *HTR2C*-Cys23Ser and 5-HTTLPR on BMI weight group. Two-locus genotype analysis of *HTR2C*-Cys23Ser and 5-HTTLPR and *HTR2C*−759C/T and BMI (B). L+ = L/L + L/S; Ser23+ = Ser23/Ser23 + Cys23/Ser23. (Reprinted from Bah J, Westberg L, Baghaei F, et al. Further exploration of the possible influence of polymorphisms in HTR2C and 5HTT on body weight. *Metabolism.* 2010;59:1156-1163, with permission from Elsevier.)

gene (*SLC6A4*) was assessed. The polymorphisms were genotyped in subjects recruited from the normal population (n = 510), and possible associations between genotype and body mass index (BMI) were assessed. The Ser23 allele was more common in underweight subjects (BMI <20) than in normal- and overweight (BMI ≥20) subjects (*P* = .006). The T allele of the −759C/T polymorphism was less common in the overweight group (BMI ≥25) (*P* = .007). Homozygosity for the short allele of 5-HTTLPR was more frequent in underweight subjects (*P* = .015). Our results are in agreement with previous studies, suggesting polymorphisms in *HTR2C* to be associated with body weight, particularly in women; and they also suggest that 5-HTTLPR may influence this phenotype. Further studies on the importance of the investigated genes for eating disorders and drug-induced weight gain are warranted (Figs 1 and 2).

▶ I liked this article because, although cross-sectional in design, it addresses a key topic that is a major drawback of the psychopharmacology and treatment of major mental disorders, namely, antipsychotic-induced weight gain. While there is to some extent an impact of the drug itself, it is also clear that increased food intake alone during therapy does not fully explain this relationship. Drug-induced obesity is far more complex, and there is now evidence that how the body regulates and handles food is crucial to the development of obesity. Genetics are key here, and in particular, the serotonin system has been strongly implicated in obesity. This important article examined polymorphisms of the serotonin system in relation to weight among 510 normal subjects. The study found that the Ser23 allele was more common in underweight subjects than in normal and overweight subjects. In contrast, the T allele of the 759C/T polymorphism in the *HTR2C* gene was less in overweight individuals. Figs 1 and 2 illustrate these effects.

This well-conducted study is important because it advances our understanding of the genetic basis of weight gain in the normal population, and this of course has direct relevance to understanding the biology of antipsychotic-induced weight gain. Antipsychotic-induced weight gain and metabolic disturbances are now the most serious side effects in treating psychosis or mood disorders. This study provides data from normal subjects that, if extrapolated to patients with mental illness and their medications, could conceivably in the future influence the choice of antipsychotic medication in a manner that is consistent with the emergence of personalized medicine in other areas of medicine. This is not too far-fetched an idea, although time will tell!

P. F. Buckley, MD

No association between the serotonin transporter gene polymorphism 5-HTTLPR and cyclothymic temperament as measured by TEMPS-A

Landaas ET, Johansson S, Halmøy A, et al (Univ of Bergen, Norway; Hankeland Univ Hosp, Bergen, Norway)
J Affect Disord 129:308-312, 2011

Background.—Temperaments are stable personality traits that can be considered subsyndromal risk factors of psychiatric illnesses. The 5-HTTLPR polymorphism of the serotonin transporter gene has been found to be associated with affective temperaments, particularly the cyclothymic temperament, as measured with the Temperament Evaluation of Memphis, Pisa, Paris and San Diego—autoquestionnaire version (TEMPS-A). In this study we have attempted to replicate this finding in a population-based sample which is five times as large as the sample used in the original study.

Methods.—The 21 items of the cyclothymic subscale of TEMPS-A was filled in by 691 individuals (404 females, 287 males, 18—40 years) randomly recruited from the general population. DNA was isolated from saliva, and the serotonin transporter polymorphism 5-HTTLPR was genotyped using the polymerase chain reaction and fragment analysis.

Results.—No significant association was found between 5-HTTLPR genotype and TEMPS-A score, neither when analysing by an additive allelic model nor when the different genotypes and allelic dominance were examined. Furthermore, no association was observed after gender stratification, or when TEMPS-A was analysed as a dichotomous measure, using a cut-off of ≥11 positive item responses.

Limitations.—Although being used in clinical settings, TEMPS-A has not been officially validated in Norway.

Conclusions.—This study suggests that there is no association between the 5-HTTLPR polymorphism and cyclothymic temperament as measured by TEMPS-A.

▶ Temperament is always hard to measure. Additionally, the relationship between temperament and distinct psychiatric disorders is contentious. Cyclothymic temperament—whether irritability or reflecting mild shifts in mood that are really part of a cyclothymic personality disorder—is also contentious. It is hardly surprising that the serotonin polymorphisms proved unrelated to temperament, especially because it is likely that the "signal" from the Temperament Evaluation of Memphis, Pisa, Paris and San Diego-autoquestionnaire measurement is too weak to generate any meaningful associations, even if they are present. This is a good attempt toward personalized medicine—understanding our proclivity to psychiatric disturbances as a function of our genetic profile. However, temperament is probably not the best area to study to advance this proposition.

P. F. Buckley, MD

Pain relief in office gynaecology: a systematic review and meta-analysis
Ahmad G, Attarbashi S, O'Flynn H, et al (Pennine Acute Trust, Greater Manchester, UK; Tameside General Hosp, Lancashire, UK; Univ Hosp of South Manchester Foundation Trust, Manchester, UK)
Eur J Obstet Gynecol Reprod Biol 155:3-13, 2011

Hysteroscopy, hysterosalpingography (HSG), sonohysterography and endometrial ablation are increasingly performed in an outpatient setting. The primary reason for failure to complete these procedures is pain. The objective of this review was to compare the effectiveness and safety of different types of pharmacological intervention for pain relief in office gynaecological procedures. A systematic search of medical databases including PubMed, EMBASE, Cochrane Central register of controlled trials, PsychInfo and CINHAL was conducted in 2009. Randomised controlled trials (RCTs) investigating the use of local anaesthetics, opioid analgesics, non-opioid analgesics and intravenous sedation for pain relief during and after hysteroscopy, HSG, sonohysterography and endometrial ablation were reviewed. Secondary outcomes included adverse effects and failure to complete procedures. Where RCTs were not identified, the best available evidence was sought. Each study was assessed against inclusion criterion. Results for each study were expressed as a standardised mean difference (SMD) with 95% confidence intervals and combined for meta-analysis with Revman 5 software. Meta-analysis revealed beneficial effect of the use of local anaesthetics during and within 30 min after hysteroscopy; SMD -0.45 (95% CI -0.73, -0.17) and SMD -0.51 (95% CI -0.81, -0.21) respectively. No beneficial effect was noted during HSG. One RCT found evidence of benefit for pain relief during hysterosalpingo-contrastsonography; SMD -1.04 [95% CI -1.44, -0.63]. There was no significant difference in failure to complete hysteroscopy due to cervical stenosis between the intervention and control groups (OR 1.31 (95% CI 0.66, 2.59)), but the incidence of failure to complete the procedure due to pain was significantly less in the intervention group (OR 0.29 (0.12, 0.69)). There is evidence of benefit for the use of local anaesthetics for outpatient hysteroscopy and hysterosalpingo-contrastsonography. Local anaesthetics may be considered when performing hysteroscopy in postmeno-pausal women to reduce the failure rate.

▶ This is an important topic, although extremely difficult to study. This particular study is a meta-analysis of available studies that addresses outpatient OBGyn procedural pain management. Although it follows the typical Cochrane reviews and compilation of studies from multiple sources, it is nevertheless evident that the insufficient number of studies as well as marked heterogeneity makes it difficult to address this important topic in any definitive manner. Additionally, the modes of analgesia vary substantially across studies. We also know less about the details regarding how pain was addressed in each study—another important consideration. All that said, the review does not provide compelling evidence for the "aggressive" use of analgesia for outpatient OBGyn procedures.

P. F. Buckley, MD

The evidence for pharmacological treatment of neuropathic pain
Finnerup NB, Sindrup SH, Jensen TS (Aarhus Univ Hosp, Denmark; Odense Univ Hosp, Denmark)
Pain 150:573-581, 2010

Randomized, double-blind, placebo-controlled trials on neuropathic pain treatment are accumulating, so an updated review of the available evidence is needed. Studies were identified using MEDLINE and EMBASE searches. Numbers needed to treat (NNT) and numbers needed to harm (NNH) values were used to compare the efficacy and safety of different treatments for a number of neuropathic pain conditions. One hundred and seventy-four studies were included, representing a 66% increase in published random-ized, placebo-controlled trials in the last 5 years. Painful poly-neuropathy (most often due to diabetes) was examined in 69 studies, postherpetic neuralgia in 23, while peripheral nerve injury, central pain, HIV neuropathy, and trigeminal neuralgia were less often studied. Tricyclic antidepressants, serotonin noradrenaline reuptake inhibitors, the anticonvulsants gabapen-tin and pregabalin, and opioids are the drug classes for which there is the best evidence for a clinical relevant effect. Despite a 66% increase in pub-lished trials only a limited improvement of neuropathic pain treatment has been obtained. A large proportion of neuropathic pain patients are left with insufficient pain relief. This fact calls for other treatment options to target chronic neuropathic pain. Large-scale drug trials that aim to iden-tify possible subgroups of patients who are likely to respond to specific drugs are needed to test the hypothesis that a mechanism-based classification may help improve treatment of the individual patients (Fig 4).

▶ This is an interesting study providing an efficacy assessment for current treat-ments for neuropathic pain. Although the study documents a 66% increase in published randomized controlled trials of drug therapies for the treatment of

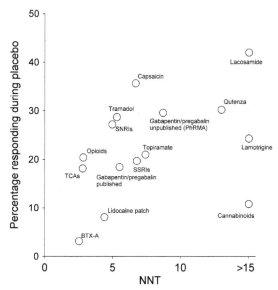

FIGURE 4.—It shows the combined numbers needed to treat (NNT) values for various drug classes and the corresponding percentage of patients reporting at least 50% pain relief during placebo treatment. (Reprinted from Finnerup NB, Sindrup SH, Jensen TS. The evidence for pharmacological treatment of neuropathic pain. *Pain*. 2010;150:573-581, with permission from International Association for the Study of Pain.)

neuropathic pain, the results of this analysis are an overall disappointment and certainly do not endorse any particular drug choice for this intractable form of pain (Fig 4). In part, this may be because of the metric used, number needed to treat (NNT); this metric is reasonable as an assessment, but they chose a stringent NNT—a 50% (or in some cases 30%) reduction in pain attributable to the medication in the randomized trial. First, this is a very high bar. Second, it might not have been adequately described in trials. Third, this sample is so resistant to therapies that this may be an overly pessimistic view of the medications in this situation. For people with intractable pain, any decrease in pain is welcome. Therefore, the efficacy here may be understated. Nevertheless, it is useful to have this objective evaluation of drug efficacy for this situation.

P. F. Buckley, MD

Vietnam's Palliative Care Initiative: Successes and Challenges in the First Five Years

Krakauer EL, Cham NTP, Khue LN (Massachusetts General Hosp, Boston; Vietnam Administration of Med Services, Hanoi)
J Pain Symptom Manage 40:27-30, 2010

In 2005, Vietnam's Ministry of Health (MoH) launched a palliative care initiative that uses the World Health Organization (WHO) public health strategy for national palliative care program development. With international financial and technical support, the initiative has made significant early progress. A rapid situation analysis in 2005 led to national Guidelines on Palliative Care in 2006, radically improved opioid prescribing regulations in 2008, the training of more than 400 physicians in palliative care by early 2010 using three curricula written especially for Vietnam, and the initiation of palliative care services in some hospitals and in the community. Yet, access to palliative care services remains very limited. Many challenges must be overcome to reach the goal of access for all to essential palliative care services that are integrated into the systems of cancer care, HIV/AIDS care, and primary care. Going forward, crucial aspects of the initiative will be continued commitment to palliative care by the MoH, careful planning and targeted funding that address each part of the WHO public health strategy, ongoing expert technical support, and collaboration among international technical and financial supporters.

▶ This brief article chronicles efforts by the World Health Organization to support the development and implementation of palliative care services in Vietnam. It is of interest because many of the issues generalize to other global health initiatives. Illustrated herein are the problems with building a competent clinical workforce and securing an overall national health care policy. These aspects resonate with many of the global health care initiatives that US academic medical centers are increasingly becoming involved with. It's a slow process, especially the efforts to develop a competent clinical workforce. As is described here, this often requires a lengthy period of mentorship and prolonged clinical oversight. Academic medical centers are required to commit personal and time resources for the long haul!

P. F. Buckley, MD

A Randomized Trial of 2 Prescription Strategies for Opioid Treatment of Chronic Nonmalignant Pain
Naliboff BD, Wu SM, Schieffer B, et al (Veteran's Affairs Greater Los Angeles Health Care System, CA; et al)
J Pain 12:288-296, 2011

The use of opioid medications for treating chronic noncancer pain is growing; however, there is a lack of good evidence regarding their long-term effectiveness, association with substance abuse, and proper prescribing guidelines. The current study directly compares for the first time in a randomized trial the effectiveness of a conservative, hold the line (Stable Dose) prescribing strategy for opioid medications with a more liberal dose escalation (Escalating Dose) approach. This 2-arm, parallel, randomized pragmatic clinical trial followed 135 patients referred to a specialty pain clinic at a Veterans Affairs Hospital for 12 months (94% male and 74% with

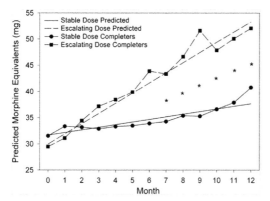

FIGURE 3.—Average Morphine Equivalents (in mg) per day for each month for the 2 treatment groups. Lines without symbols are mean predicted values for each month from the mixed model. Mean monthly values for the subjects who completed the study are shown for comparison purposes (lines with symbols). Asterisks indicate months in which there was a significant ($P < .05$) difference in opioid dose between the groups. (Reprinted from The Journal of Pain, Naliboff BD, Wu SM, Schieffer B, et al. A randomized trial of 2 prescription strategies for opioid treatment of chronic nonmalignant pain. *J Pain.* 2011;12:288-296. Copyright 2011 with permission from the American Pain Society.)

musculoskeletal pain). Primary outcomes included monthly or quarterly evaluations of pain severity, pain relief from medications, pain-related functional disability, and opioid misuse behaviors. All subjects received identical pain treatment except for the application of treatment group specific strategies for opioid prescriptions. No group differences were found for primary outcomes of usual pain or functional disability although the Escalating Dose group did show a small but significantly larger increase in self-rated pain relief from medications. About 27% of patients were discharged over the course of the study due to opioid misuse/noncompliance, but there were no group differences in rate of opioid misuse.

Perspective.—The results of this study demonstrate that even in carefully selected patients there is a significant risk of problematic opioid misuse. Although in general there were no statistically significant differences in the primary outcomes between groups, the escalating dose strategy did lead to small improvements in self-reported acute relief from medications without an increase in opioid misuse, compared to the stable dose strategy.

▶ This is a thorough study from the US Department of Veterans Affairs (VA). It uses all the value of the VA's superb electronic medical records to track medication and other outcomes over an extended period of time. The study is well conducted (Table 1). The article is well written. The topic is extremely interesting. The result will not be favored by drug-seeking chronic pain patients; more opioids, given under therapeutic guidance, do not seem to induce any dramatically better outcome despite greater drug exposure over time (Fig 3).

TABLE 1.—Demographic and Initial Values for Primary and Secondary Outcomes at the Time of Randomization. Morphine Equivalents Are Daily Amounts Prescribed

Characteristic	Stable Dose Group	Escalating Dose Group
Age, years: Mean (SD)	52.4 (7.1)	52.7 (7.9)
Gender: n (%)		
Female	1 (1)	7 (11)
Male	69 (99)	57 (89)
Marital status: n (%)		
Single/never married	7 (10)	11 (17)
Married	25 (36)	17 (27)
Cohabiting	9 (13)	2 (3)
Divorced/separated	25 (36)	28 (44)
Widowed	4 (6)	4 (6)
Uncertain	0 (0)	2 (3)
Pain problem: n (%)		
Musculoskeletal	54 (77)	50 (78)
Neuropathic	13 (19)	12 (19)
Complex	3 (4)	2 (3)
Initial morphine equivalents [mg]		
Mean (SD)	32.2 (23.1)	29.2 (19.6)
Outcome variables: mean (SD)		
Usual pain (0-10)	6.7 (1.8)	7.0 (1.9)
Worst pain (0-10)	8.0 (1.7)	8.4 (1.2)
Mood (0-10)	5.3 (2.3)	5.7 (2.7)
Pain interference (0-10)*	6.0 (2.6)	6.9 (2.2)
Days relief (0-7)	3.0 (2.1)	2.4 (2.0)
Pain relief from medications (0-10)	5.3 (2.2)	5.1 (2.4)
Satisfaction with pain Tx (0-7)	3.8 (1.3)	3.7 (1.2)
ABC (0-20)	1.6 (2.1)	1.5 (2.0)
ODI (%)	47.8 (14.0)	48.6 (12.6)

Abbreviations: ABC, Addiction Behaviors Checklist; ODI, Oswestry Disability Index; n, number of subjects; Tx, treatment.
*There was a significant ($P = .03$) difference between the groups at baseline on Pain Interference but no other group differences (all, $P > .1$).

These results are salutary. They may also generalize to other patient populations, not just the VA.

P. F. Buckley, MD

Other Conditions

Serotonergic Activity Influences the Cognitive Appraisal of Close Intimate Relationships in Healthy Adults
Bilderbeck AC, McCabe C, Wakeley J, et al (Oxford Univ, UK; et al)
Biol Psychiatry 69:720-725, 2011

Background.—Close supportive relationships protect against psychological disorders and also facilitate recovery. However, little is known about the neurochemical mechanisms that mediate these effects. Variation in serotonin function influences affiliative behavior in humans and nonhuman primates. Here, we used tryptophan depletion in healthy adults to investigate the role of serotonin in the cognitive appraisal of close personal relationships.

Methods.—Twenty-two healthy adults drank an amino acid drink without tryptophan, and 19 healthy adults drank an amino acid drink containing tryptophan. Participants were presented with color photographs of heterosexual "couples" standing apart or making affiliative touch gestures and rated the couples for descriptors that capture qualities of close personal relationships. Trait attachment style and state affect of participants were also measured.

Results.—Tryptophan depletion reduced the judged intimacy and romance of photographed couples. Tryptophan-depleted women rated men as more dominant in relationships and touching couples as more able to resolve their conflicts, when compared with nondepleted women. These effects were not due to changes in mood and remained statistically reliable when the marked impact of attachment style upon relationship judgments was statistically controlled.

Conclusions.—Our results suggest that central serotonin activity influences the appraisal of close intimate partnerships, raising the possibility that serotonergic dysfunction contributes to altered cognitions about relationships in psychiatric illnesses.

▶ This is a fascinating report. It is an experimental design that relates well to the public interest in over-the-counter "relationship enhancing" and "quasi-aphrodisiac" agents that are sold at stores and gas stations. The results suggest a powerful influence of tryptophan depletion—which is an indirect measurement of serotonergic activity—on human perceptions with regard to intimacy. There is interesting literature describing the relationships between serotonergic activity/dysfunction and social cues, fear, and, of course, depression. So although we think of social relationships with respect to human and ontogenesis of social dominance, these study findings do indicate a neurobiological basis to pretty fundamental human expressions. This study does not address whether this effect is selective to the serotonergic system or involves other central nervous systems; the latter is likely.

P. F. Buckley, MD

Mood Disorders

Brain-derived neurotrophic factor and serotonin transporter gene-linked promoter region genes alter serum levels of brain-derived neurotrophic factor in humans

Bhang S, Ahn J-H, Choi S-W (Univ of Ulsan College of Medicine, Republic of Korea)
J Affect Disord 128:299-304, 2011

Background.—Polymorphisms in the brain-derived neurotrophic factor (BDNF) val66met and serotonin transporter gene-linked promoter region (5-HTTLPR) are associated with alterations in mood and BDNF protein, but the effects of two genetic variations on the serum level of BDNF is unclear. Therefore, we sought to explore the effects of two polymorphisms on serum levels of BDNF in healthy subjects.

Methods.—One hundred healthy Korean subjects were genotyped. Serum levels of BDNF were measured with enzyme-linked immunoassay, and factors (sex, age, body mass index, alcohol and smoking) that can affect BDNF level were evaluated. The effects of these two genetic variations on serum levels of BDNF were tested using an analysis of covariance.

Results.—We found that serum levels of BDNF were significantly affected by the factor 'genotype' (*met* carrier vs. *val* homozygote) (F = 4.618, $p = 0.034$) and (*s* homozygote vs. *l* carrier) (F = 3.965, $p = 0.049$), respectively. Moreover, subjects with *s* homozygosity at the 5-HTTLPR and BDNF *met* carriers (16.2 ± 7.9 ng/ml) had lower serum levels of BDNF as compared with those with *l* carriers of the 5-HTTLPR in combination with BDNF *val* homozygosity (21.7 ± 4.4 ng/ml) ($p = 0.024$).

Limitations.—A larger study will be needed to confirm this additive effect of both risk genotypes.

Conclusions.—In this study, we report for the first time that healthy subjects who were homozygous for *s* at 5-HTTLPR and the *met* allele of the BDNF val66met polymorphism displayed significantly lower serum levels of BDNF. Our findings might contribute to a better understanding of the effect of BDNF and 5-HTTLPR gene on serum BDNF level in humans.

▶ This study explores the genetic influences and reciprocity between serotonin receptor gene polymorphisms and brain-derived neurotrophic factor (BDNF) polymorphisms. This is in a healthy sample—important because the report associations could be otherwise distorted in a clinical sample. The study population is adequate in size and is of homogeneous composition, although the entirely Korean focus might limit the generalizability of the study findings. The impact of homozygosity upon BDNF levels appears a robust finding (Table 2) and is an interesting association. Clearly there is considerable literature of serotonergic

TABLE 2.—Serum level of BDNF (ng/ml) for BDNF *met* carriers vs. *val* Homozygotes and *l* Carriers vs. *s* Homozygotes

Met Carrier	S Homozygote	Mean ± Standard Errors
met+	ss− (n = 28)	19.6 ± 5.8
	ss+ (n = 43)	16.2 ± 7.9*
	Total (n = 71)	17.5 ± 7.3
met−	ss− (n = 11)	21.7 ± 4.4*
	ss+ (n = 18)	19.8 ± 7.8
	Total (n = 29)	20.5 ± 6.7
Total	ss− (n = 39)	20.2 ± 5.5
	ss+ (n = 61)	17.3 ± 8.0
	Total (n = 100)	18.4 ± 7.2

Post-hoc comparisons of Fisher's least significant difference revealed that subjects with *s* homozygosity at 5-HTTLPR and BDNF *met* carriers exhibited lower levels of BDNF (16.2 ± 7.9 ng/ml) as compared with those who were *l* carriers at the 5-HTTLPR and also homozygous for *val* at the BDNF locus (21.7 ± 4.4 ng/ml) * ($p = 0.024$). *met* carrier + *l* carrier vs. *met* carrier + *s/s* ($p = 0.051$), *val/val* + *l* carrier vs. *val/val* + *s/s* ($p = 0.492$), *met* carrier + *l* carrier vs. *val/val* + *l* carrier ($p = 0.409$), *met* carrier + *l* carrier vs. *val/val* + *s/s* ($p = 0.919$), *met* carrier + *s/s* vs. *val/val* + *s/s* ($p = 0.072$): not significant. BDNF, brain-derived neurotrophic factor; 5-HTTLPR, the serotonin transporter gene-linked promoter region; met+, met carriers; met−, val homozygotes; ss−, l carriers; ss+, s homozygotes.

dysfunction in mood disorders, especially in depression. There is also a growing literature showing BDNF medications that appear related to (causality is yet to be determined) mood status. This study adds to this story.

P. F. Buckley, MD

Association of Plasma Interleukin-18 Levels with Emotion Regulation and µ-Opioid Neurotransmitter Function in Major Depression and Healthy Volunteers

Prossin AR, Koch AE, Campbell PL, et al (Univ of Michigan Med School, Ann Arbor; et al)

Biol Psychiatry 69:808-812, 2011

Background.—Alterations in central neurotransmission and immune function have been documented in major depression (MDD). Central and peripheral endogenous opioids are linked to immune functioning in animal models, stress-activated, and dysregulated in MDD. We examined the relationship between µ-opioid receptor (OR)-mediated neurotransmission and a proinflammatory cytokine (interleukin [IL]-18).

Methods.—We studied 28 female subjects (14 MDDs, 14 control subjects) with positron emission tomography and $[^{11}C]$ carfentanil (µ-OR selective) during neutral and sadness states. With a simple regression model in SPM2 (Wellcome Trust, London, England) we identified brain regions where baseline µ-OR availability (nondisplaceable binding potential $[BP_{ND}]$) and sadness-induced changes in µ-OR BP_{ND} were associated with baseline IL-18.

Results.—Baseline IL-18 was greater in MDDs than control subjects $[t(25) = 2.13, p = .04]$. In control subjects IL-18 was correlated with negative emotional ratings at baseline and during sadness induction. In MDDs, IL-18 was positively correlated with baseline regional µ-OR BP_{ND} and with sadness-induced µ-opioid system activation in the subgenual anterior cingulate, ventral basal ganglia, and amygdala.

Conclusions.—This study links plasma IL-18 with sadness-induced emotional responses in healthy subjects, the diagnosis of MDD, and µ-opioid functioning, itself involved in stress adaptation, emotion regulation, and reward. This suggests that IL-18 represents a marker associated with emotion regulation/dysregulation at least in part through central opioid mechanisms.

▶ Central opioid dysfunction has been linked to major depression. Additionally, there is a complex, yet nevertheless robust, relationship between immune dysfunction and major depression. This study extends and links these disparate lines of inquiry through the rubric of neuroimaging with positron emission tomography. Of course, the immune system is inordinately complex in itself, and reducing the measurement to a single metric—in this instance, interleukin-18, although it appeared to work out here—is still somewhat reductionist. We know that multiple immune parameters are disturbed in depression, and indeed this is so in other conditions as well. Selecting which of these biomarkers—and which aggregate of them—is potentially useful in depression is a major challenge.

P. F. Buckley, MD

The Serotonin Transporter Promoter Variant (5-HTTLPR), Stress, and Depression Meta-analysis Revisited: Evidence of Genetic Moderation

Karg K, Burmeister M, Shedden K, et al (Univ of Wuerzburg, Germany; Univ of Michigan, Ann Arbor)

Arch Gen Psychiatry 68:444-454, 2011

Context.—Two recent meta-analyses assessed the set of studies exploring the interaction between a serotonin transporter promoter polymorphism (5-HTTLPR) and stress in the development of depression and concluded that the evidence did not support the presence of the interaction. However, even the larger of the meta-analyses included only 14 of the 56 studies that have assessed the relationship between 5-HTTLPR, stress, and depression.

Objective.—To perform a meta-analysis including all relevant studies exploring the interaction.

Data Sources.—We identified studies published through November 2009 in PubMed.

Study Selection.—We excluded 2 studies presenting data that were included in other larger studies.

Data Extraction.—To perform a more inclusive meta-analysis, we used the Liptak-Stouffer z score method to combine findings of primary studies at the level of significance tests rather than the level of raw data.

Data Synthesis.—We included 54 studies and found strong evidence that 5-HTTLPR moderates the relationship between stress and depression, with the 5-HTTLPR s allele associated with an increased risk of developing depression under stress ($P = .00002$). When stratifying our analysis by the type of stressor studied, we found strong evidence for an association between the s allele and increased stress sensitivity in the childhood maltreatment ($P = .00007$) and the specific medical condition ($P = .0004$) groups of studies but only marginal evidence for an association in the stressful life events group ($P = .03$). When restricting our analysis to the studies included in the previous meta-analyses, we found no evidence of association (Munafò et al studies, $P = .16$; Risch et al studies, $P = .11$). This suggests that the difference in results between meta-analyses was due to the different set of included studies rather than the meta-analytic technique.

Conclusion.—Contrary to the results of the smaller earlier meta-analyses, we find strong evidence that the studies published to date support the hypothesis that 5-HTTLPR moderates the relationship between stress and depression (Table 1).

▶ This study, in addition to its important findings, illustrated the scientific power of the meta-analytic strategy to clarify the research landscape. Our

TABLE 1.—Description of 5-HTTLPR, Stress, and Depression Studies Included in the Overall Meta-Analysis

Source, Year	No. of Participants	Female, %	Mean Age, y	Study Design	Stressor	Stress Assessment Method	Depression Measure	Reported Findings[a]	Averaged 1-Tailed P Value[b]	Liptak-Stouffer P Value After Study Exclusion
Mössner et al,[51] 2001	72	46	NA	Exposed only	Parkinson disease	Objective	Hamilton Depression Rating Scale	Positive	.0125	1.90×10^{-5}
Caspi et al,[1] 2003	845	48	26	Longitudinal	Child maltreatment	Objective	Diagnosis of depression	Positive	.0100	4.20×10^{-5}
Eley et al,[72] 2004	374	58	16	Case-control	Adverse family environment	Self report questionnaire	MFQ	Partially positive	.2575	1.95×10^{-5}
Grabe et al,[73] 2005	973	69	52	Cross-sectional	Number of chronic diseases	Self-report questionnaire	von Zerssen Complaints Scale	Partially positive	.2503	2.16×10^{-5}
Kendler et al,[19] 2005	549	NA	35	Longitudinal	Stressful life events	Interview	Diagnosis of depression	Positive	.0070	3.27×10^{-5}
Nakatani et al,[28] 2005	2509	25	64	Exposed only	Acute myocardial infarction	Objective	Zung Self-Rating Depression Scale	Positive	.0075	1.62×10^{-4}
Jacobs et al,[20] 2006	374	100	27	Longitudinal	Stressful life events	Self-report questionnaire	SCL-90	Positive	.0200	2.51×10^{-5}
Kaufman et al,[18] 2006	196	51	9	Cross-sectional	Child abuse	Objective	MFQ	Partially positive	.0225	2.12×10^{-5}
Ramasubbu et al,[30] 2006	51	35	60	Exposed only	Stroke	Objective	Diagnosis of depression	Positive	.0130	1.86×10^{-5}
Sjöberg et al,[21] 2006	198	63	17	Cross-sectional	Psychosocial circumstances in family	Interview	Depression Self-Rating Scale	Partially positive/opposite	.4721	1.76×10^{-5}
Surtees et al,[74] 2006	4175	47	60	Cross-sectional	Childhood adversities/stressful life events	Self-report questionnaire	Diagnosis of depression	Negative	.5000	1.33×10^{-6}
Taylor et al,[63] 2006	110	57	21	Cross-sectional	Childhood adversities	Self-report questionnaire	BDI	Partially positive	.0268	1.95×10^{-5}
Wilhelm et al,[75] 2006	127	67	48	Longitudinal	Stressful life events	Interview	Diagnosis of depression	Partially positive	.1178	1.89×10^{-5}

(Continued)

Table 1.—(Continued)

Source, Year	No. of Participants	Female, %	Mean Age, y	Study Design	Stressor	Stress Assessment Method	Depression Measure	Reported Findings[a]	Averaged 1-Tailed P Value[b]	Liptak-Stouffer P Value After Study Exclusion
Zalsman et al,[64] 2006	79	68	38	Case-control	Stressful life events	Interview	Hamilton Depression Rating Scale	Partially positive	.2233	1.81×10^{-5}
Cervilla et al,[76] 2007	737	72	49	Case-control	Stressful life events	Self-report questionnaire	Diagnosis of depression	Positive	.0143	3.62×10^{-5}
Chipman et al,[61] 2007	2094	52	23	Cross-sectional	Stressful life events	Self-report questionnaire	Goldman Depression Scale	Negative	.3400	1.60×10^{-5}
Chorbov et al,[77] 2007	236	100	22	Longitudinal	Traumatic events	Self-report questionnaire	Diagnosis of depression	Opposite	1.0000	1.10×10^{-5}
Cicchetti et al,[22] 2007	339	46	17	Cross-sectional	Child abuse	Objective	ASEBA	Partially positive	.2518	1.94×10^{-5}
Dick et al,[35] 2007	956	NA	NA	Family-based association study	Problems with work, relationship, or health	Self-report questionnaire	Diagnosis of depression	Positive	.0040	5.37×10^{-5}
Kilpatrick et al,[14] 2007	589	64	≥ 60 (77%)	Cross-sectional	Hurricane exposure + low social support	Objective	Diagnosis of depression	Positive	.0015	3.94×10^{-5}
Kim et al,[78] 2007	732	NA	≥ 65	Cross-sectional	Stressful life events	Interview	Diagnosis of depression	Negative	0.0385	3.11×10^{-5}
Kraus et al,[36] 2007	139	49	42	Exposed only	Interferon alfa treatment	Objective	Hospital Anxiety and Depression Scale	Negative	.5650	1.73×10^{-5}
Mandelli et al,[15] 2007	670	68	48	Case-only	Stressful life events	Interview	Diagnosis of depression	Positive	.0112	3.50×10^{-5}
Middeldorp et al,[79] 2007	367	68	39	Longitudinal	Stressful life events	Self-report questionnaire	Anxiety-Depression Rating Scale	Negative	.5000	1.73×10^{-5}
Otte et al,[29] 2007	557	15	68	Exposed only	Coronary disease	Objective	Diagnosis of depression	Partially positive	.0275	2.86×10^{-5}
Scheid et al,[16] 2007	568	100	20-34	Cross-sectional	Stressful life events	Self-report questionnaire	CES-D	Negative	.0800	2.50×10^{-5}

Study				Study design	Exposure	Measurement	Depression measure	Direction		
Brummett et al,[37] 2008	288	75	58	Cross-sectional	Alzheimer caregiving	Objective	CES-D	Positive	.0015	2.64×10^{-5}
Kohen et al,[26] 2008	150	37	60	Exposed only	Stroke	Objective	Geriatric Depression Scale	Positive	.0225	2.03×10^{-5}
Lazary et al,[38] 2008	567	79	31	Cross-sectional	Stressful life events	Self-report questionnaire	Zung Self-Rating Depression Scale	Positive	.0025	3.67×10^{-5}
Lenze et al,[27] 2005	23	87	77	Exposed only	Hip fracture	Objective	Diagnosis of depression	Positive	.0068	1.81×10^{-5}
Power et al,[80] 2010	1421	NA	≥65	Cross-sectional	Stressful life events	Self-report questionnaire	MINI, CES-D	Negative	.6200	1.10×10^{-5}
Wichers et al,[39] 2008	394	100	18-64	Cross-sectional	Childhood trauma	Self-report questionnaire	SCL-90; SCID depressive symptoms	Negative	.2000	2.03×10^{-5}
Aguilera et al,[23] 2009	534	55	23	Cross-sectional	Childhood trauma	Self-report questionnaire	SCL-90-R	Positive	.0001	4.63×10^{-5}
Araya et al,[34] 2009	4334	NA	7	Longitudinal	Stressful life events	Self-report questionnaire	SDQ emotional symptom 5-item subscale	Negative	.5000	1.03×10^{-6}
Aslund et al,[40] 2009	1482	48	17-18	Cross-sectional	Parental fighting and maltreatment	Self-report questionnaire	Depression Self-Rating Scale	Positive	.0078	7.68×10^{-5}
Bull et al,[41] 2009	98	36	46	Longitudinal	Interferon alfa and ribavirin treatment	Objective	Zung Self-Rating Depression Scale/BDI	Positive	.0150	1.95×10^{-5}
Coventry at al,[42] 2010	3243	60	32	Longitudinal	Stressful life events	Self-report questionnaire	Diagnosis of depression	Negative	.5000	4.33×10^{-6}
Bukh et al,[43] 2009	290	66	39	Case-only	Stressful life events	Interview	Diagnosis of depression	Negative	.0350	2.25×10^{-5}
Kim et al,[25] 2009	521	55	72	Longitudinal	No. of chronic health problems	Self-report questionnaire	Diagnosis of depression	Positive	.0050	3.27×10^{-5}
Laucht et al,[62] 2009	309	54	19	Cross-sectional	Stressful life events	Self-report questionnaire	Diagnosis of depression, BDI	Partially negative/opposite	.7375	1.57×10^{-5}
Lotrich et al,[33] 2009	71	27	48	Exposed only	Interferon alfa treatment	Objective	BDI	Positive	.0250	1.88×10^{-5}
McCaffery et al,[44] 2009	977	21	59	Exposed only	Cardiovascular disease	Objective	BDI	Negative	.5000	1.57×10^{-5}

(Continued)

Table 1.—(Continued)

Source, Year	No. of Participants	Female, %	Mean Age, y	Study Design	Stressor	Stress Assessment Method	Depression Measure	Reported Findings[a]	Averaged 1-Taile[b] P Value	Liptak-Stouffer P Value After Study Exclusion
Ressler et al,[81] 2010	926	62	≥18	Cross-sectional	Childhood trauma	Self-report questionnaire	Diagnosis of depression (partially), BDI	Partially positive	.5000	1.59×10^{-5}
Ritchie et al,[82] 2009	942	58	65-92	Cross-sectional	Childhood adversities	Self-report questionnaire	Diagnosis of depression, CES-D, treatment with antidepressants	Partially opposite	.5390	1.51×10^{-5}
Wichers et al,[83] 2009	502	100	27	Longitudinal	Stressful life events	Self-report questionnaire	Diagnosis of depression, SCL-90-R	Partially positive	.3803	1.84×10^{-5}
Zhang et al,[45] 2009	792	54	33	Case-control	Stressful life events	Self-report questionnaire	Diagnosis of depression	Opposite	.9975	5.24×10^{-6}
Zhang et al,[84] 2009	306	38	NA	Exposed only	Parkinson disease	Objective	CES-D	Negative	.5000	1.74×10^{-5}
Hammen et al,[13] 2010	346	62	24	Longitudinal	Negative acute life events, chronic family stress	Interview	BDI	Partially positive	.3763	1.86×10^{-5}
Benjet et al,[46] 2010	78	100	12	Cross-sectional	Relational aggression	Self-report questionnaire	Children's Depression Inventory	Positive	.0050	1.94×10^{-5}
Goldman et al,[50] 2010	984	45	66	Longitudinal	Stressful life events	Interview	CES-D	Partially positive	.0203	4.19×10^{-5}
Grassi et al,[85] 2010	145	100	56	Exposed only	Breast cancer	Objective	Hospital Anxiety and Depression Scale	Negative	.5000	1.75×10^{-5}
Kumsta et al,[47] 2010	125	NA	11/15	Longitudinal	Institutionalization in Romanian orphanages	Objective	CAPA, Rutter Child Scale, SDQ	Positive	.0117	2.02×10^{-5}

Sen et al,[48] 2010	268	58	28	Longitudinal	Medical internship	Self-report questionnaire	PHQ	Positive	.0020	2.54×10^{-5}
Sugden et al,[49] 2010	2017	51	12	Longitudinal	Bullying victimization	Interview	ASEBA	Negative	.1603	2.94×10^{-5}
Total	40 749									
Average sample size	755									.00002

Abbreviations: ASEBA, Achenbach System of Empirically Based Assessment; BDI, Beck Depression Inventory; CAPA, Child and Adolescent Psychiatric Assessment; CES-D, Center for Epidemiologic Studies Depression Scale; MFQ, Mood and Feelings Questionnaire; MINI, Mini International Neuropsychiatric Interview; NA, not available; PHQ, Patient Health Questionnaire; SCID, Structured Clinical Interview for *DSM* Disorders; SCL-90, Symptom Checklist 90; SCL-90-R, Symptom Checklist 90 Revised; SDQ, Strengths and Difficulties Questionnaire.

Editor's Note: Please refer to original journal article for full references.

[a] "Positive" indicates a significant (*P*<.05) interaction effect with the *s* allele, "Negative" indicates no interaction effect (*P*>.05), and "Opposite" indicates a significant (*P*<.05) interaction effect with the *l* allele.

[b] One-tailed *P* value, with smaller values indicating greater stress sensitivity among *s* allele subjects.

field moves through an iterative process of discovery, replication, reputation, and, ultimately, consolidation. This leads to establishing each nugget of scientific foundational evidence. The early findings of the association between the serotonin transporter promoter gene and both anxiety and depression promoted a very encouraging response with our field (indeed, one of the original articles on anxiety was voted the major article in science several years ago). However, as could always be anticipated, perhaps subsequent studies (even though very well conducted) did not uniformly uphold this initial seminal finding (Table 1). So this meta-analysis of all appropriate available studies does confirm the original observation of a robust relationship between anxiety-depression and the serotonin transporter gene.

P. F. Buckley, MD

Life stress, 5-HTTLPR and mental disorder: findings from a 30-year longitudinal study
Fergusson DM, Horwood LJ, Miller AL, et al (Univ of Otago, Christchurch, New Zealand)
Br J Psychiatry 198:129-135, 2011

Background.—Recent meta-analyses have raised concerns about the replicability of gene × environment interactions involving the serotonin transporter gene (5-HTTLPR) in moderating the associations between adverse life events and mental disorders.

Aims.—To use data gathered over the course of a 30-year longitudinal study of a New Zealand birth cohort to test the hypothesis that the presence of short ('s') alleles of 5-HTTLPR are associated with an increased response to life stress.

Method.—Participants were 893 individuals from the Christchurch Health and Development Study who had complete data on: the 5-HTTLPR genotype; psychiatric disorders up to the age of 30; and exposure to childhood and adult adverse life events.

Results.—A series of 104 regression models were fitted to four mental health outcomes (depressive symptoms, major depression, anxiety disorder and suicidal ideation) observed at ages 18, 21, 25 and 30 using 13 measures of life-course stress that spanned childhood and adult stressors. Both multiplicative and additive models were fitted to the data. No evidence was found that would support the hypothesis that 's' alleles of 5-HTTLPR are associated with increased responsivity to life stressors.

Conclusions.—The present findings add to the evidence suggesting that it is unlikely that there is a stable gene × environment interaction involving 5-HTTLPR, life stress and mental disorders.

▶ When the Caspi study of the Dunedin population was reported in *Science* in 2003, it was almost automatically hailed as a landmark study. In brief, the study found that polymorphisms of the serotonin transporter gene modulated the impact of social adversity in contributing to anxiety and depression. The study drew great attention and has substantially moved our field forward. Inevitably, replications and failures to replicate followed the Caspi article. This study is quite similar in sample and methodology to the Caspi study; indeed, the follow-up and measures of adversity are more robust than in the Caspi study. However, despite the intent and rigor of the investigation, this study did not replicate these initial findings. Surprisingly, the authors address more why their study might have failed to detect the anticipated effect rather than being more definitive in their conclusions.

P. F. Buckley, MD

Serotonin Receptor Imaging: Clinically Useful?
Parsey RV (Columbia Univ, NY)
J Nucl Med 51:1495-1498, 2010

Serotonin is a modulatory neurotransmitter in the human brain that regulates mood, anger, reward, aggression, and appetite and plays a central role in brain development. These effects are mediated through the interaction of serotonin with at least 15 different receptor molecules. Through the development and careful characterization of novel radiotracers, we have been able to visualize and quantify in vivo many of the key molecular sites—including serotonin receptors, reuptake transporters, and enzymes—responsible for serotonin metabolism. The clinical goals of serotonin imaging are to aid in determining the pathophysiology of brain disorders, to determine novel therapeutic strategies, to predict treatment, to estimate risk, and to determine individualized dosing strategies. Despite the contradictory results of early studies, the field as a whole has made significant progress on nearly all of these fronts, and advances in methodology suggest paths toward coherence. Through concerted, directed, and cooperative efforts, the routine use of serotonin imaging in the clinic will most likely be achieved in the next decade.

▶ This article has a provocative title—no is the answer! Nevertheless, the brief article provides a *Reader's Digest* overview of the incredibly complex world of positron emission tomography (PET) imaging on neuroreceptor function in psychiatry. The article is extremely well written and does not assume expert knowledge in advance. Its brief description of pitfalls in methodology is helpful for those who are interested in reading other "state-of-the-art" PET imaging studies. For those who are not interested in this work, this article will hold little appeal. That said, it must be acknowledged that the Columbia group is "first rate" and has contributed seminal findings to our understanding of the neurobiology—and, via PET, the in vivo neurochemistry—of effective disorders.

P. F. Buckley, MD

Interaction of 5-HTTLPR and a Variation on the Oxytocin Receptor Gene Influences Negative Emotionality

Montag C, Fiebach CJ, Kirsch P, et al (Univ of Bonn, Germany; Goethe Univ, Frankfurt, Germany; Central Inst of Mental Health, Mannheim, Germany)
Biol Psychiatry 69:601-603, 2011

Background.—Pharmacological studies indicate a functional interaction between the serotonergic and oxytocinergic system.

Methods.—This study tested for an interaction of the prominent serotonin transporter polymorphism (SLC6A4) and an oxytocin receptor gene variation on individual differences in negative emotionality in healthy Caucasians ($n = 750$).

Results.—Participants carrying both the homozygous LL-variant of the serotonin transporter polymorphism and the TT variant of the single nucleotide polymorphism rs2268498 on the oxytocin receptor gene showed lowest scores on the personality dimensions Fear and Sadness of the Affective Neuroscience Personality Scales, as well as on an underlying factor Negative Emotionality.

Conclusions.—The observed interaction effect provides converging evidence from human molecular genetics that serotonergic and oxytocinergic neurotransmission are entwined and play a crucial role for human personality with implications for affective disorders.

▶ This is a German study of affective traits/expression, focusing on fear and sadness, in relation to both serotonin and oxytocin receptor polymorphisms. Unlike other studies, this report documents that a relationship between homozygosity for both neurotransmitter systems is associated with higher scores on a dimensional scale that evaluates sadness and fear. The dimensionality aspect is an important distinction because it greatly increases the statistical power to detect a potential association. The strength of the association reported here is impressive.

P. F. Buckley, MD

Evolving Concepts of the Pathogenesis of Irritable Bowel Syndrome: To Treat the Brain or the Gut?

Camilleri M (Mayo Clinic, Rochester, MN)
J Pediatr Gastroenterol Nutr 48:S46-S48, 2009

Recent in-depth studies of irritable bowel syndrome (IBS) that assessed multiple physiological endpoints in large patient cohorts confirm evidence of abnormal motility, sensation, and psychosocial disturbances. However, the proportion with hypersensitivity has dropped from the time of the original claim that it is a "biological marker" of IBS. Discomfort thresholds in male and female IBS patients normalize over time, whereas IBS symptoms persist, and increased colonic sensitivity in IBS is strongly influenced by a psychological tendency to report pain and urge rather than increased neurosensory sensitivity. The objectives of this article are to review the classical pathophysiology of IBS, the putative roles of infection, inflammation, and bacterial flora; consider mimics of IBS; assess the evidence that IBS is a serotonergic disease; evaluate recent advances in membrane biology and neuroscience related to IBS; consider genetic association with IBS and its endophenotype; and discuss whether to treat the gut or the brain.

▶ This is a useful commentary and brief overview on a vexing issue, especially vexing if you happen to be a gastroenterologist. The review focus falls just short of saying "it's all in your head," and the evidence for clear neurobiologic abnormalities is pretty unconvincing. Well, at least there is no "smoking gun" here. Irritable bowel syndrome is a nightmare to treat. The article mentions antidepressant treatment but makes essentially no reference to biofeedback or other nonpharmacologic approaches. These, in selective samples, have been shown to be of benefit.

P. F. Buckley, MD

Article Index

Chapter 1: Child and Adolescent Psychiatry

Chapter 2: Psychotherapy

Chapter 3: Alcohol and Substance Abuse

Chapter 4: Psychiatry and the Law

Chapter 5: Hospital and Community Psychiatry

Chapter 6: Clinical Psychiatry

Chapter 7: Biological Psychiatry

Author Index

Printed and bound by CPI Group (UK) Ltd, Croydon, CR0 4YY

08/05/2025

01864678-0013